Henry B. Parsons.

Pharmacy Class of

MATERIA MEDICA,

FOR

THE USE OF STUDENTS.

BY

JOHN B. BIDDLE, M.D.,

PROFESSOR OF MATERIA MEDICA AND GENERAL THERAPEUTICS IN THE JEFFERSON MEDICAL COLLEGE, MEMBER OF THE AMERICAN PHILOSOPHICAL SOCIETY, FELLOW OF THE COLLEGE OF PHYSICIANS, ETC., ETC.

SIXTH EDITION, REVISED AND ENLARGED,

WITH ILLUSTRATIONS.

PHILADELPHIA:
LINDSAY & BLAKISTON,
1874.

HENRY B. ASHMEAD, PRINTER.

PREFACE

TO THE SIXTH EDITION.

ALTHOUGH little more than a year has elapsed since the publication of the fifth edition of the *Materia Medica*, the author is gratified to find that it has been entirely exhausted. He has bestowed unusual care upon the preparation of the present edition, having recast and often rewritten the *therapeutical* articles, and remodelled the chemical descriptions. The new method of chemical *notation* is now so universally used, that it has been adopted in this edition. Many new articles have been introduced, and the work has been, in every respect, revised.

The illustrations of the book comprise, as in previous editions, representations of most of the important indigenous and naturalized plants, as well as diagrams of instruments employed in the atomization of liquids, in the new operation of pneumatic aspiration, and in the transfusion of blood.

The author has aimed in this, as in previous editions, to present a succinct account of the articles of the Materia Medica, in general use in the United States, and discussed in the courses of lectures delivered upon the subject, to which he trusts the work will be found, as heretofore, to furnish a suitable text-book. He takes pleasure in renewing his dedication of it to the gentlemen in attendance upon the various medical schools of North America.

PHILADELPHIA, June, 1874.

CONTENTS.

MATERIA MEDICA.

THE agents employed in the treatment of diseases are denominated REMEDIES, and the branch of medicine which is devoted to their consideration is termed MATERIA MEDICA. Remedies may be divided into *Hygienic*, *Mechanical*, *Imponderable*, and *Pharmacological* agents.

HYGIENIC REMEDIES are usually treated of in works specially devoted to the subject.

PART I.

MECHANICAL REMEDIES.

MECHANICAL REMEDIES belong chiefly to Surgery. A few agents of this class are, however, employed in the practice of medicine, and are included in the Materia Medica. They are *bloodletting* (general and local), *setons*, *issues*, *bandages*, *friction*, *acupuncture*, and *aspiration*.

1. GENERAL BLOODLETTING is performed principally by *venesection* or *phlebotomy*, which is usually practised on the median-cephalic or basilic veins of the arm—sometimes also on the external jugular and other veins. *Arteriotomy* is occasionally resorted to, on the temporal artery, in cerebral affections.

Bloodletting is employed, to moderate vascular excitement, reduce inflammatory action, relieve congestion, allay spasm and pain, relax the muscular system, promote absorption, and arrest hemorrhage; and for these purposes it has long been considered a valuable therapeutical resource. So powerful and exhausting an agent is, however, always to be resorted to with caution and discrimination; is not to be unduly repeated, even in inflammatory cases; and is seldom or never proper in diseases of a typhoid tendency, or where a tubercular diathesis is suspected, or in extreme infancy and old age.

2. The Local Abstraction of Blood is practised by means of *leeches*, *cups*, and *scarification*. The leech (*hirudo*) is an annulated aquatic worm, with a flattened body, tapering towards each end and terminating in circular flattened disks, which is found throughout Europe, America, and India. The European leech (*h. medicinalis*, termed also *sanguisuga officinalis*), is of a blackish or grayish-green colour on the back, from two to three or four inches in length, and is characterized by six longitudinal dorsal ferruginous stripes, the four lateral ones being interrupted or tesselated with black spots. The American leech (*h. decora*), is usually from two to three inches long, and is of a deep green colour, with three longitudinal dorsal rows of square spots. Both the imported and indigenous leech are employed in this country, but the latter makes a smaller incision, and is preferable in infantile cases. When the discharge of blood from leech-bites is excessive, it may be arrested by pressure, by compresses of lint, the application of alum, creasote, solution of subsulphate of iron, and other styptics, by cauterizing the wounds with nitrate of silver or a red-hot probe; and, if these means fail, the wounds may be sewed.

In the operation of *cupping*, cupping-glasses and a scarificator are employed. The removal of atmospheric pressure, by the application of glasses partially exhausted of air, produces a determination of blood to the capillaries of a part, and it is afterwards readily drawn by scarification. When blood is not abstracted, the operation is termed *dry cupping*, and is a valuable revulsive agent. The topical abstraction of blood by leeches and cut cups combines the advantages of depletion and revulsion. Leeches are employed in external inflammations, in situations where cups are inadmissible, and in infantile cases. Cups are generally preferable in internal inflammations, from their more decided revulsive influence. When blood is drawn by leeches, its continued flow may be promoted by the application of warm fomentations to the wounds.

Scarifications are slight incisions made in inflamed parts, to relieve the engorged capillary vessels; they are often employed with benefit in inflammations of the conjunctiva and of the tonsils.

3. SETONS (*Setacea*) and ISSUES (*Fonticuli*), are employed when a permanent counter-irritant effect is desired. A *seton* is established by passing through the integument a seton-needle, armed with a skein of silk, or, a piece of tape or a strip of sheet-lead may be used for the purpose. An *issue* is made with a cauterant, usually potassa; and after the slough has separated, a discharge is maintained by the introduction of an issue-pea, for which purpose a common dried pea is used, or a dried unripe Curaçoa orange, or a small round ball, made of Florentine orris-root.

4. BANDAGES are employed, in the practice of medicine, to promote the absorption of dropsical effusions. For the same purpose, strips of adhesive plaster may be applied to the chest, in chronic pleurisy and empyema, in the manner in which they are employed in the treatment of fractured ribs.

5. FRICTIONS are useful as revellents, and as local stimulants. They may be employed either with the dry hand, or with horse-hair gloves, or with liniments.

6. ACUPUNCTURE consists in the introduction into the body of fine, well-polished, sharp-pointed needles. It is a useful

remedy in rheumatism, neuralgia, local paralysis, &c., and is sometimes conjoined with electricity, when the operation is known as ELECTRO-PUNCTURE.

7. PNEUMATIC ASPIRATION is the employment of an instrument termed an ASPIRATOR (invented by Dieulafoy), for the removal by suction of pathological fluids.

The Aspirator consists of—

1. A Glass Bottle or Reservoir, A, mounted with a two-way stop-cock, B, and having an opening at the bottom for the insertion of the tube, C.
2. An exhausting syringe, D, with elastic connecting tube, H.
3. A tubular needle, E, to be attached to the reservoir by an india-rubber tube, F.

A syringe and stop-cock for injecting astringents or other fluids is supplied if desired. The stop-cock is in such cases fixed to the tube F at its juncture with stop-cock B. Thus the tube can be detached from the aspirator without any chance of air entering the morbid cavity.

Directions for Use.—Adjust the aspirator as figured in the diagram with the stop-cock B turned vertically, that is, open to the bottle; close the stop-cock in the tube C, and form a vacuum by a few upward and downward movements of the piston of the exhausting syringe D.

Insert one of the needles beyond the two eyes, attach tube F to it, turn the stop-cock B towards the needle, namely, horizontally, and continue the insertion of the needle until fluid is seen to flow through the short glass tube G into the reservoir.

To empty the latter turn stop-cock B vertically, detach the syringe tube, and open the stop-cock in tube C.

The presence of fluid having been established by the use of one of the fine needles, it is recommended for more quickly emptying the cavity to use one of the larger needles or trocars.

The introduction of the needle into the tissues requires some precautions. In place of endeavoring to penetrate by pressure as with an ordinary trocar, it is preferable to combine pressure

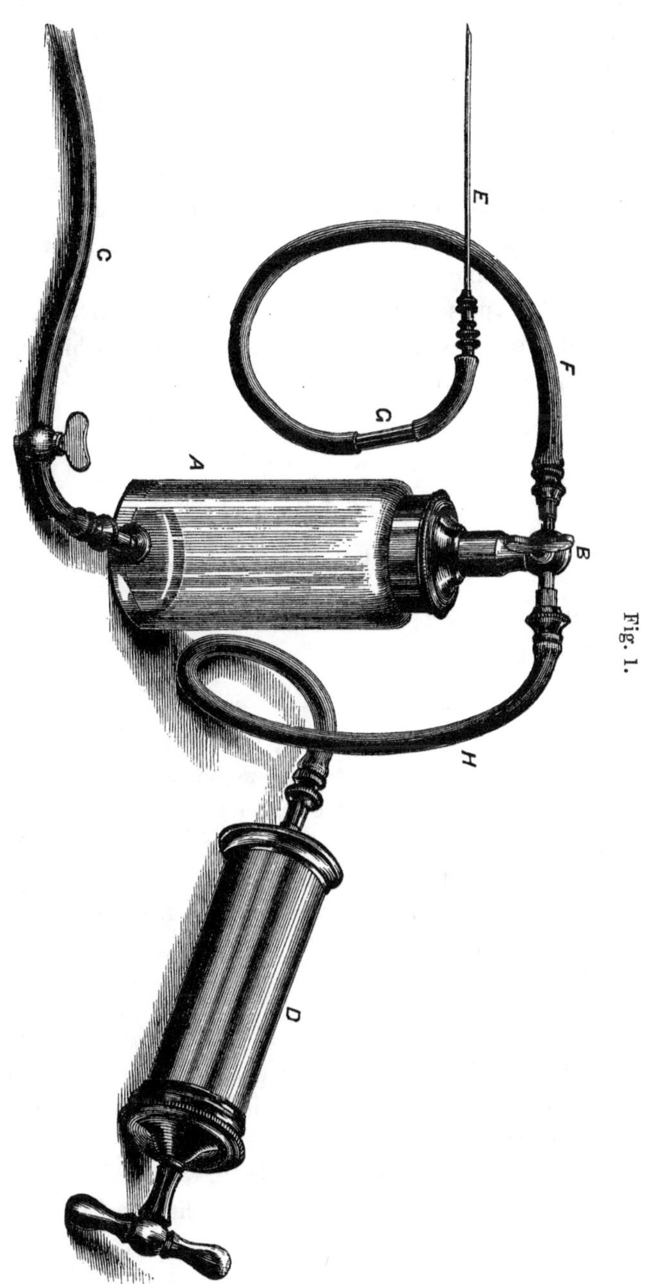

Fig. 1.

with rotation, by taking the needle in the forefinger and thumb, and rolling it between them. Such a manœuvre is rendered necessary by the extreme fineness of the needle, which would be liable to bend or twist if driven in by direct pressure. Before using a needle it is well to be assured of its permeability.

Aspiration has been employed with safety and success in the removal of intrathoracic effusions (as in chronic pleurisy, empyema, and pericarditis), of the fluid of hydrocephalus, ascites, cysts and abscesses of the liver, of the urine in retention, and of poisonous liquids from the stomach. It is also applicable to the diagnosis and treatment of morbid fluids, and to the arrest of internal hemorrhage.

PART II.

IMPONDERABLE REMEDIES.

UNDER this head are included *Light*, *Heat*, *Cold*, and *Electricity*.

1. LIGHT (*Lux*), exercises an important influence in the organized world as a vivifying stimulus. It is useful as a therapeutic agent, in diseases dependent on imperfect nutrition and sanguification; and the exposure of the surface of the body to its action, as far as nudity is compatible with proper warmth, promotes the regular development and strength of the organs. On the other hand, in many diseases the action of light is injurious, and *darkness* is resorted to as a sedative and tranquilizing agent.

2. HEAT (*Calor*), applied to the human system in moderate amount, acts, both locally and generally, as a stimulant; in intense degree, it destroys vitality and organization. It is employed as a *local* excitant and revulsive, by means of hot bottles, hot bricks, the hot foot-bath, &c., and as an application to painful and inflamed parts in the form of elastic bags containing hot water, and of poultices and fomentations. As

a *general* application, heat is chiefly resorted to in the form of the water-bath and vapour-bath. The *warm bath*, at a temperature from 92° to 98° F., is used as a relaxant in dislocations, herniæ, spasm, infantile convulsions, croup, &c., and also for its action on the skin in rheumatic and chronic cutaneous affections. The *hot bath* has a temperature of from 98° to 112°, and is a powerful excitant in cases of exhaustion, asphyxia, or suffocation, and is employed also in old paralytic and rheumatic cases. The *hot air-bath*, at a temperature of from 98° to 130°, is useful as an excitant, diaphoretic, and revellent, and is employed in cases of internal congestion, to produce vicarious action from the skin, where the secretion from other organs, as the kidneys, is suspended, and in rheumatic, neuralgic, and cutaneous affections. The *hot vapour-bath*, is adapted to the same class of cases as the hot air-bath, and exerts a more marked diaphoretic and relaxing influence.

The destructive agency of heat is resorted to for the purpose of *vesication*, as by the application to the skin of a metallic plate heated to 212° by immersion in boiling water; and of *cauterization*, by the employment of red-hot iron, or of moxa. Hot iron (known as the *actual cautery*), is used chiefly as a styptic. The term *moxa* is applied to small masses of combustible matter (as cottonwool), which are burnt slowly in contact with the skin, with a view to a revulsive effect in deep-seated inflammations, nervous affections, &c.

3. Cold (*Frigus*).—The application of cold to living bodies produces a reduction of the temperature and volume of the part, with contraction of the bloodvessels and other tissues, and suspension of the secretions and exhalations. The application of excessive or prolonged cold is followed by the torpor and death of the part. When it is applied in moderation and for a short period, reaction generally takes place, with a return and even increase of temperature, volume, colour, and sensibility.

Cold is employed therapeutically, with a view to both its primary and secondary effects. The *primary* action of cold is used, 1. To lessen vascular and nervous excitement, and preternatural heat, as by the use of cold lotions and spongings in fevers, the ice-cap in cerebral affections, the shower-bath in insanity, the bladder filled with ice to the spine in epilepsy, the ether spray to the spine in chorea, &c. 2. To constringe the tissues, promote the coagulation of the blood, and lessen the volume of parts; hence the local application of ice or cold water to abate inflammation, check hemorrhage, cure aneurism, and reduce strangulated hernia. 3. To produce local anæsthesia in surgical operations, by means of a freezing mixture topically applied.

The *secondary* effects of cold are obtained by the employment of a less intense degree of cold. They are resorted to, 1. To invigorate the system, as with the cold shower-bath, and plunge-bath. 2. To rouse the system, as by cold affusions in coma, asphyxia, syncope, and the narcotism from opium, chloroform, hydrocyanic acid, alcohol, &c. 3. In spasmodic diseases, as laryngismus stridulus, chorea, &c. 4. To recall the vital properties to frost-bitten parts. 5. To effect local excitation, as by the application of the cold douche to rheumatic and paralyzed limbs.

The cold bath, or packing in a cold wet sheet, is employed in sun-stroke, and in fevers, where the temperature of the body is very high, as scarlet fever.

The icebag is sometimes applied along the spine in convulsive diseases, as epilepsy, tetanus, and infantile convulsions, and even in diseases of the secreting organs.

Cold liquids and ice are taken into the stomach as refrigerants in fevers. They are introduced into the rectum and vagina, to check hemorrhage and allay irritation; and cold water, injected into the impregnated uterus, is among the most certain means of inducing premature delivery.

4. Electricity (*Electricitas*).—The electric current acts as an excitant to the nerves both of sensation and motion. It influences to some extent, also, the secretions, through its action on the nerves distributed to the secreting organs; it may

promote the function of absorption, through an effect on the absorbents; and it affects the circulation by inducing contractions of the heart. A powerful charge of electricity produces violent and frequently fatal effects on the central nervous system.

For medicinal purposes, electricity is obtained from three sources:

1. FRICTION or STATIC electricity.
2. GALVANIC electricity.
3. FARADIC, INDUCED, MAGNETIC, or VOLTAO-MAGNETIC electricity.

FRICTION electricity may be applied in three modes. 1. By the electric bath, when the patient, placed upon an insulated stool, and connected with the prime conductor of an electrical machine, is *charged* with electricity. 2. By a *spark* to a particular part. Or, 3, a *shock* through a charged Leyden jar may be directed through the part which it is desired to affect.

GALVANISM is that form of electricity which is developed by chemical decomposition, and is known as the continuous, Voltaic, or *battery* current. It is characterized by relatively low intensity of action, but it is developed in considerable quantity, and produces chemical and thermic results, that are not reached by the friction electricity.

FARADIZATION, FARADISM, INDUCED or MAGNETO-ELECTRIC electricity, is applied by means of electro-magnetic machines. It is inferior in chemical and thermal influence to galvanism, but it produces more marked contraction of muscles and a more powerful action on the nerves both of sensation and motion.

Electricity is employed in medicine both for *diagnostic* and *therapeutic* uses. Thus, in the *diagnosis* of spinal paralysis: when a muscle is merely separated from the influence of the spinal cord, by destruction of its nerve, or by destructive disease of the cord at the origin of its nerve, it loses its electric irritability to all forms of electric irritation; in cerebral paralysis, on the other hand, there is no diminution in the contractility of the paralyzed muscle to the electric current, and there may be even an increase. In malingering, real may be distinguished from feigned paralysis, as, after railway accidents, faradization, by showing a marked difference in the contractility of the two sides, establishes the fact of an actual morbid condition. In recent *hysterical* paralysis, the contractility of the muscles is unimpaired.

Therapeutically, electricity may be employed, either to arouse or increase the action of a nerve or muscle, as in paralysis of sensation or of motion, or to reduce or even temporarily abolish this action, as in pain, neuralgia, and spasm, either tonic or clonic. It is chiefly useful in cases of local or functional paralysis, which are independent of lesion of the nervous centres, or in lead palsy, after the elimination of lead from the system. In anæmic and hysterical paralysis, as hysterical aphonia, static electricity is often very useful.

Electricity has been prescribed also as an emmenagogue, to produce contraction of the uterus in post-partum hemorrhage, to overcome constipation, to promote the biliary secretion, and to heal ulcers. It has been also resorted to with success to induce the absorption of tumours and indurations. In the form of electro-magnetism, it is a powerful excitant in the coma resulting from narcotic poisons, and in asphyxia generally, and is probably the most active remedy that can be exhibited in these cases.

PART III.

PHARMACOLOGICAL REMEDIES.

Pharmacological Remedies, or Medicines, are substances, not essentially alimentary, which, when applied to the body, so alter or modify its vital functions, as to be rendered applicable to the treatment of diseases.

The designation, Materia Medica, or Pharmacology, is *strictly speaking* limited to the consideration of medicines. The application of medicines to the treatment of diseases is termed Therapeutics. Pharmacy is the department of Materia Medica which treats of the collection, preparation, preservation, and dispensation of medicines.

To the student of medicine, the objects of examination in relation to medicines are,—the sources from which they are derived; the mode in which they are prepared and brought to market; their sensible qualities, and also their chemical composition and relations; their physiological effects, or the effects which they are capable of producing in healthy individuals; their therapeutical effects, or those which they produce in morbid states of the system; and, lastly, the doses, modes of administration, and preparations (extemporaneous and officinal), under which they are administered.

To facilitate a uniform nomenclature and dispensation of medicines, authoritative works have been issued in different countries, termed Pharmacopœias. The Pharmacopœia of the United States was first promulgated by the authority of a convention held at Washington, in 1820, and it has been since revised decennially. It furnishes a list of articles which are in general use, sets forth the weights and measures which are employed in dispensing and preparing them, and supplies formulæ for such preparations as should be kept in the shops, and which are thence termed *officinal*, from the Latin word *officina*, a shop. It is divided into three portions: a *primary* list of the *materia medica*, containing articles of assured reputation, a *secondary* list of articles of less importance, and a division of *preparations*.

The effects of medicines take place either in the parts to which they are applied, or in distant parts of the system. The former are termed *local* or *topical effects;* the latter, *remote* or *constitutional effects.*

MODUS OPERANDI OF MEDICINES.

The medium through which the influence of medicines is exerted on remote parts of the body, or their *modus operandi* (as it is usually termed), was long a contested point. Until within a comparatively recent period, it was maintained that the impressions of medicines and poisons were transmitted from the parts receiving them to distant parts, by means of a *communication through the nerves.* But it is now generally admitted, that the *absorption* or passage of the medicinal or poisonous molecules into the blood is necessary to their action on parts remote from the seat of impression.

While, however, it is well established, that the *characteristic* action of medicines is transmitted to the parts influenced, exclusively through the medium of the circulation, it is undeniable that the functions of the nervous system may be *secondarily* excited by a local medicinal impression. The number of agents which operate in this manner is, however, very limited.

The action of medicines by absorption is proved by a variety of facts.

They are detected in many parts of the system remote from that to which they have been applied, having been found in the blood, the solids, and the excretions, after being taken into the stomach. If the circulation be interrupted, the influence of a poison cannot be transmitted; while its effects have been obtained, when applied to a wound in the foot of an animal, after all parts of the extremity have been severed, except the artery and vein. In confirmation of the doctrine of absorption may be cited also the admitted facts, that the remote effects of medicines or poisons are promoted or retarded by circumstances which promote or retard absorption; that the blood of poisoned animals is found to possess poisonous properties; that the fluids and solids acquire medicinal properties after the use of medicines (as the milk of nurses); that the specific effects of medicines are produced by their injection into the blood; and that medicines disappear from closed cavities into which they are introduced.

After their absorption into the blood, medicines circulate with it, penetrate through the capillaries to the various organs, and are afterwards thrown out of the system with the excretions. Some medicines produce changes in the condition of the circulating fluid. Others have a specific action upon some one or other of the organs of the body. And in passing out of the system, most medicines act as excitants of the organs by which they are thrown out.

The absorption of medicines is effected principally by the veins, and in some degree also by the lymphatics and lacteals. The medicinal particles penetrate or soak through the interstices of the tissue with which they are placed in contact, and are thence diffused through the circulation. To a limited extent, medicinal substances probably penetrate all the tissues of the part to which they are applied, and in this way the activity of medicines is most decided upon the organs contiguous to the seat of application.

The absorption of insoluble substances cannot take place until they are previously rendered soluble. In the stomach, this is accomplished partly by the agency of the acids of digestion, and partly by the albuminoid constituents of the gastric fluid. Some substances are dissolved by the alkaline liquids of the small intestine.

It is objected to the theory of the operation of medicines by absorption, that certain poisons act with a rapidity incompatible with their previous introduction into the circulation. This is, however, not the fact, as the action of the most violent poisons (hydrocyanic acid, for example), is never wholly instantaneous; and careful experiments have shown that the velocity of the circulation is sufficient to diffuse a poison through the blood in a shorter space of time than its effects are ever observed on the system.

CIRCUMSTANCES WHICH MODIFY THE EFFECTS OF MEDICINES.

The circumstances which modify the effects of medicines relate both to the medicines and to the human system.

1. The properties of medicines are modified by the soil in which they grow, by climate, cultivation, age, and the season of the year at which they are gathered.

2. Medicines are more active, because more readily absorbed, in a state of solution than in a solid state.

3. Soluble medicines are often rendered inert by a chemical reaction which converts them into insolubles; in this way antidotes modify the effects of poisons.

4. Differences in dose greatly modify the effects of medicines.

5. Pharmaceutical modifications have an important influence on the efficacy of medicines. They may be exhibited in the solid, semi-solid, liquid, and aëriform states:

In the *solid* state they are administered in the shape of powders, pills, lozenges, confections, and papers.

In the *liquid* state, they are administered in the shape of mixtures, solutions, medicated waters, infusions, decoctions, tinctures, spirits, wines, juices, vinegars, honeys, syrups, and glycerites.

In the *semi-solid*, or soft state, they are employed internally, in the form of suppositories, and externally, in that of liniments, ointments, cerates, plasters, and cataplasms.

In the form of *gases* and *vapours*, medicines are used for purposes of inhalation.

SOLIDS.

POWDERS (*Pulveres*). The form of powder is usually selected for the administration of medicines, which are not very bulky, nor of very disagreeable taste, which have no corrosive property, and which do not deliquesce rapidly on exposure. Deliquescent substances, and such as contain a large proportion of fixed or volatile oil, should always be recently pulverized, as they deteriorate when kept. Most substances, employed in the form of powder, are usually pulverized on a large scale. For the purpose of pulverizing drugs in small quantity, the physician makes use of a *pestle* and *mortar*, of iron, brass, glass, Wedgewood-ware, or marble, the finer particles being afterwards separated from the coarser, by a sieve. In some cases, a stone slab and muller are used. Some powders are obtained by *precipitation;* and the finer particles of a powder are often separated from the coarser, by a process termed *elutriation*, in which the powder is diffused through water, the heavier portions being first allowed to subside, and, the liquid being poured off, the finer particles settle separately.

Salts of difficult pulverization are often *granulated*, by making a hot saturated solution of the salt, filtering and stirring the filtered liquid, until cool. Of late years, *granulated effervescing* salts have been used in imitation of the waters of mineral springs, the effervescence being produced by the addition of carbonate of sodium and tartaric or citric acid.

The lighter powders may be administered in water or other thin liquid. The heavier powders require a more consistent vehicle, as syrup, treacle, or honey.

PILLS (*Pilulæ*), are small globular masses, of a semi-solid consistence, and of a size that can be conveniently swallowed.

The form of pill is suitable for the exhibition of medicines which are not bulky, and are of disagreeable taste or smell, or insoluble in water. Deliquescent substances should not be made into pills, and those, which are efflorescent, should be previously deprived of their water of crystallization.

Some substances are readily made into pills, with the addition of a little water or spirit. Very soft or liquid substances require the addition of some dry inert powder, as bread-crumb, or powdered gum Arabic, to reduce them to a proper consistence. Wax is a good excipient for oils.

Heavy powders are mixed with some soft solid, as confection of rose, plasma, manna, &c., or with a tenacious liquid, as treacle or syrup. When the pilular mass is properly prepared, it is rolled with a spatula into a cylinder of uniform thickness, and is then divided into the required number of pills, with the hand, or, more accurately, with a pill-tile, or with a pill-machine. The pills are rolled into spherical form between the fingers; and, to prevent adhesion, are dusted with some dry powder, as powdered liquorice-root, orris-root, starch, or carbonate of magnesium. They should not weigh above six grains; a large pill is termed a *bolus*. To conceal the taste and smell of pills, they are sometimes coated with gelatin, collodion, mucilage, sugar,

&c. When they are designed to be of slow operation, the modern practice of sugar-coating pills answers very well. But, when they are intended to act quickly, the coating is objectionable, as it retards the solution of the pills in the gastric fluids. Pills, which have been long kept, may pass unchanged through the stomach and bowels, and are therefore objectionable.

Troches or Lozenges (*Trochisci*), are small, dry, solid masses, made of powders with sugar and mucilage, and intended to be held in the mouth and allowed to dissolve slowly. Mucilage of *tragacanth* is usually employed in preparing lozenges.

Confections (*Confectiones*), are soft solid preparations, made with some saccharine matter. They are subdivided into *Conserves* and *Electuaries:* the former consist of combinations of recent vegetable substances and refined sugar, beat into a uniform mass; the latter are extemporaneous mixtures of medicines, usually dry powders, with syrup, honey, or treacle.

Papers (*Chartæ*), are preparations designed for external application, which are made by spreading mixtures of medicinal substances, as cantharides or mustard, upon paper.

LIQUIDS.

Mixtures (*Misturæ*), are preparations of *insoluble* substances, suspended in water by means of gum Arabic, sugar, the yolk of eggs, or other viscid matter. When the suspended substance is oleaginous, the mixture is termed an *emulsion.*

Solutions (*Liquores*), are solutions (chiefly aqueous) of non-volatile substances, which are wholly soluble in the menstruum employed. In making solutions, and all other aqueous preparations, the water used should be fresh river, rain, or distilled water, and free from saline impurities.

Medicated Waters (*Aquæ*), are preparations consisting of

water holding volatile or gaseous substances in solution. Many of them, having been made by distilling water from plants containing volatile oil, were formerly termed *distilled waters.* In place of distillation, trituration with carbonate of magnesium (afterwards separated by filtration) is now employed to impregnate water with volatile oils.

INFUSIONS (*Infusa*) are partial solutions of vegetable substances in water, obtained without the aid of ebullition. They are made with both hot and cold water; the former extracts the soluble principle more rapidly and in larger proportion; the latter is preferred, when the active principle would be injured by heat, or when it is desirable not to take up some matter, insoluble at a low temperature. Infusions have been usually made by pouring water upon the substances to be infused, and allowing it to remain upon them for some time in a tightly-covered vessel; when the process takes place at a heat of from 60° to 90°, it is termed *maceration;* when at a heat of from 90° to 100°, *digestion.* Of late years, a more efficient mode of extracting the medicinal virtues of plants has been introduced, termed *percolation* or *displacement.* In this operation, the medicinal substance is coarsely powdered, and placed in a conical or nearly cylindrical instrument called a *percolator,* in the lower part of which is fitted a porous or colander-like partition or diaphragm. The powder is then saturated with water or other menstruum, till it will absorb no more; and, after they have remained for some time in contact, fresh portions of the menstruum are added, till the required quantity is employed. The fresh liquid, as it is successively added, percolates the solid particles of the medicinal substance, driving the previously saturated liquid before it; and in this way completely exhausts the substance to be dissolved. An ordinary glass funnel answers very well for percolation; and a circular piece of muslin or lint, pressed into the neck by means of a cork with notched sides, forms a good diaphragm—care being taken to interpose a similar piece of muslin, moistened slightly with the menstruum, between the diaphragm and powder.

Decoctions (*Decocta*), are partial solutions of vegetable substances in water, in which the active principles are obtained by ebullition. This is a more rapid and active mode of extracting the virtues of plants than by infusion. But it is objectionable, when the proximate principles are volatile at a boiling heat, or undergo decomposition by ebullition. In making decoctions, ebullition should be continued for a few minutes only, and the liquid should be allowed to cool slowly in a close vessel. As they are apt to spoil, they should be prepared only when wanted for use.

Tinctures (*Tincturæ*), are solutions of medicinal substances in alcohol or diluted alcohol. Ammonia and ethereal spirit are also sometimes employed as solvents; and solutions in these menstrua are called *ammoniated* tinctures and *ethereal* tinctures. Alcohol or rectified spirit (of a sp. gr. 0.835, according to the U. S. Pharmacopœia), is employed in making tinctures of substances nearly or quite insoluble in water, as the resins, essential oils, iodine, &c. Diluted alcohol or proof spirit (consisting of equal measures of officinal alcohol and water) is preferred, when the substance is soluble both in alcohol and water, or when some of its ingredients are soluble in the one menstruum and some in the other. Tinctures have been usually prepared by maceration or digestion, more commonly by the former process, and a period of two weeks is recommended for its duration. It should be conducted in well-closed glass vessels, which should be frequently shaken; and when the maceration is completed, the tincture should be separated from the dregs by filtration. The U. S. Pharmacopœia now recommends percolation in making most tinctures, and, in the hands of skilful pharmaceutists, this process is preferable, as the most thorough mode of exhausting medicinal substances; but, where the operator cannot trust himself, it is better to recur to the old process of maceration. Tinctures should be kept in bottles accurately stoppered, to prevent evaporation, which might seriously increase their strength.

The form of tincture is adapted to the exhibition of medicines, which are to be given in small quantity, and it affords a convenient mode of graduating doses. In prescribing large and continued doses of tinctures, the stimulating effects of the alcohol which they contain must be borne in mind.

SPIRITS (*Spiritus*), are alcoholic solutions of volatile or gaseous principles, properly speaking procured by distillation, but now usually prepared by dissolving the volatile principles in alcohol or diluted alcohol. The spirits of the aromatic vegetable oils are used to give a pleasant odour and taste to mixtures, to correct the nauseating and griping effects of cathartics, and also as carminatives and stomachics.

WINES (*Vina*), are solutions of medicinal substances in Sherry or other white wine. They are more liable to decomposition than tinctures, and are of variable strength; but they are in some cases preferred from the less stimulating character of the menstruum, which has also sometimes an increase of solvent power, from the acid which it contains.

JUICES (*Succi*), are the expressed juices of fresh plants, preserved by the addition of one-fifth their measure of alcohol.

VINEGARS (*Aceta*), are infusions or solutions of medicinal substances in distilled vinegar or diluted acetic acid, which is a particularly good solvent of many vegetable principles, as the organic alkalies.

HONEYS (*Mellita*,) are preparations of medicinal substances in honey. In *oxymels*, a combination of honey and vinegar is employed. The latter preparations are not now officinal.

SYRUPS (*Syrupi*), are preparations of medicinal substances in concentrated solutions of sugar. The term *syrup* (*syrupus*), or *simple syrup*, is applied to a solution of sugar (thirty-six troyounces) in water (Oij f℥xij), dissolved with the aid of heat. *Medicated* syrups are usually made by incorporating refined sugar with vegetable infusions, decoctions, expressed juices, fermented liquors, or simple aqueous solutions. They may also be prepared by adding a tincture to simple syrup, and afterwards evaporating the alcohol; or, by mixing the tincture with sugar in coarse powder, and dissolving the impregnated sugar, after evaporation, in the necessary proportion of water. Syrups are apt to be spoiled by heat, and should be made in small quantities at a time.

By the evaporation of the solutions of vegetable principles, a very useful class of preparations termed *Extracts* (*Extracta*), is obtained. They are prepared from infusions, decoctions, tinctures, and vinegars; and sometimes, in the case of recent vegetables, from the expressed juices of plants, usually diluted with water. Extracts, prepared by the agency of water, are termed *watery extracts;* those by means of alcohol, *alcoholic extracts;* those by means of acetic acid, *acetic extracts.* The evaporation of extracts is generally continued, till they have a pilular consistence. Within a few years, however, these preparations have been employed in the liquid form, under the name of *Fluid Extracts* (*Extracta Fluida*), which have the advantage of convenience of administration, and of being prepared at a less degree of heat. They are more liable than the solid extracts to spontaneous decomposition; and this difficulty is usually counteracted by means of sugar. In making the fluid extracts, alcohol and glycerin are the menstrua chiefly resorted to. The portion of the solvent, which remains after evaporation, contributes in some degree to the preservation of the preparation.

GLYCERITES (*Glycerita*), are solutions of medicinal substances in glycerin, made by rubbing them together in a mortar.

The OLEORESINS (*Oleoresinæ*), are extracts obtained by the agency of ether, which consist of fixed or volatile oils, holding resins and sometimes other active matters in solution. They retain a liquid or semi-liquid state, upon the evaporation of the liquid employed in their preparation, and have the property of self-preservation.

SEMI-SOLIDS.

SUPPOSITORIES (*Suppositoria*), are soft solids, made by mixture of a medicinal substance with the oil of theobroma, usually in a conical form, of a weight of thirty grains, and designed for introduction into the rectum. They are employed with a view both to a local effect on the lower bowel and also to the gradual absorption of the medicinal substance. As the solvent action of the fluids of the rectum is much less than that of those of the stomach, only readily soluble medicines should be introduced in this way, for a constitutional effect; absorption, too, takes place less rapidly from the rectum than from the stomach.

LINIMENTS (*Linimenta*), are oily preparations designed for external use, usually, thicker than water, but always liquid at the temperature of the body.

OINTMENTS (*Unguenta*), are preparations of a consistence like that of butter, made with lard or some other fatty substance. They are fitted for application to the skin by friction or inunction. Most of the ointments become rancid, when long kept, and it is therefore best to prepare them only as wanted for use. The term, *ointment* (*unguentum*), is applied to a mixture of one part of yellow wax and four parts of lard.

CERATES (*Cerata*), are made of oil or lard, mixed with wax, spermaceti, or resin, with the addition of various medicinal substances. They are of harder consistence than ointments, and do not melt when applied to the skin. The term, *cerate* (*ceratum*), is applied to a mixture of one part of white wax and two parts of lard.

PLASTERS (*Emplastra*), are adhesive at the temperature of the body, and must generally be heated to be spread. Some substances have sufficient consistence and adhesiveness to be made into plasters. Usually, however, medicinal substances when employed in this form, are mixed with *Lead Plaster* or

Litharge Plaster (*Emplastrum Plumbi*), a compound of olive oil and litharge. Plasters are prepared for use by spreading them upon sheepskin, linen, or muslin, with a margin a quarter or half inch broad.

Cataplasms, or Poultices (*Cataplasmata*), are soft, moist substances, intended for external use. The common emollient poultice, employed to relieve inflammation and promote suppuration, is made by mixing bread-crumbs with boiling milk, or powdered flaxseed with boiling water. A fabric, termed *spongio-piline,* consisting principally of sponge, has lately been used as a substitute for the old poultice, and, when saturated with hot water, is a good vehicle of heat and moisture.

GASES AND VAPOURS.

When employed in this form, medicines are administered by *inhalation.* This may be effected either by diffusing the gas or vapour through the air to be respired by the patient; or by inclosing it in a bag or bottle with a suitable tube, through which the patient may breathe; or, when ethereal vapours are employed, by saturating a sponge or handkerchief with the ether, and applying it to the mouth and nostrils of the patient; or the fumes of burning medicinal substances may be inhaled, by means of cigarettes or pipes, variously contrived.

WEIGHTS AND MEASURES.

In prescribing and dispensing medicines, the following are the *weights* and *measures* employed in the United States, with their signs annexed.

TROY OR APOTHECARIES' WEIGHT.

The pound, ℔	contains	Twelve ounces, ℥.
The ounce	contains	Eight drachms, ʒ.
The drachm	contains	Three scruples, ℈.
The scruple	contains	Twenty grains, gr.

The term *pound* should be avoided in formulæ, owing to the danger of mistakes from confounding the troy pound with the heavier avoirdupois pound, and large weights should be expressed in *troyounces*. The drachm and scruple are also now disused by the United States Pharmacopœia, and are replaced by their equivalents in grains. The troyounce contains 480 grains; the drachm, 60 grains.

In France and other parts of the continent of Europe, a system of metrical weights is employed, the relation of which to those used in the United States, is as follows: 1 *grain* = 6.479 *centigrammes;* 1 *scruple* = 1.295 *grammes;* 1 *drachm* = 3.887 *grammes;* 1 *ounce* = 3.1103 *decagrammes;* 1 pound = 3.7324 *hectogrammes;* or, 1 *centigramme* = about $\frac{1}{6}$ *grain;* 1 *decigramme* = about $1\frac{1}{2}$ *grain;* 1 *gramme* = about 15 *grains;* 1 *decagramme* = about $2\frac{1}{2}$ *drachms;* 1 *hectogramme* = about 3 *troyounces* and 5 *scruples;* 1 *kilogramme* = about 2 *pounds* and 8 *troyounces;* 1 *myriagramme* = about 26 *pounds*, 9 *troyounces*, and 4 *drachms*. The GRAMME is the weight of a cubic centimetre of water at 4° C.

COMPARATIVE TABLE OF DECIMAL WITH TROY WEIGHTS.

NAMES	EQUIVALENT IN GRAMMES.	EQUIVALENT IN GRAINS.	EQUIVALENT IN TROY WEIGHT.			
			℔	℥	ʒ	gr.
Milligramme,	.001	.0154				
Centigramme,	.01	.1543				
Decigramme,	.1	1.5434				1.5
Gramme,	1	15.4340				15.4
Decagramme,	10	154.3402			2	34.0
Hectogramme,	100	1543.4023		3	1	43.0
Kilogramme,	1000	15434.0234	2	8	1	14.
Myriagramme,	10000	154340 2344	26	9	4	20.

WINE OR APOTHECARIES' MEASURE.

The gallon, C	contains	Eight pints, O.
The pint	contains	Sixteen fluidounces, f℥.
The fluidounce	contains	Eight fluidrachms, fʒ.
The fluidrachm	contains	Sixty mimins, ♏.

The term *gallon* is not used by the U. S. Pharmacopœia, that measure being always expressed in pints.

Liquid measures are sometimes prescribed by *drops*, which, however, vary in quantity according to the nature of the liquid, the shape and size of the vessel from which it is dropped, and even the amount of liquid which the vessel contains. (Thus, a fluidrachm of distilled water contains only 45 drops, while this measure of alcohol and of most tinctures contains 120 drops, and of chloroform, 220 drops or even more.) Approximate measurements are also frequently employed in prescribing the less powerful liquids: thus a *teacup* is used for f℥iv, or a gill; a *wineglass* for f℥ij; a *tablespoon* for f℥ss; a *teaspoon* for fʒj.

The French measures, although not adopted by the U. S. Pharmacopœia, are now a good deal used: 1 fluidounce = 31 cubic centimetres; 1 c. c. or 1 gramme = 15½ grains of distilled water.

FRENCH MEASURE OF CAPACITY—APOTHECARIES' MEASURE.

1 millilitre or cubic centimetre = 16.2318 minims.
10 millilitres = 1 centilitre = 2.7053 fl. drachms.
100 millilitres = 10 centilitres = 1 decilitre = 3.3816 fl. ounces.
1000 millilitres = 100 centilitres = 10 decilitres = 1 litre = 2.1135 pints.
10,000 millilitres = 1000 centilitres = 100 decilitres = 10 litres = 1 decalitre = 2.6419 gallons.
100,000 millilitres = 10,000 centilitres = 1000 decilitres = 100 litres = 10 decalitres = 1 hectolitre = 26.4190 gallons.
1,000,000 millilitres = 100,000 centilitres = 10,000 decilitres = 1000 litres = 100 decalitres = 10 hectolitres = 1 kilolitre = 264.1900 gallons.

A variety of circumstances, relating to the human organism, modify the effects of medicines.

Age exerts a most important influence in this particular. Children are more susceptible than adults; and in advanced age, also, smaller doses are required than in the prime of life. No general rule can be laid down for the adaptation of the doses of medicines to different ages, as the different susceptibilities to the influence of different medicines are unequal at the same age. Thus, infants are peculiarly alive to impressions from opium, while, in the cases of calomel and castor oil, they will bear much larger proportional doses.

Dr. Young's scheme for graduating the doses of medicines to different ages answers very well in prescribing: For children under twelve years, the doses of most medicines must be diminished in the proportion of the age to the age increased by 12; thus, at two years to $\frac{1}{7}$, viz.: $\frac{2}{2+12}=\frac{1}{7}$. At 21, the full dose may be given.

A good practical rule for graduating doses is that of Dr. Cowling: "The proportional dose for any age under adult life is represented by the number of the following birth-day divided by twenty-four;" for one year, $\frac{2}{24} = \frac{1}{12}$; for three years, $\frac{4}{24} = \frac{1}{6}$; for eleven years, $\frac{12}{24} = \frac{1}{2}$.

Sex, temperament, and *idiosyncrasy*, all modify the effects of medicines. Women require somewhat smaller doses than men; and during menstruation, pregnancy, and lactation, all active treatment, which is not imperatively demanded, should be avoided. To persons of a sanguine temperament, stimulants are to be administered with caution, while in cases of nervous temperament, the same care is to be observed in the employment of evacuants. Mercurials are called for where the bilious temperament exists, but, on the other hand, they are generally injurious where the lymphatic temperament is strongly marked. Idiosyncrasy renders many individuals peculiarly susceptible or insusceptible to the action of particular medicines, as mercury, opium, &c.

In *disease*, an extraordinary tolerance of the action of many medicines is established. In tetanus, immense quantities of opium are borne and required; in typhoid fever, alcohol is freely administered without inducing narcotism; in pneumonia, tartar emetic may be taken in large doses, without nausea.

The *time of administration* modifies the action of medicines. Where a rapid effect is desired, they are to be given on an empty stomach; on the other hand, irritant substances, as the arsenical or iodic preparations, are best borne, when the stomach is full; and the insoluble chalybeates, requiring the gastric fluid to dissolve them, should be taken with the food.

The *condition of the stomach* is to be considered in prescribing medicines. In the black vomit of yellow fever, absorption cannot take place by the stomach, and in the second stage of cholera, endosmosis by the bowels is impossible; here, the hypodermic medication is invaluable.

Habit diminishes the influence of many medicines, especially narcotics.

The influence of *race*, *climate*, *occupation*, and the *imagination*, upon the effects of medicines is often decided, and deserves attention in prescribing.

PARTS TO WHICH MEDICINES ARE APPLIED.

Medicines are applied to the skin, to mucous membranes, to serous membranes, to wounds, ulcers, cysts, and abscesses, and they are injected into the veins.

1. *To the Skin.*—Medicines are applied to the skin for both a local and a general effect. As their influence on *distant* organs is the result of their absorption, this function is usually assisted by friction, or by removal of the cuticle, when medicines are applied to the skin to affect remote parts of the system.

The application of medicines to the skin by *friction* is occasionally resorted to, but its results are slow and uncertain; and, when we wish to affect the system through the agency of the skin, the preferable method is to apply the medicine to the dermis denuded of the cuticle.

This is termed the *endermic method*, and the cuticle is usually removed by means of a blister. The medicine is applied to the denuded dermis in the form of powder, or, if very irritating, it may be incorporated with gelatine, lard, or cerate. This method is useful in cases of irritability of the stomach, of inability to swallow, or where we desire to influence the system rapidly, and by every possible avenue, or where it is of importance to apply the medicine near the seat of disease. The dose is to be two or three times the amount which is administered by the stomach.

Another method of applying medicines through the skin is

by injection into the subcutaneous cellular tissue. This method is termed the *hypodermic* method, and is of recent introduction into therapeutics. Medicines are injected hypodermically, for both a local and a general effect. A constitutional impression can be produced by this means much more rapidly and efficiently than by the introduction of medicines into the stomach. It is particularly adapted to the speedy relief of pain, to the treatment of diseases in which it is desirable to influence the system with the greatest possible rapidity and effect, and also to cases where the internal administration of medicines is interfered with. The substances, proper for hypodermic injection, are those which are small in bulk and are of perfect solubility, such as the vegetable alkaloids. Substances of imperfect solubility should not be injected hypodermically, dangerous results having followed therefrom, as from the use of the salts of quinia. The dose, particularly in first injections, should be one half the ordinary dose by the stomach, and for females about a third.

The instrument used for injection is a small syringe armed with a small, sharp lancet, and, for the better regulation of the dose, it is desirable that the syringe should be graduated. It is important to avoid the puncture of a vein, lest a suddenly overwhelming effect be produced; and, with this view, the syringe-needle should not be pushed too deeply into the tissues, and should be withdrawn a little, to allow a wound of a vein to close from elasticity. When a constitutional effect only is aimed at, a good spot for injection is at the insertion of the deltoid muscle in the arm, and, where repeated operations are practised, it is well to vary the point of injection.

2. *To Mucous Membranes.*—Medicines are applied to all the gastro-pulmonary and genito-urinary mucous surfaces.

a. To the *conjunctiva*, they are applied for local effects only, and are termed *collyria*, or eye-washes.

b. To the *nasal* or *pituitary membrane*, they are applied usually for local purposes; sometimes, however, to irritate, and excite a discharge, when they are termed *errhines;* sometimes, also, to produce sneezing, with a view to the expulsion of foreign bodies from the nasal cavities, when they are termed *sternutatories.*

c. To the *mucous membrane of the mouth and throat*, medicines are applied almost exclusively for local purposes. When in solution, they are termed *gargarismata* or *gargles*. Powders are introduced by insufflation.

d. To the *Eustachian tubes*, washes are applied in local affections.

e. On the *aërial* or *tracheo-bronchial membrane*, medicines produce a very decided influence, both local and general. Liquid substances are introduced into the air-passages by means of a sponge or syringe, in the treatment of chronic inflammations of the larynx. Various substances are inhaled with advantage in phthisis, chronic bronchitis and laryngitis, asthma, &c., while the most powerful effects are produced on the system, by the absorption of ethereal vapours and gases through the pulmonary surface.

Within the last few years, liquids have been introduced into the air passages, for the treatment of diseases of the respiratory organs, in the form of a *fine spray*. This mode of application, termed the *pulverization*, *nebulization*, or *atomization* of fluids, has proved very valuable, particularly in the relief of throat affections. Various instruments have been resorted to in the atomization of liquids. The *hand-ball atomizer*, which is usually employed, consists of two glass tubes, with capillary openings, placed at right angles to each other,

Fig. 2.

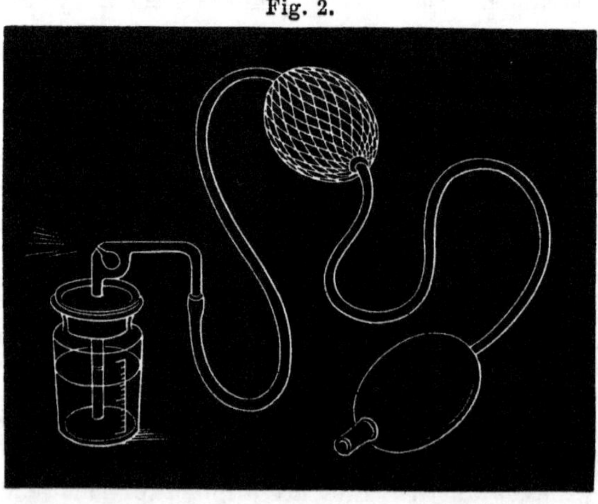

the vertical tube being dipped in a bottle containing the fluid to be atomized, while at the other end it is close to and about opposite to the centre of a capillary opening in the horizontal tube. This connects with an elastic tube, intercepted by two elastic balls, one in the middle, the other, which is furnished with the valves, at the end of the tube. The upper ball acts as a reservoir, into which a current of air is forced from the lower ball by pressure with the hand. The air in the vertical glass tube being rarified, the liquid rises to the capillary opening, and is there pulverized by the current of air from the horizontal tube. The *atomizer* is used also to produce local anæsthesia, and as a deodorizer.

As modified by Winterich, the spray can be readily gener-

Fig. 3.

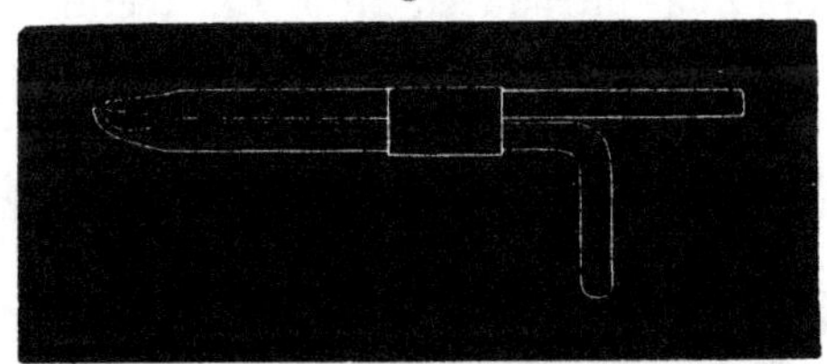

ated within various parts of the body, as the back of the throat, nostril, meatus of the ear, &c. Instead of air, steam has been substituted as the forcing power in the apparatus known as Siégle's. In this instrument, as modified by Da

Fig. 4.

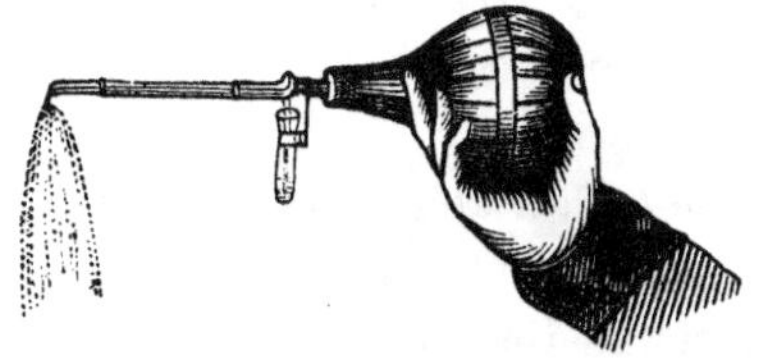

Costa, inhalation can be practised without fatigue or assistance, and the warmth of the spray is also an advantage in many diseases of the respiratory organs.

f. The *gastro-intestinal mucous membrane*, of all parts of the body, is most employed for the exhibition of medicines. The stomach, from its great susceptibility, its active absorbing power, and the numerous relations which it has with almost every part of the body, is the chief recipient of medicinal agents. The rectum is, however, also frequently employed for various purposes, as to relieve disease of this or of neighbouring organs, to occasion revulsion, to produce alvine evacuations, to destroy ascarides, and when, for any reason, it is desirable to spare the stomach.

It is usually recommended, that the dose of medicines, introduced into the rectum for constitutional effects, should be two or three times greater than when taken into the stomach. In the case of active, soluble medicines, however, especially narcotics, it is most prudent to give the same amount by the rectum as by the mouth.

Solid substances introduced into the rectum are termed *suppositories.* Liquids introduced into the rectum are termed *clysters, lavements, injections,* and *enemata.* Soluble substances, when thus applied, are usually dissolved in water; insoluble substances are suspended in some mucilaginous vehicle. When the enema is to be retained, it should be from one to four fluidrachms in quantity. When it is introduced to act upon the bowels, its bulk may be from twelve to sixteen fluidounces, for an adult, six to eight fluidounces for a youth of twelve, three to four fluidounces for a child of one to five years, and a fluidounce for a newly-born infant. Various instruments are used for the administration of enemata, as the pipe and bladder, the ordinary syringe, the self-injecting apparatus, and the elastic bottle and tube. Gaseous matters have also been thrown into the rectum—tobacco-smoke, for example,—to relieve obstructions of the bowels.

g. To the *urino-genital* and *vagino-uterine membranes*, applications are made exclusively for local purposes. Within a few years, intra-uterine medication has been a good deal employed in local affections of the uterus, but, in the injection of fluids into the uterus, there is danger of peritonitis.

3. To *Serous Membranes.* Irritating solutions are injected into he cavity of the tunica vaginalis testis, in hydrocele; into the hernial sac, in hernia; and even into the pleural cavity, in pleurisy, for the purpose of producing adhesion of the sides of the sacs.

4. To *Ulcers*, *Wounds*, and *Abscesses*, medicines are applied chiefly for their local effects. The absorbing power of these surfaces is to be kept in mind in such applications. *Cysts* are sometimes cured by injections, as of iodine into cysts of the thyroid gland.

5. *The Injection of medicines into the Veins* has been occasionally practised. The operation is, however, objectionable, from the danger of introducing air into the circulation; and it is seldom resorted to, except in the case of *transfusion of blood* after uterine or other hemorrhage, or exhausting disease.

Transfusion will often be found an efficient remedy, although there is always risk of coagulation of the blood in the veins. The more direct and immediate the transfusion, the safer the operation, as by Aveling's apparatus, which consists of an India-rubber bulb, oblong in shape, and of sufficient size to contain two fluidrachms; India-rubber tubes six or seven

Fig. 5.

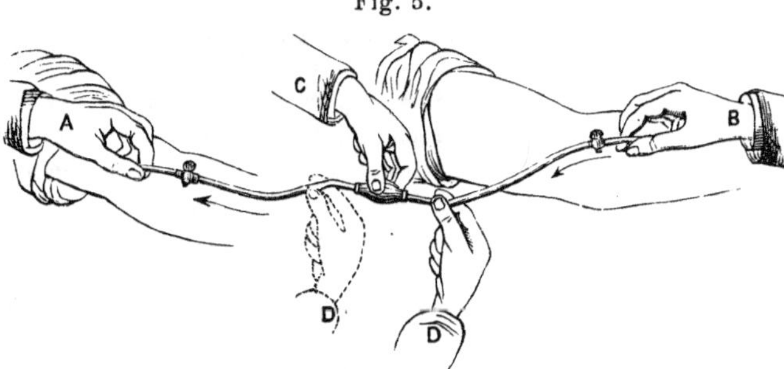

inches in length attached to the extremities of the bulb; and stop-cocks attached to the outer extremities of the tubes. Also, two silver tubes: one, bevel-pointed, called the afferent tube (seen at A), which is to be inserted into the vein in the arm of the patient; the other round-pointed, called the efferent tube (seen at B), which is to be inserted into the vein in the arm of the donor. Also, a pair of fine forceps and a scalpel.*

* The mode of operation is as follows:

First, place the apparatus in a basin of tepid water, and, while completely under the water, for the purpose of filling it and insuring its cleanliness, compress and expand the bulb until the air contained within the bulb and rubber tubing is completely expelled. When the air has been completely expelled, and while the apparatus is yet remaining beneath the

THE CLASSIFICATION OF MEDICINES.

In treating the articles of the Materia Medica, some writers have classified them according to their natural properties, others,

surface of the water, turn the stop-cocks at both extremities of the rubber tubing in such a manner as to entirely preclude the possibility of air gaining access to its cavity. The patient having been brought to the side of the bed and the arm made bare, a fold of skin over a vein at the bend of the arm is to be raised, transfixed, and divided. The vein now brought into view is to be seized with the fine forceps, slightly raised, and a small opening made into it for the reception of the bevel-pointed silver or afferent tube. This tube, which has been lying in the basin of tepid water, should carefully be kept filled with water when it is removed, by placing the thumb or finger over its larger opening.

The tube, now being filled with water, has its bevel-pointed extremity at once inserted into the opening already made in the vein, and is then entrusted to the care of an assistant (A), who carefully compresses the edges of the wound around the tube, and at the same time holds his thumb or finger over its larger opening to prevent the escape of the water.

While the operator is performing this part of the operation, an assistant should prepare the arm of the blood-donor in the same manner as for venesection. An opening is then made into the vein, and the round-pointed or efferent tube at once inserted with its point towards the fingers. The donor should then be seated in a chair at the bedside of the patient. It is better not to secure the tubes in the veins by ligatures. B represents the hand of an assistant holding the efferent tube carefully compressed within the lips of the wound, in the same manner as with the afferent tube at A.

The India-rubber portion of the apparatus, thoroughly cleansed, air perfectly expelled, and completely filled with water, is now to be carefully and closely adjusted to the two tubes in the veins. When adjusted, the stop-cocks are turned straight, and transfusion is commenced by first compressing the India-rubber tube on the efferent side (donor's) and then squeezing the bulb which forces two drachms of water into the afferent vein. Next, while the bulb is compressed, shift the hand and compress the India-rubber tube upon the afferent (patient's) side. Then allow the bulb to expand slowly, and blood will be drawn into it from the donor's vein. When the tubing and bulbs are filled, bring the hand back, compress the tube, follow this by compression of the bulb, and two drachms of blood will be thrown into the afferent vein. In this manner the process can be repeated any number of times desired, rapidly or slowly, and the exact amount of blood transfused can be known by counting the number of times the bulb has been emptied, one being subtracted which accounts for water first used.

according to their action on the human system. To the student of medicine, a classification, based upon the sensible qualities or natural affinities of medicines, can be of little value, since it associates articles of the most opposite remedial properties. A classification of medicines, founded on a similarity of action on the animal economy, is more desirable and useful, and various arrangements of the Materia Medica have been attempted on this basis. They are all, to some extent, necessarily imperfect, owing partly to the diversified effects of medicines, and partly to our ignorance of the real nature of many of the modifications which they produce upon the tissues. Still, the advantages of some arrangement of this kind are so numerous, that it cannot well be dispensed with.

The following classification will be found to include the more ordinary and generally received divisions of the Materia Medica, and to present the articles in convenient groups for therapeutic application.

Medicines may be divided into—

I. Those which have a special action on the nervous system, or *Neurotics* (from νευρον, a nerve).	Narcotics, Anæsthetics, Antispasmodics, Tonics, Astringents, Stimulants, Sedatives, Spinants.
II. Those which have a special action on the secretions, or *Eccritics* (from εκκρισις, secretion).	Emetics, Cathartics, Diaphoretics, Diuretics, Blennorrhetics, Emmenagogues.
III. Those which modify the blood, or *Hæmatics* (from αιμα, the blood).	Hæmatinics, Alteratives, Antacids.
IV. Those which act topically.	Irritants, Demulcents, Colouring Agents, Anthelmintics.

CLASS I.—NEUROTICS.

ORDER I.—NARCOTICS.

Narcotics (from ναρκεω, to *stupefy*), are medicines which impair or destroy nervous action. The primary effect of narcotics, is, however, of a stimulant character, and their therapeutic efficacy is in a great degree due to this action. They are often administered, too, for a true narcotic or sedative influence on the motor, sensor, and intellectual functions. In diseased conditions, a marked tolerance of this class of medicines is established, and they can be exhibited in large doses without inducing narcosis. They are employed, chiefly, to remove muscular spasm, relieve pain, allay cerebral or spinal irritability, and procure sleep.

When employed to relieve pain, they are termed *anodynes;* when employed to procure sleep, *hypnotics* or *soporifics.*

When this class of medicines is resorted to for any length of time, with a view to a *narcotic* effect, their influence upon the system is much diminished, and constantly increased amounts are called for, to maintain the same effect.

OPIUM.

Opium (from οπος, *juice*), is the CONCRETE JUICE of the unripe capsules of Papaver somniferum (*Nat. Ord.* Papaveraceæ). The opium-poppy is a native of Persia, but is cultivated in various parts of Asia, in Europe, and in the United States. It is an annual plant, with a round, leafy stem, from two to four feet or more in height, and large four-petaled flowers. There are two prominent varieties of this species: the *black* poppy, with violet-coloured or red flowers, brown or blackish seeds, and globular capsules; and the *white* poppy, with white flowers and seeds, and ovate capsules; but these varieties run into each other under cultivation.

The NEARLY RIPE CAPSULES (PAPAVER) are from an inch and a half to two inches or more in diameter, and contain a good deal of opium. They are sometimes given to children in the form of *syrup*, and are applied externally as an anodyne emollient, in the form of *decoction*. The seeds are destitute of narcotic properties, and are used in Europe as an article of diet, and for the manufacture of an oil.

Opium is obtained from incisions in the half-ripe capsules. The juice, which exudes from the incisions, is allowed to evaporate spontaneously, and is scraped off after drying, generally with more or less of the epidermis, and is sometimes sent into the market unmixed, as a choice variety. The opium of commerce is, however, commonly made by adding the dried juice, obtained by incision, to an extract prepared from a decoction of the leaves, the whole being kneaded together, formed into cakes, and wrapped in fresh poppy leaves.

The commerce of the United States is supplied with opium almost exclusively from Asiatic Turkey. This is known in the market as *Smyrna* or *Turkey* opium, and comes in irregularly rounded or flattened cakes, covered with the capsules of a species of Rumex.

A large amount of opium is produced in British India, for consumption in India and China, but it is not found in our markets. The Persian opium is another variety, but it does not reach the United States. Much opium was formerly obtained from Upper Egypt, in the neighbourhood of Thebes, but its production was for a long time abandoned, though within the last thirty years again introduced. Successful attempts have been made with the cultivation of the poppy in England and other parts of Europe, which have resulted in the production of opium. During the civil war in the United States, a good deal of opium was made in the Southern States, from poppies of almost every variety; samples of this opium have yielded about the same amount of morphia as that obtained from Turkey opium, and even in New England, very good opium has lately been produced. The great source of our supply of opium has, however, long been, and still is, the Turkish dominions.

The best opium should have a fine chestnut colour, an aromatic, strong, peculiar smell, and a dense consistence—becoming, however, harder and darker by being kept. It should be moderately ductile, break with a deeply notched fracture, and, when drawn across white paper, should leave an interrupted stain. The taste is very bitter and somewhat acrid, and when chewed it excites irritation in the mouth and throat. It is inflammable, and imparts its virtues to water, alcohol, and diluted acids—but not to ether.

Chemical Constituents.—Opium contains a great variety of chemical constituents, the most important of which is the alkaloid MORPHIA. Other principles found in opium are the alkaloids, *narcotina*, *codeia*, *narceia*, paramorphia, papaverina, opiana, cryptopia, meconin, meconic and thebolactic acids, porphyroxin, gum, extractive, resin, oil, &c., and, in very minute amounts, alkaloids, termed meconidia, laudamia, codamia, pseudormorphia, apomorphia, lanthopia, rhœadinia, and rhœagenia. Morphia is the principle upon which the narcotic effects of opium essentially depend, and, with its salts, is officinal in all the pharmacopœias.

MORPHIA exists in opium chiefly in combination with meconic acid. The meconate of morphia is separated from the other constituents of the drug, by successive macerations with water. Alcohol and water of ammonia are then added to the aqueous solution, by which the salt is decomposed, the ammonia precipitating the morphia, and the alcohol seizing the colouring matter as soon as it is separated from the alkali. The crystals of morphia, which are formed, are afterwards boiled in alcohol, and the solution is filtered through animal charcoal. Good samples of opium, when dried, should yield at least ten per cent. of morphia.

Morphia ($C_{17}H_{19}NO_3,H_2O$), occurs in colourless, rhombic, prismatic crystals, without smell, but of a very bitter taste. It is very slightly soluble in water and ether, nearly insoluble in chloroform, partially soluble in cold, and more soluble in boiling alcohol. Acetic ether is the best solvent for it. From the insolubility of the alkaloid, the *salts* of morphia are preferred for medicinal use; they are freely soluble in water and diluted alcohol, but are insoluble in ether and chloroform. *Tests:* 1. *Concentrated nitric acid* strikes with morphia and its salts a rich orange-red colour, slowly fading to yellow. 2. *Chloride* or *tersulphate of iron* colours them deep blue. 3. *Iodic acid* is deoxidized by morphia, and, if a solution of starch is added with heat, dark blue starch-iodide is produced; this is a very delicate test. 4. *Sulphomolybdic acid* (made by dissolving, with a gentle heat, 5 or 6 grains of molybdate of ammonium in 2 drachms of strong sulphuric acid), when rubbed with morphia, produces an intense purplish or crimson colour, changing to green, and finally to sapphire blue. 5. *Iodic acid* in solution, mixed with *sulphide of carbon*, produces, when added to morphia, a pink or red colour, owing to the liberation of the iodine and its solution by the sulphide. Other tests are recommended, but these are the best.

Narcotina ($C_{22}H_{23}NO_7$) exists in opium chiefly in the free state, and, being insoluble in water, is left behind when the drug is macerated in this menstruum. It occurs in white, tasteless, inodorous, needle-like crystals, which are soluble in ether, alcohol, and still more so in chloroform. At one time it was thought to possess a portion of the narcotic properties of opium, but it is now admitted to be inert in this respect. Its salts, which are bitter, have been used in India as febrifuge tonics, in the treatment of intermittent fevers.

Codeia ($C_{18}H_{21}NO_3,H_2O$) exists in opium combined like morphia with meconic acid, and is extracted in the process for obtaining the latter alkaloid, from which it may be separated by an alkaline solution, which dissolves the morphia and leaves the codeia. It occurs in colourless octohedral crystals, of a bitter taste, soluble in water, alcohol, ether, and chloroform. It has been found to possess narcotic powers, with an especial direction to the great sympathetic nerve, and has been used in gastrodynia and dyspepsia, in the dose of half a grain or more. It is, however, too expensive an article for general use.

Narceia ($C_{23}H_{29}NO_9$) is obtained from the mother liquid left after crystallizing out the salts of morphia. It has been asserted that it possesses valuable medicinal properties, but experience in the United States has not confirmed the statements made in Europe as to its efficacy.

Paramorphia, known also as *Thebaia* ($C_{19}H_{21}NO_3$), has been lately said to be a tetanizing toxic agent, analogous in its effects to strychnia; two grains, given hypodermically, have killed a dog.

Papaverina ($C_{20}H_{21}NO_4$) is said to produce some soporific action, with a sedative influence on the pulse; its strength is from one-eighth to one-fourth of that of morphia.

Cryptopia ($C_{21}H_{23}NO_5$) is thought to produce an hypnotic influence, analogous to that of morphia, though a much feebler agent.

Apomorphia ($C_{17}H_{17}NO_2$) a recently discovered alkaloid, possesses marked emetic properties: $\frac{1}{10}$ of a grain, injected hypodermically, or $\frac{1}{4}$ of a grain, taken by the stomach, will produce prompt emesis, and the muriate has been recommended to relieve rigidity of the os uteri in labour.

Meconic acid is inert, but is interesting as affording the most delicate test for opium; chloride or tersulphate of iron strikes with even very diluted solutions of opium a blood-red meconate of iron, which is not dissolved by diluted acids or corrosive sublimate.

Incompatibles.—Alkalies, and astringent infusions containing tannic acid, are incompatible with opium; the former precipitate morphia from its soluble combination, while the latter form with it an insoluble compound. Many of the mineral salts are also decomposed by opium, as the acetate of lead, (meconate of lead and acetate of morphia being formed when these articles are prescribed together).

Physiological Effects.—Opium exerts a marked therapeutic action in the relief of pain, spasm, wakefulness, nervous irritability, and certain forms of morbid discharge, especially from the alimentary canal, by a primary stimulant action, antecedent to any narcotic influence. In such conditions, a tolerance of of its effects is established, and very large amounts may be taken, without inducing narcosis. Its first physiological action is shown in a moderate excitation of the circulation, an increase in the temperature of the skin, and an agreeable exhilaration of the intellectual functions. This state, although generally termed the stage of excitement, is really one of incipient narcosis, and is usually of short duration. The pulse soon sinks below the normal standard, susceptibility to external impressions is diminished, the faculties of the mind become confused, and consciousness is finally lost in sleep. All the secretions are diminished, except that of perspiration, which is heightened; the mouth and throat become dry, with thirst; muscular contraction is lessened; and in some persons nausea and vomiting are produced; occasionally an itching and miliary eruption of the skin occur.

When a poisonous dose is taken, the stage of excitement is wanting; giddiness and stupor rapidly come on, with diminution in the frequency, though not in the fullness of the pulse; and these symptoms are soon followed by an irresistible tendency to sleep, and finally by coma. The breathing is heavy and stertorous, the pulse slow and oppressed, and the *pupils are contracted.* If relief is not afforded, the pulse sinks, the muscular system becomes relaxed, and death ensues, preceded sometimes in children by violent convulsions.

In cases of poisoning from opium or its preparations, the stomach should be immediately evacuated by the stomach pump, if possible, or by emetics. Owing to the torpor of the stomach, emetics are to be given in double the ordinary doses, and the direct emetics are to be preferred, as the sulphate of zinc (20 to 30 grains), or the sulphate of copper (5 to 10 grains). A large tablespoonful of mustard flour or of powdered alum, answers very well as an emetic. Every means should be taken to arouse the patient from his lethargy; he should be kept awake, and made to walk as long as possible; afterwards cold affusions, counter-irritation to the nape of the neck and extremities, flagellation to the palms of the hands and soles of the feet, and, best of all, when the coma is profound, the *electro-magnetic battery*, should be resorted to. Artificial inflation of the lungs is also to be practised. The use of strong coffee has proved efficacious; and stimuli may be given to support the system. Of late years, it has been found that belladonna exercises a powerful influence as a physiological antidote against narcotism from opium, and the administration of this substance by the stomach, or still better, the hypodermic injection of a solution of atropia, is one of the most available remedies that can be employed in poisoning from opium. The poisonous action of opium appears to be entirely directed to the nervous system, no local lesions being found after death.

Opium is largely used as an habitual narcotic in Oriental countries, and to some extent in Europe and the United States. The effects of indulgence in this species of intoxication are of the most destructive character upon both the physical and mental faculties.

Medicinal Uses.—Of all the articles of the Materia Medica, opium enjoys the widest range of therapeutic application. From its properties of assuaging pain and inducing sleep, it is useful in almost all diseases; and it is positively contraindicated, only where there is a tendency to apoplexy or coma, or where there exists an idiosyncrasy with respect to its effects. As an *anodyne* in painful and malignant ulcers and severe injuries, and in resisting surgical *shock*, we have no substitute for opium; and, as an *hypnotic* in mania-a-potu, and in the wakefulness and cerebral irritability of fever, mania, &c., it is equally invaluable. From its power of relaxing muscular spasm, it is our most efficient resource in tetanus, colic, and spasm of the stomach, bowels, biliary ducts, ureters, neck of the bladder, &c. In dysentery and cholera it forms the basis of every variety of treatment, partly for its diaphoretic effects, but principally for its action in arresting both the secretions and peristaltic motion of the bowels. For the relief of the cough of pulmonary affections, opium has no equal in the Materia Medica. In cerebro-spinal meningitis and in puerperal fever, it has been found more successful than any other remedy. In gastric irritability, to check vomiting, in colica pictonum, peritonitis, rheumatism, gout, neuralgia, typhus, gangrene, convulsive diseases, diabetes, &c., it is also constantly employed.

Administration.—The ordinary dose of opium as an anodyne and hypnotic is one grain. Much larger doses are, however, called for in many diseases; and, when it is administered for a length of time, as a narcotic, the dose must be gradually increased. To infants and very old persons, it is to be given with great caution.

Opium is administered in the form of *powder* or *pills*. It is easily powdered when thoroughly dried, and the pills, as well as all the other preparations of opium, should always be made from the powder. The powder is sometimes used endermically and is sprinkled on irritable ulcers. In the form of *suppositories* it is also applied to the rectum.

The following are the officinal preparations of opium:

PILULÆ OPII (*Pills of Opium*). *Twenty-four grains* of opium, made into twenty-four pills, with *six grains* of soap. Each pill contains a grain of opium. They are kept in the shops, as hard old opium pills are sometimes preferred in cases of irritable stomach.

PILULA SAPONIS COMPOSITA (*Compound Pill of Soap*). *Sixty grains* of opium made into a pilular mass, with water and *half a troyounce* of soap. Useful for the administration of small doses. Five grains of the mass contain one grain of opium.

CONFECTIO OPII (*Confection of Opium*). Opium beaten up with honey and spices (opium, 270 grains, aromatic powder, 6 troyounces, and clarified honey, 14 troyounces). Dose, gr. xxxvj.

EXTRACTUM OPII (*Extract of Opium*). Made by evaporating the aqueous solution (opium, 12 troyounces dissolved in 5 pints of water). Dose, gr. ½.

TROCHISCI GLYCYRRHIZÆ ET OPII (*Troches of Liquorice and Opium*). Much used in Philadelphia under the name of *Wistar's cough lozenges.* Made with extract of opium, 24 grains, liquorice, 2 troyounces, gum arabic, a troyounce, sugar, 3 troyounces, and oil of anise, 15 minims. The mass is to be divided into 480 troches. Each troche contains one-twentieth of a grain of extract of opium.

EMPLASTRUM OPII (*Opium Plaster*). Made by mixing extr. opium, a troyounce, with 3 fluidounces of water, and evaporating to a fluidounce and a half; and adding this to Burgundy pitch, 3 troyounces, and plaster of lead, 12 troyounces, previously melted together.

SUPPOSITORIA OPII (*Suppositories of Opium*), are made by incorporating extr. opium, 12 grains, with oil of theobroma, 348 grains; each suppository, weighing 30 grains, contains 1 grain of extr. opium.

SUPPOSITORIA PLUMBI ET OPII (*Suppositories of Lead and Opium*), contain each half a grain of extr. opium, and 3 grains of acetate of lead. Useful in diarrhœa and dysentery, and in hæmorrhoids and other diseases of the rectum.

PULVIS IPECACUANHÆ COMPOSITUS (*Compound Powder of Ipecacuanha*). This powder, well known under the name of *Dover's Powder*, is made by rubbing up *sixty grains* of opium and ipecacuanha each, with *a troyounce* of sulphate of potassium, the salt being employed to promote the minute division and thorough intermingling of the opium and ipecacuanha. Dover's Powder is a most valuable anodyne diaphoretic, extensively prescribed in diarrhœa, dysentery, rheumatism, bronchitis, pneumonia, &c. Dose, gr. x, containing gr. j of opium and ipecacuanha each.

TINCTURA OPII (*Tincture of Opium*). *Laudanum.* Prepared by macerating *two troyounces and a half* of powdered opium for three days in a pint of water, then adding a pint of alcohol, and, after three days of further maceration, introducing the whole into a percolator, and adding diluted alcohol until two pints of tincture are obtained. This is the most commonly employed of all the officinal preparations of opium. When long kept, particularly if exposed to the air, it becomes thick from evaporation of the alcohol, and its strength is much increased. Dose, ♏xiij, or 25 drops, equivalent to a grain of opium. There are 120 drops in f℥j. Laudanum is much used in the form of enema.

TINCTURA OPII CAMPHORATA (*Camphorated Tincture of Opium*). *Paregoric Elixir.* Prepared by macerating *sixty grains* of opium in diluted alcohol Oij, with benzoic acid, *sixty grains*, oil of anise, *a fluidrachm*, clarified honey, *two troyounces*, and camphor, *forty grains*. Dose, f℥ss, or a tablespoonful, containing rather less than a grain of opium. A favorite preparation for children. 5 to 20 drops may be given to an infant.

Tinctura Opii Deodorata (*Deodorized Tincture of Opium*) contains the same proportion of opium as laudanum. In preparing it, a liquid watery extract of opium is first made, which is then washed with ether. The ether is afterwards separated, the residue dissolved in water, and mixed with enough alcohol to preserve it. *Two troyounces and a half* of opium are macerated with *half a pint* of water and expressed; the operation is twice repeated with the same quantity of water; the expressed liquids are mixed, and the mixture is evaporated to *four fluidounces*, and shaken, when cold, with *half a pint* of ether; the ethereal solution, when it has separated by standing, is poured off, and the remaining liquid is evaporated, until all traces of the ether have disappeared; this is mixed with *twenty fluidounces* of water and filtered; water enough is added to make the filtered liquid measure *a pint and a half;* lastly, *half a pint* of alcohol is added, and the liquids are mixed together. The narcotina as well as the odorous and many other injurious ingredients of opium are thus got rid of. A new but valuable preparation. Dose, the same as that of laudanum.

Tinctura Opii Acetata (*Acetated Tincture of Opium*). Prepared by macerating *two troyounces* of opium, in distilled vinegar, f℥xij, and alcohol Oss. Dose, ♏x, or 20 drops.

Acetum Opii (*Vinegar of Opium*). *Black Drop*. Prepared by macerating powdered opium, *five troyounces*, nutmeg, *a troyounce*, sugar, *eight troyounces*, in a pint of diluted acetic acid, and afterwards percolating with the same menstruum, till two pints are obtained. Black drop is twice the strength of laudanum, and is to be given in half the dose of that preparation.

Vinum Opii (*Wine of Opium*). *Sydenham's Laudanum*. Prepared by macerating *two troyounces* of opium in Sherry wine, *fifteen troyounces*, with cinnamon and cloves, each sixty grains; and afterwards adding wine enough to make a pint. Dose, ♏viij, or 16 drops.

Morphiæ Sulphas (*Sulphate of Morphia*), Morphiæ Acetas (*Acetate of Morphia*), Morphiæ Murias (*Muriate of Morphia*), are the officinal salts of morphia, made by saturating the alkaloid with sulphuric, acetic, and muriatic acids. The sulphate and muriate occur in the form of snow-white feathery crystals, the acetate as a white powder. They have a bitter taste; are all freely soluble in water and alcohol, and produce analogous medicinal effects, the sulphate being, however, most employed in this country. The salts of morphia possess the anodyne, hypnotic, antispasmodic, and diaphoretic properties of opium, and are considered less apt to produce headache and nausea, or other unpleasant effect. They are peculiarly adapted to the *hypodermic* and *endermic* methods of application. Dose, one-sixth to one-fourth of a grain. *A Solution of the Sulphate of Morphia* is officinal, and is much prescribed (*Liquor Morphiæ Sulphatis*). It contains one grain to f℥j of distilled water; dose, f℥j–ij. Majendie's solution, used hypodermically, contains sixteen grains to f℥i.

Troches of Morphia and Ipecacuanha (Trochisci Morphiæ et Ipecacuanhæ), are made with sulphate of morphia, 12 grains, ipecacuanha, 40 grains, sugar, 10 troyounces, oil of gaultheria, 5 minims, formed into a mass, with mucilage of tragacanth, which is to be divided into 480 troches; each troche contains $\frac{1}{40}$ of a grain of sulphate of morphia. *Suppositories of Morphia* (*Suppositoria Morphiæ*), contain, each, $\frac{1}{6}$ of a grain of sulphate of morphia.

CHLORAL.

This interesting compound, although discovered by Liebig in 1832, has attracted attention as a therapeutic agent, only since the statements of Liebrich, a physician of Prussia, published in May, 1869. It is prepared by passing dried chlorine gas through pure anhydrous alcohol, afterwards heating with concentrated sulphuric acid, the crude chloral which is separated being rectified over lime: the reaction, upon which the formation of chloral depends, in this process, is complicated, chloral and hydrochloric acids being the chief products. Anhydrous chloral (C_2HCl_3O) is a limpid, oily, colourless liquid, with a fatty taste, and a strong caustic smell, producing lachrymation. It has a sp. gr. of 1.502, a boiling point of 203° F., and mixes in all proportions with water, alcohol, and ether. With water it combines to form a HYDRATE (C_2HCl_3O,H_2O), which crystallizes in a mass of snow-white needles, soluble in their own weight of water; and, as pure chloral readily undergoes decomposition, the more stable hydrate is the form which is employed for medicinal use. It is incompatible with the alkalies, which decompose it into formic acid and chloroform.

Chloral combines also with alcohol, forming a compound termed *Chloral Alcoholate*, which resembles the hydrate, but is distinguishable by its insolubility in water and its solubility in cold chloroform.

Effects and Uses.—Chloral, in doses of 20 grains, is a most reliable hypnotic, with no influence on the secretion from the bowels, and a slight diuretic action. The sleep which it induces is usually quiet and refreshing; and the pulse is not affected. Generally, no unpleasant effects follow its employment, though occasionally slight headache and even nausea supervene. When larger amounts are given, the sleep is deeper and may pass into coma; the respiration is slower; the pulse is reduced in fullness and frequency; the temperature is lowered; the muscular system is relaxed; and both sensibility and reflex action are diminished. Large amounts may be taken without fatal result, as 460 grains have been given without unpleasant effects, though 50 grains have proved poisonous; the symptoms of poisoning are diminished frequency of the respiration and circulation, redness of the conjunctiva, contraction of the pupils, lividity of the lips, and falling of the jaw, with occasionally eruptions of the skin. Death takes place from sudden failure of the heart's action, or of the respiration, or of both. The treatment of chloral-poisoning is the same as that pursued in opium-poisoning; artificial respiration is always to be resorted to. It is asserted that chloral is decomposed in the blood with the liberation of chloroform, but this is scarcely probable, and its effects are certainly not identical with those of chloroform.

Chloral is a most valuable hypnotic remedy in all the forms of insomnia, in hysterical excitement, in acute mania, and in delirium tremens. As an antispasmodic, larger doses are required, but it has been used with advantage in infantile convulsions, and even in puerperal and uræmic convulsions, both by the mouth and hypodermically, and it is especially recommended in the relief of rigid os during labour. In whooping cough, chorea, tetanus, &c., it has also been employed with advantage. As an anodyne, it is available, but only in narcotic amounts. The dose of chloral is 20 grains, which may be safely repeated every hour or two, till three doses have been taken, or sleep occurs.

Chloral is administered only in aqueous solution, and the addition of mucilage or syrup, particularly of the syrup of orange-peel, will disguise its unpleasant taste. It is not well adapted to the hypodermic method, as painful phlegmons sometimes follow its repeated use. Locally, in dilution (gr. x to f℥i of water), it is a good stimulant and deodorizing application to foul and fœtid indolent ulcers; and, injected into subjects for the dissecting room, and in the preservation of anatomical preparations, it has lately been found useful.

Croton-Chloral Hydrate, recently introduced, is made by the action of chlorine upon aldehyde, and occurs in small, shining, tabular crystals, only slightly soluble in water. It is highly recommended as an anodyne in neuralgia, in doses of from 10 to 20 grains, in syrup.

LACTUCARIUM.

Lactucarium (sometimes called *lettuce-opium*), is the concrete juice of Lactuca Sativa, the garden lettuce (*Nat. Ord.* Cichoraceæ), and is obtained from incisions in the plant, in the stem, during the period of inflorescence. Another and inferior mode of procuring it is by expression and evaporation of the expressed juice. Two varieties are found in the market: *English lactucarium*, which occurs in small, irregular lumps, of a reddish-brown colour externally, an opiate smell, and a bitter, unpleasant taste, and *German lactucarium* (which is inferior), in four-sided pieces, from an inch to an inch and a half thick, with one side convex and the three other sides flat, the convex surface darkish-brown, and the flat surfaces light yellowish-brown. An active principle termed *lactucin* is said to have been isolated. Lactucarium, prepared from the juice of the Lactuca elongata, American or wild lettuce, has been found to possess effects similar to those of the officinal article.

Effects and Uses.—Lactucarium possesses the *anodyne* and *hypnotic* qualities of opium with a slight sedative action on the circulation, but it is an uncertain preparation. It may be given where opium disagrees, from idiosyncrasy in the patient. Dose, gr. x. The *syrup* is the most eligible form of administration. It is made by rubbing a troyounce of lactucarium with sufficient diluted alcohol to bring it to a syrupy consistence, then percolating with diluted alcohol till half a pint of tincture has passed, afterwards evaporating to two fluidounces, and finally mixing the tincture with fourteen fluidounces of syrup. Dose, two or three fluidrachms.

BELLADONNA.

Belladonnæ Folia, Belladonna Leaves; Belladonnæ Radix, Belladonna Root.

Atropa Belladonna, or Deadly Nightshade (*Nat. Ord.* Solanaceæ), is a European perennial plant, with herbaceous, branched, downy stems, about three or four feet high, large ovate leaves, of a dull-green colour, and drooping, bell-shaped, purple flowers. The whole plant possesses narcotic properties, but the LEAVES and ROOT only are officinal. When fresh, the leaves have an unpleasant smell, and a sweetish, subacrid, slightly nauseous taste. When dried, they retain this taste, but have scarcely any odour. The root should be obtained from plants more than two years old; the dried root is long, round, from one to several inches in thickness, branched, of a reddish brown colour, of little odour, and a feeble sweetish taste.

The narcotic properties of belladonna depend on the presence of an alkaloid termed *atropia*, which is found in all parts of the plant. It is officinal, and is prepared from the root, by exhaustion with alcohol, afterwards adding sulphuric acid, precipitating with potassa, dissolving the atropia in chloroform, and then evaporating the chloroform. *Atropia* ($C_{17}H_{23}NO_3$) occurs in the form of yellowish-white, silky, prismatic crystals, without smell, but of a bitter, acrid taste, soluble in alcohol, more so in ether, still more so in chloroform, but only partially soluble in water. Perchloride of gold gives with atropia solution a yellow precipitate, and cyanogen gas passed through its alcoholic solution strikes a deep red colour; the best test is bromine, in hydrobromic acid, which produces a yellow amorphous precipitate, soon becoming crystalline; the physiological test should also be applied, by dilating the pupil of a rabbit or cat by local application to the eye. It is a most energetic poison, producing analogous effects to those of belladonna, but much more powerful. Latterly, atropia has been a good deal employed medicinally as a substitute for belladonna, on account of its greater certainty. The dose to begin with for internal use is about one-thirtieth of a grain in solution, one-sixtieth of a grain for hypodermic injection. As a collyrium, *to dilate the pupil*, a solution of a grain in four fluidrachms of water, with a few drops of acetic acid, may be employed, and a drop of the solution applied to the eye. A tincture (atropia gr. j, diluted alcohol f℥ss) is used for the same purpose—dose, for internal use, 8 drops. The *sulphate of atropia* is also officinal; it is made by adding a mixture of sulphuric acid and alcohol to an ethereal solution of atropia, and is deposited in the form of a white, slightly crystalline powder, very soluble in water and alcohol, but insoluble in ether—dose the same as that of atropia.

Physiological Effects of Belladonna.—In small doses, the effects of belladonna are those of an anodyne stimulant, with little or no action on the circulation, or on any of the secretions, except a peculiar dryness of the mouth and throat. In larger doses it causes *dilatation of the pupils*, loss of vision, giddiness, constriction of the throat, difficulty of deglutition and articulation, increased heart-action, quickened respiration, elevation of temperature, marked diuresis, nausea, with occasional vomiting and purging, and sometimes a red eruption. When excessive doses are taken, the temperature of the body falls, the muscular system is relaxed, sensation is impaired, the pulse fails, and maniacal delirium sets in, followed by coma, syncope, and death, often preceded by convulsions. Belladonna is eliminated chiefly by the urine. Dissections show that the action of the poison is not confined to the cerebro-spinal system, but that it is attended by inflammation of the digestive organs. Cases of poisoning from belladonna are to be treated by evacuation of the stomach, cathartics, and, if coma occurs, by the electro-magnetic battery. Opium may be given as a physiological antidote, or hypodermic injections of solutions of the salts of morphia may be administered. As atropia and its salts are decomposed and rendered inert by prolonged contact with caustic alkalies, the solutions of potassa and soda are recommended as antidotes for belladonna, and are to be considered also as medicinally incompatible with it; lime-solution is said to have the same action. Applied to the eyebrow, belladonna causes dilatation of the pupil; and accompanying its mydriatic action are paralysis of accommodation and a diminished intra-ocular pressure.

Medicinal Uses.—Belladonna is one of our most highly esteemed anodyne and antispasmodic remedies. It is destitute of hypnotic effect, and, on the contrary, has a tendency to occasion wakefulness. In the treatment of neuralgia, it ranks at the head of the narcotics, and is extensively employed both alone and in combination with the sulphate of quinia. It should be given until dryness of the throat, dilatation of the pupil, and some disorder of vision are produced. Its powers of allaying spasm have been found very efficacious in the treatment of whooping-cough and asthma. In lead colic, spasmodic constriction of the bowels generally, dysmenorrhœa, laryngismus stridulus, chorea, and tetanus, belladonna ranks among the best antispasmodic remedies. In spasmodic stricture of the urethra, the local application of belladonna ointment to the urethra by a bougie, is very efficacious. As a discutient of cancerous indurations, belladonna has enjoyed some reputation, but any good effects, in these cases, have probably been owing to an anodyne and not a resolvent influence. In mania, and many diseases of the cerebro-spinal system, especially epilepsy, it has been occasionally employed with advantage. Its action on the kidneys renders it useful in chronic Bright's disease; and, by its influence in relieving irritability of the bladder, it is probably the best remedy for the nocturnal incontinence of urine of children. In constipation, iritis, and as a prophylactic against scarlatina, it is also resorted to. As a preventive of scarlatina, it was originally proposed from its power of affecting the throat and skin, and respectable authority is not wanting in confirmation of its efficacy in this particular. It is used too, in cases of poisoning by opium. Lately, hypodermic injections of $\frac{1}{60}$ to $\frac{1}{80}$ of a grain of atropia have been found useful in checking colliquative night-sweats.

As a topical remedy, belladonna is employed as an anodyne, and also to relieve rigidity of the os uteri in labour. The local use of atropia in diseases of the eye is of the greatest importance; solutions of the alkaloid or its sulphate may be dropped into the conjunctival sac, to relieve the pain and photophobia of conjunctivitis, to determine the refraction of the eye from its influence on accommodation, in the diagnosis of suspected cataract, in operations for cataract, in iritis, prolapsus iridis, and ulcers of the cornea generally. Gelatine wafers, containing $\frac{1}{50}$ to $\frac{1}{150}$ of a grain of atropia are sometimes used to dilate the pupil for ophthalmoscopic purposes.

Administration.—The dose of the *powder* of the root or leaves is gr. j, to be repeated and increased till dryness of the throat, dilatation of the pupil, and dimness of vision are produced. It is most frequently exhibited in the form of *extract* (or inspissated juice) of the fresh leaves. Dose, $\frac{1}{4}$ to $\frac{1}{2}$ a grain, to be repeated and increased. The *tincture* (four troyounces of the leaves to diluted alcohol Oij—dose, 15 to 30 drops) and the *alcoholic extract* are also officinal. The *fluid extract of belladonna root* contains a troyounce of root in a fluidounce of extract —dose, 2 to 5 drops. *Suppositories of belladonna* (made with alcoholic extract of belladonna, 1 part, and oil of theobroma 59 parts), contain each half a grain of extract. For external use, a plaster (*Emplastrum Belladonnæ*), made by adding melted resin plaster to an alcoholic extract of belladonna root, and an ointment (*Unguentum Belladonnæ*), made by rubbing sixty grains of the extract first with water, *half a fluidrachm*, and then with lard, *a troyounce*, are employed.

STRAMONIUM.

Stramonii Folia, Stramonium Leaves; Stramonii Semen, Stramonium Seed.

Fig. 6.

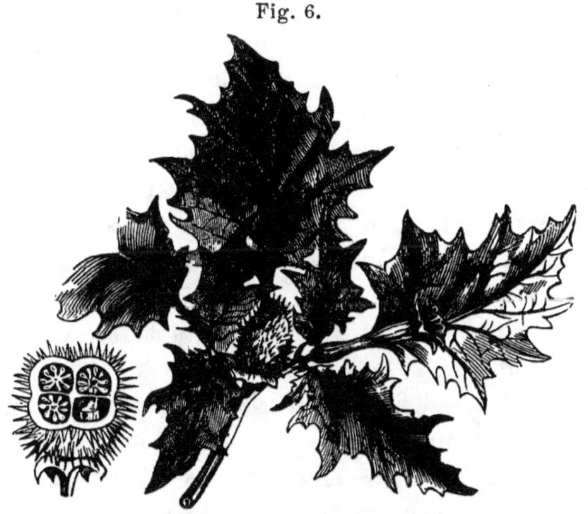

Datura Stramonium, or Thorn-Apple, sometimes called Jamestown weed (*Nat. Ord.* Solanaceæ), is an annual indigenous plant, which grows very abundantly in waste grounds in all parts of the world. It has a forked, branching stem, from three to six feet high, ovate, toothed leaves, large funnel-shaped white or purplish flowers, which appear in midsummer, and ovate capsules, filled with numerous kidney-shaped, brownish-black seeds. The odour of the plant is strong and disagreeable, and its taste bitter and nauseous. It loses these properties very much when dried, but the process does not appear to weaken its narcotic qualities. The LEAVES and SEEDS are officinal, but the seeds are most powerful from containing most daturia.

The active principle of Stramonium is an alkaloid termed *daturia*, which possesses properties analogous to those of atropia.

The *physiological effects* of stramonium are closely allied to those of belladonna, with a more marked action on the secretions. From its common occurrence in every part of the country, cases of poisoning from this weed are very frequent, particularly with children, who are fond of swallowing the seeds. The treatment laid down for the relief of poisoning from belladonna is applicable to these cases.

The *medicinal uses* of stramonium are similar to those of belladonna. It is prescribed internally in neuralgia, whooping-cough, mania, and epilepsy; and in spasmodic asthma, cigarettes of the leaves are smoked with great relief. The practice is, however, dangerous in aged or apopletic persons. Topically, stramonium is used by oculists to *dilate the pupils* and diminish the sensibility of the retina to light; and it is an excellent anodyne application, in the form of cataplasm and ointment, to inflammatory tumours, irritable ulcers, bed-sores, and hemorrhoids.

Administration.—The dose of the *powdered leaves* is gr. ij; of the *seeds*, a grain, to be repeated and gradually increased till narcotic effects are produced. Dose of the *extract of the leaves*, gr. j, to commence with; of the *extract of the seed*, gr. $\frac{1}{2}$. The *tincture* (*four troyounces* of the seeds to diluted alcohol Oij, dose 20 to 40 drops), and the *ointment* made by mixing the extract of the leaves with lard (according to the formula for ointment of belladonna), are also officinal.

HYOSCYAMUS.

Hyoscyami Folia, Hyoscyamus Leaves; Hyoscyami Semen, Hyoscyamus Seed.

Hyoscyamus niger, or Henbane (*Nat. Ord.* Solanaceæ), is a native of Europe, and is naturalized in the northern parts of the United States. It grows to the height of about two feet, with large, sinuated, pale-green leaves, and flowers of a straw-yellow colour. The whole plant has narcotic properties; but the LEAVES and SEEDS only are officinal. Henbane should be gathered when in flower; and, when fresh, has a strong, offen-

Fig. 7.

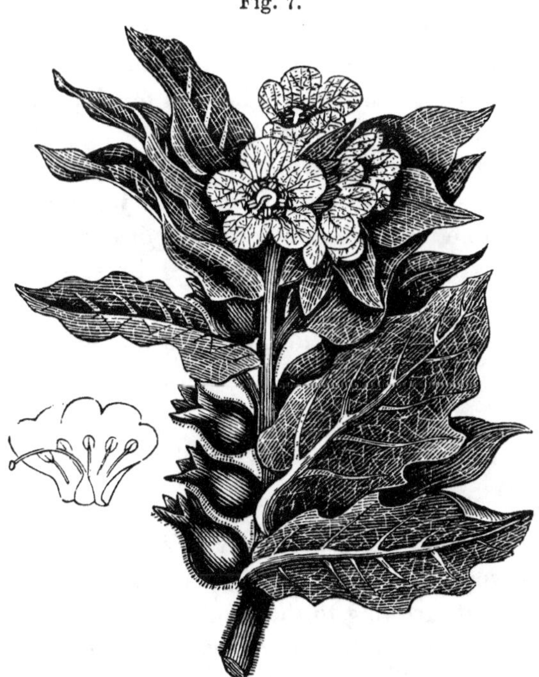

sive narcotic odour, and a mucilaginous, unpleasant, slightly acrid taste; but it loses most of these qualities in drying. The seeds are of a yellowish-gray colour, with something of the odour of the plant, and have an oleaginous, bitter taste. The active properties of the plant depend upon a peculiar alkaloid principle, termed *hyoscyamia* ($C_{18}H_{23}N_2O_3$), nearly identical in its action with atropia, but more soluble in water.

Effects and Uses.—The effects of henbane on the system much resemble those of belladonna. They differ from those of opium in their comparatively feeble hypnotic effect, and in their relaxing influence on the bowels. In large doses it causes *dilatation of the pupil*, delirium, loss of vision, &c. In cases of poisoning, the same treatment is to be pursued as for belladonna and stramonium. Henbane may be used remedially, in the same diseases, as belladonna and stramonium, than which it is, however, less active. It has been administered also, from the earliest days, to palliate cough, where opium is objectionable from its constipating or nauseating influence. Externally, it is employed in the form of cataplasm or fomentation to painful swellings and ulcers; and it may be used to dilate the pupil, in the same manner as belladonna.

Dose of the powdered leaves, gr. v to gr. x; of the seeds, somewhat less. The *extract* (an inspissated juice of the leaves) is the preferable form of administration; it is of a dark olive colour, and extremely variable quality. Dose, gr. v to gr. x. *Tincture* (four troyounces to diluted alcohol Oij), dose f℥j. An *alcoholic extract*, and a *fluid extract* (dose 10–20 drops), are also officinal.

TABACUM—TOBACCO.

Nicotiana Tabacum, or Virginia Tobacco (*Nat. Ord.* Solanaceæ), is a native of the warm countries of America, but is now extensively cultivated in most parts of the world. It is an annual plant, growing to the height of from three to six feet, with large, oblong, pointed, hairy, pale-green leaves, and light-greenish, funnel-shaped flowers, expanding above into rose-coloured segments. The DRIED LEAVES are the portion used. They have a yellowish-brown colour, a strong, peculiar, narcotic odour, and a bitter, nauseous taste. The darker-coloured leaves are the strongest.

The virtues of tobacco are imparted to alcohol and water, and depend on the presence of an alkaloid called *nicotia* ($C_{10}H_{14}N_2$), which is found in all parts of the plant. It is a colourless, oily, volatilizable, alkaline liquid, highly soluble in water, alcohol, ether, chloroform, the fixed oils, and oil of turpentine, of a feeble odour, when cold, but irritant, when heated, of an acrid, burning taste, and is a most energetic poison. From the dried leaves are also obtained a concrete volatile oil, termed *nicotianin*, which is probably the odorous principle of the plant, and an *empyreumatic oil*, which gives the peculiar smell to old tobacco pipes. Both of these principles are poisonous; the *oil* (*oleum tabaci*), is officinal.

Physiological Effects.—On persons unaccustomed to its use, tobacco, in small doses, produces a slight sedative action, with nausea, swimming of the head, increased flow from the kidneys, and sometimes, also, from the bowels. In larger doses, it induces vomiting and purging, a sensation of sinking at the pit of the stomach, giddiness, disorder of vision, the pupils, however, being little affected, depression of the circulation, great relaxation of the muscular system, coldness of the surface, and other symptoms of prostration; and, when excessive doses have been taken, these symptoms become more violent, and are followed by convulsions, paralysis, coma, and death. Cases of poisoning are to be treated on the principles applicable to other cases of narcotic poisoning; the diffusible stimuli are to be freely given.

The habitual use of tobacco as an exhilarant is well known. When taken to excess, it frequently develops disorders of the stomach, heart, and nervous system.

Medicinal Uses.—Tobacco is employed in medicine, chiefly with a view to its action on the muscular system—its anodyne and hypnotic properties being relatively feeble. In various spasmodic diseases, particularly in colic, ileus, strangulated hernia, constipation from spasmodic constriction, tetanus, spasm of the neck of the bladder and the glottis, and asthma, it is a remedy of great value. It has been also successfully applied to the treatment of poisoning by strychnia. Internally, tobacco is to be employed with caution, as it occasionally acts with dangerous energy. Stupes of an infusion of tobacco (half an ounce to a pint of water), have been found an efficacious application to wounds, in cases of traumatic tetanus.

Administration.—Tobacco is not given by the stomach, owing to its emetic properties. It is usually administered by the rectum, in the form of *infusion* (ʒj—Oj of boiling water, one-third to be given at a dose), or tobacco-smoke may be introduced into the rectum. It may also be smoked for medicinal effect, or applied locally in the form of cataplasm. *Ointment of Tobacco* (*Unguentum Tabaci*), is made by mixing a watery extract, prepared from *half a troyounce* of finely powdered tobacco, with *eight* troyounces of lard; it is a useful application to indolent ulcers and some cutaneous affections, particularly tinea capitis, but the external application of tobacco to abraded surfaces of considerable extent has occasioned dangerous consequences. The *Wine of Tobacco* (*Vinum Tabaci*) is made by macerating a *troyounce* of tobacco in a pint of Sherry wine for seven days; it is occasionally used as a diuretic—dose 20–30 drops. The *Oil* is sometimes mixed with ointments.

LOBELIA.

Lobelia inflata, or Indian tobacco (*Nat. Ord.* Lobeliaceæ), is a very common annual or biennial indigenous plant, growing to the height of from six inches to two feet, with a fibrous root, an erect, hairy stem, ovate, serrated leaves, pale-blue flowers, and ovoid, inflated capsules. It flowers from July till the appearance of frost, and should be gathered about August and September. All parts of it are active, but the LEAVES and TOPS only are officinal. It has an unpleasant smell, and, when chewed, an acrid, burning, nauseous taste, which is at first faint, but soon becomes excessive. Water and alcohol extract the virtues of lobelia, which contain a volatile alkaloid principle, *lobelina* (analogous to nicotia), lobelic acid, fixed and volatile oil, gum, chlorophyl, &c. Lobelina is a yellowish liquid, lighter than water, of an aromatic odour, an acrid taste, soluble in water, but more so in alcohol and ether.

Physiological Effects.—Lobelia produces effects on the system analogous to those of tobacco, acting in small doses as a sedative, nauseant, diuretic, and diaphoretic; in larger doses

Fig. 8.

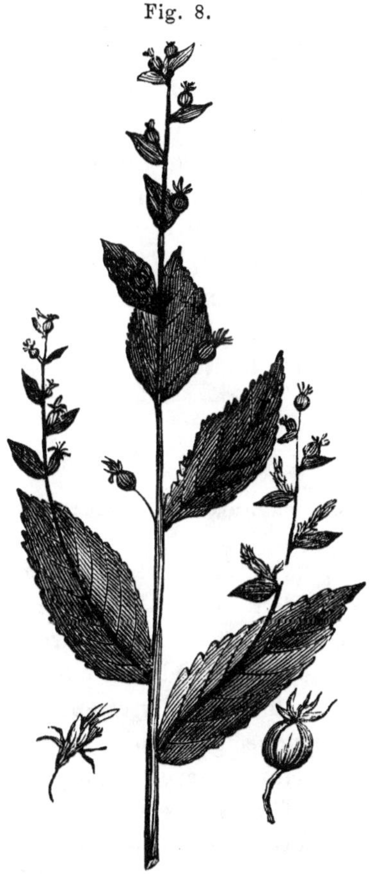

as an energetic emetic; and in still larger doses as an active acro-narcotic poison, resembling tobacco in its influence. It was employed by the aborigines, and has always been a popular empirical remedy.

Medicinal Uses.—Lobelia is sometimes classed among emetics, but its action in this particular is too violent for its safe administration. It is chiefly employed, by regular practitioners, with a view to its antispasmodic properties, for the relief of asthma, angina pectoris, and cardiac dyspnœa, and is given in small doses, gradually increased, until headache or nausea ensue. It may also be used as an enema, to fulfil the same indications as tobacco.

Administration.—Lobelia is given in substance, tincture, and infusion. The dose of the *powder* as an antispasmodic, is gr. j to gr. iij; as an emetic, gr. v to gr. xx. The best form, particularly in asthma, is the *tincture* (four troyounces to diluted alcohol Oij), which may be given in the quantity of f℥j, to be repeated as occasion may require.

ACETUM LOBELIÆ (*Vinegar of Lobelia*), made with diluted acetic acid, is a good preparation, in which the alkaloid is fixed by the acetic acid; it is of the same strength, and may be given in the same doses as the tincture.

CONIUM.

Conii Folia, Conium Leaves; Conii Fructus, Conium Seed.

Conium maculatum, or Hemlock (*Nat. Ord.* Apiaceæ), is a biennial European plant, naturalized in many parts of the United States. Its stem is erect, from three to five feet high, round, smooth, and often spotted with purple. The leaves are large, bright-green, and repeatedly compound; the flowers are small, white, and arranged in umbels, appearing in June and July. The whole plant is narcotic and virulent, and has a fetid, heavy odour. The LEAVES and SEEDS are the only portions used. The leaves should be gathered when the plant has done flowering, and kept in vessels from which the air and light are excluded. Plants grown in sunny situations and warm climates are most active. When well preserved, the dried leaves have a fine green colour, and the characteristic smell and bitterish taste of the fresh herb, though less powerfully. The seeds should be gathered while yet green, and carefully dried. They have a yellowish-gray colour, a feeble odour, and a bitterish taste; they are roundish-ovate, a line and a half in length by a line in breath.

The active principle of hemlock is a peculiar alkaloid, termed *conia* ($C_8H_{15}N$), which exists in larger proportion in the seeds

Fig. 9.

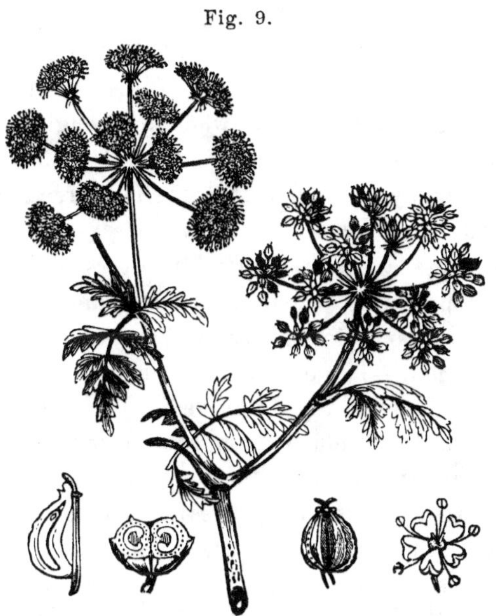

than the leaves. It is a colourless, transparent, volatile, oily fluid, of a peculiar, repulsive, suffocating, mouse-like odour, and a bitterish taste, sparingly soluble in water, and freely so in alcohol, ether, and chloroform; it is a highly energetic poison, even in very small doses.

Physiological Effects.—The action of hemlock in small medicinal doses is considered to be alterative and even tonic. Resolvent properties, in cases of glandular enlargement, have been attributed to it, and atrophy of the mammæ and testicles is said to have resulted from its continued employment. It is usually classed with the sedative narcotics, paralyzing the nerves of motion rather than those of sensation. In large doses, it causes nausea, vertigo, dimness of vision, relaxation of the muscles;

and, in poisonous quantities, dilatation of the pupils, difficulty of speech, delirium or coma, paralysis, and finally convulsions and death. It has no direct hypnotic effect. In cases of poisoning, alcoholic stimuli are to be given.

Medicinal Uses.—It is employed chiefly as a general and topical anodyne, to relieve the pain of malignant tumours; and, even if destitute of the deobstruent powers which have been ascribed to it, it certainly exerts a remarkably palliative influence upon painful chronic indurations. It has been also recommended as an antispasmodic in whooping-cough and asthma; as an anodyne in neuralgia; as an adjuvant to other remedies in mania, especially melancholia; to relieve irritability of the sexual organs; in diabetes; and it is used externally as a cataplasm to cancers and other irritable ulcers. Conium is the *cicuta* of Hippocrates, Galen, and Pliny, and is supposed to have been the poison administered to Socrates and Phocion.

Administration.—The dose of the *powdered leaves* is gr. iij to gr. iv, twice a day, to be rapidly increased, till vertigo or nausea ensue. The seeds are much stronger and more uniform in their effects than the leaves. Dose, half a grain to a grain. The *extract* (inspissated juice of the leaves) may be given in the same doses; it is an uncertain preparation, and should be rejected unless it have a strong and penetrating odour. A *tincture* (four troyounces of the leaves to diluted alcohol Oij, dose, f℥ss, f℥j), an *alcoholic extract* of the leaves, and a *fluid extract* are also used; of the *fluid extract* (a fluidounce of which contains a troyounce of the seeds), the dose is four or five minims. All the preparations made from the *dried* leaves are, however, comparatively feeble, and the best form in which to prescribe conium is the *Succus Conii* (Juice of Conium), (which is prepared by adding one measure of alcohol to five measures of the recently expressed juice of the fresh plant), dose f℥i–ij.

ACONITUM—ACONITE.

Aconiti Folia, Aconite Leaves; Aconiti Radix, Aconite Root.

Aconitum Napellus, Aconite, Wolfsbane, or Monkshood (*Nat. Ord.* Ranunculaceæ), is a native of the mountainous parts of Europe. It is a perennial, herbaceous plant, with a fusiform root, a simple erect stem, growing usually to the height of from two to four feet, palmate, deeply cleft leaves, and large, dark, violet-blue flowers. The LEAVES and ROOT are both used, but the root is the more powerful. They have little or no smell; but their taste is bitterish and acrid, and when chewed they occasion a peculiar feeling of tingling and numbness in the tongue and interior of the mouth. These properties are impaired by long keeping, and the plant loses its medicinal efficacy. Other species of aconite possess similar poisonous qualities to those of the A. Napellus. The active principle of aconite is an alkaloid named *aconitia*, which is officinal.

ACONITIA ($C_{30}H_{47}NO_7$) is prepared from an aqueous solution of an alcoholic extract of aconite root, by the addition of sulphuric acid (which converts the natural salt of aconitia into a sulphate); it is then freed from its oily and resinous portions by means of ether; the alkaloid is subsequently precipitated with ammonia, then redissolved by ether, and again separated from this menstruum by evaporation. It is a white amorphous powder, with a tinge of yellow (though it has been obtained in crystals), without smell, of a bitter acrid taste, and produces in the mouth a sense of numbness. It is partially soluble in water, and is readily dissolved by alcohol and chloroform, less readily by ether. There are no *characteristic* chemical tests of aconitia, and, in medico-legal cases, the physiological test, by producing numbness and tingling of the lips or skin, must be resorted to.

Aconitia is an exceedingly virulent poison, more powerful when pure than hydrocyanic acid. It is scarcely adapted to internal use, as even one-fiftieth of a grain has produced alarming results. As a topical agent in neuralgia and rheumatism, it has been employed with great success, in alcoholic solution (gr. i–ij to f℥j), or as an ointment (gr. ij to lard ℥j, rubbed up with alcohol, gtt. vj).

Physiological Effects.—Taken in small doses, aconite produces a sensation of numbness in the head, face, and extremities, with a sedative action on the circulation, and more or less nausea and muscular debility. In larger doses, its effects are those of an acro-narcotic poison; gastric irritation, purging, contraction or expansion of the pupils, numbness or paralysis of the limbs, syncope, convulsions, and death. In case of poisoning, the stomach is to be thoroughly evacuated, and stimulants, externally and internally, are to be freely administered.

Medicinal Uses.—Aconite is a powerful and valuable remedy, in the treatment of neuralgia, chronic rheumatism, gout, and other painful diseases, as might be inferred from its *benumbing* effects on the system. From its influence on the circulation, it is employed to reduce inflammatory action, to moderate an excessively rapid pulse in scarlatina and other fevers, and as a remedy in hypertrophy and other cases of irregular or excessive action of the heart. In controlling abnormal cardiac action, aconite is perhaps the most available article we possess, but its employment requires caution. As a *topical* anodyne, in neuralgia, it has no superior.

Administration.—The dose of the *powdered leaves* is gr. j to gr. ij; of the *root*, gr. ½ to gr. i; of the *alcoholic extract* of the dried leaves, gr. ½ to gr. j; of the *tincture* of the root, which is by far the best preparation (twelve troyounces to alcohol Oij), 5 to 10 drops. These doses are to be repeated twice or thrice daily, and cautiously increased, till the effects of the medicine are apparent. The tincture may be used externally; but for external application, the *liniment* (*linimentum aconiti*), which contains 8 troyounces of the powdered root in 7 fluidounces of alcohol and a fluidounce of glycerin, or the *plaster* (*emplastrum aconiti*), made by mixing 16 troyounces of alcoholic extract of aconite root with melted resin plaster enough to make the mixture weigh 16 troyounces, are to be preferred.

CANNABIS AMERICANA—AMERICAN HEMP, CANNABIS INDICA—INDIAN HEMP.

Cannabis sativa, or Hemp (*Nat. Ord.* Cannabinaceæ) is a native of Persia and the northern parts of India, and is cultivated in Europe, and in the United States. Narcotic virtues were formerly thought to exist only in the Cannabis Indica or Indian variety of the plant, but recent investigation seems to show that the hemp plants, raised in the Southern States, as Kentucky, are active, and might replace the East Indian drug.

The FLOWERING TOPS of both varieties are officinal. By evaporating concentrated alcoholic solutions of these, EXTRACTS are obtained (*extractum cannabis Americanæ* and *extractum cannabis Indicæ*), which are the forms usually employed. *Extract of hemp* is of a dark, olive-green colour, a fragrant narcotic odour, and a bitter, acrid taste. It is soluble in alcohol and ether, but not in water. The resin, which is the active principle, has received the name of *cannabin.*

Effects and Uses.—The medicinal properties of Extract of Cannabis are narcotic and antispasmodic, and in India both the herb and resin are extensively used as intoxicating exhilarants, under the name of *haschisch.* In large doses it is sedative, producing relaxation of the muscles, confusion of thought, heavy sleep, and abatement of pain, without much affecting the secretions, except that from the kidneys, which it increases; the pupils are dilated and the pulse is quickened. It has been chiefly extolled as an antispasmodic in traumatic tetanus, and has been employed with success in other spasmodic diseases, chorea, hysteria, &c., to relieve cerebral irritability in diabetes, and as an anodyne in rheumatism, gout, neuralgia, &c. It has also been given with advantage as an hypnotic both in mania and mania-a-potu; and its powers of exciting uterine contractions, and of checking uterine hemorrhagic discharges, are highly spoken of. Dose, from half a grain to two or more grains. The *tincture* is made by dissolving *three hundred and sixty grains* of the *extract of Indian Hemp* in a pint of alcohol; forty drops of this are about equal to a grain of the extract.

HUMULUS—HOPS.

Hops are the STROBILES of Humulus lupulus, or Hop-vine (*Nat. Ord.* Urticaceæ), a climbing vine, indigenous in Europe, and probably also in North America, with serrated, rough leaves, and greenish-yellow flowers. The medicinal portion is the fruit, or STROBILES, which are also largely employed in the preparation of malt liquors, and are known as *hops*. They consist of thin, somewhat translucent, veined, leaf-like bracts or scales, of a greenish-yellow colour, a strong, fragrant, narcotic odour, and a bitter, aromatic, slightly astringent taste. Near their base are two small, round, dark seeds, covered with aromatic glands or grains, which are the active portion of the hops, and are termed *lupulin*. They are separated by threshing, rubbing, and sifting the scales, and constitute about a sixth part of the weight of hops.

LUPULIN (*lupulina*) is officinal, and consists of rounded or reniform, rather transparent grains, of a cellular texture, and a golden-yellow colour. It is slightly soluble in water, and completely so in alcohol, and is composed of a volatile oil, a bitter principle termed *lupulite*, resin, tannic acid, and other matters. The scaly bracts contain a small portion of lupulinic matter.

Effects and Uses.—Hops are narcotic and tonic. The narcotic properties probably reside in the volatile oil, and the tonic properties in the bitter principle. They are said, also, to possess antaphrodisiac properties, and sometimes prove diuretic. The odorous emanation is employed as an hypnotic by means of the hop-pillow. Internally, they are given to relieve restlessness, induce sleep, and allay pain, and are also much employed for their stomachic and tonic effect. The combination of tonic and narcotic virtues renders hops an excellent remedy in mild forms of mania-a-potu. Topically, they are employed in the form of fomentation or poultice, as a resolvent or discutient, in painful swellings and tumours.

Administration.—Hops are given in the form of *infusion* (half a troyounce to boiling water Oj), and *tincture* (five troyounces to diluted alcohol Oij), dose f℥j to f℥iij.

The best preparation for internal use is LUPULIN, in the dose of gr. v to gr. xij, in powder or pills. The *tincture of lupulin* (four troyounces to alcohol Oij) may be given in the dose of f℥j to f℥ij. The *fluid extract* is a concentrated tincture, containing the virtues of an ounce of lupulin in a fluidounce. The *oleoresin* also is officinal—dose, gr. ij to v.

DULCAMARA—BITTERSWEET.

The YOUNG BRANCHES of Solanum Dulcamara, the Woody Nightshade, or Bittersweet (*Nat. Ord.* Solanaceæ), a European vine, naturalized in the United States, possess combined narcotic and diaphoretic properties. They are of a greenish-gray colour, about the thickness of a quill, and have, when fresh, an unpleasant odour, which they lose by drying. Their taste is at first bitter, afterwards slightly acrid and sweet. The active principle is a poisonous alkaloid termed *solania* ($C_{43}H_{70}NO_{16}$), which has been found also in Solanum tuberosum, or common potato, and S. nigrum, or black nightshade.

Effects and Uses.—In small doses, the most obvious effects of Bittersweet are an increase in the secretions from the skin and mucous surfaces, with some diminution of sensibility. In excessive doses it is an acro-narcotic poison. It is principally used in the form of decoction (a troyounce boiled in a pint of water for fifteen minutes, and water enough afterwards added to make the decoction measure a pint),* dose, f℥i–ij, in painful cutaneous affections, and also in chronic catarrh, rheumatism, and gout. An extract (*alcoholic*), (dose, ten to twenty grains), and *fluid extract* (of which a fluidounce represents a troyounce of the stalks), are both officinal.

* This is the usual formula for the decoctions, and is the mode of preparation of all those which are stated to be of the strength of an ounce to a pint of water.

ACIDUM HYDROCYANICUM DILUTUM—DILUTED HYDROCYANIC ACID.

Hydrocyanic acid, known also as cyanhydric acid, and *prussic* acid, is derived from a variety of vegetable substances, as the bitter almond, peach kernels and leaves, wild cherry, cherry laurel, &c. It is employed in medicine only in a state of extreme dilution; and the diluted acid is obtained by the action of sulphuric acid and water on the ferrocyanide of potassium, or, when wanted for immediate use, by the action of muriatic acid and water on cyanide of silver.

Diluted hydrocyanic acid is a colourless, volatile liquid, with a peculiar odour, and a cooling, somewhat irritating taste. It undergoes decomposition if exposed to the light, and should be kept in bottles covered with black paint or paper. It contains two per cent. of the anhydrous or concentrated acid.

The anhydrous acid (HCy, or HNC) is a colourless, transparent, very volatile and decomposable liquid, with a powerful, peculiar odour, and a cooling, afterwards burning taste. Both water and alcohol dissolve it readily. It consists of one eq. of cyanogen and one of hydrogen. Its presence in a suspected mixture may be detected by the addition of a solution of nitrate of silver, which throws down a white, curdy precipitate of cyanide of silver, distinguishable by its exhaling the peculiar odour of prussic acid on the addition of muriatic acid, and by being wholly soluble in boiling nitric acid, (the silver test is the most delicate, when applied to prussic acid in the state of *vapour*); or, by adding to the suspected solution a little liquor potassæ, and then a mixed solution of protosulphate and tersulphate of iron, a dirty greenish-blue precipitate is thrown down, which, on the addition of a few drops of pure hydrochloric acid, becomes *Prussian* blue; or (the best liquid test) the hydrocyanic acid may be converted into sulphocyanide of ammonium by the addition of sulphide of ammonium, and the salt thus formed yields a deep blood-red colour upon the addition of a sesquioxide salt of iron, (the sulphur test may be advantageously employed as a vapour test); or, fourthly, by the copper test, (which may be also used in the form of vapour), the liquid is first rendered slightly alkaline by liquor potassæ, and, on adding a dilute solution of sulphate of copper, a greenish-white precipitate is thrown down.

Physiological Effects.—When taken in medicinal doses, gradually increased, hydrocyanic acid occasions a bitter taste, increased flow of saliva, irritation in the throat, nausea, headache, giddiness, faintness, disorder of the vision, and tendency to sleep. The pulse is sometimes accelerated, but more commonly depressed. In a poisonous dose, hydrocyanic acid arrests life with fearful rapidity, and is one of the most energetic poisons known, one or two drops of the pure acid being sufficient to destroy a dog in a few seconds. When not immediately fatal, it produces great and sudden prostration, trismus, difficult and spasmodic respiration, dilatation and immobility and sometimes contraction of the pupils, convulsions, &c. The best *antidotes* are chlorine, and a mixture of sulphate of iron (gr. x to water fʒj), tincture of chloride of iron (fʒj), and carbonate of potassium (℈j), in water (f℥j or ij); inhalations of ammonia or its carbonate, and (if the patient can swallow), alcoholic stimuli are to be employed, and at the same time cold affusions and artificial respiration are to be also resorted to. The subcutaneous injection of the sulphate of atropia has been also found available, acting as a physiological antidote.

Medicinal Uses.—Hydrocyanic acid is a valuable agent in allaying spasm, pain, and nervous irritability, in a variety of disorders, and is much used to relieve cough, particularly in phthisis pulmonalis, and for its antispasmodic virtues in asthma and whooping-cough. It is, moreover, a most efficacious remedy in gastrodynia, and in neuralgic affections of the bowels, and also in chronic vomiting. Topically, it is employed as an anodyne in neuralgia, and in various forms of cutaneous disease (fʒj to water Oj–Ojss).

Dose of the officinal acid, one or two drops, to be repeated and gradually increased by a drop, till some effect is perceptible. When it is taken for a length of time, care should be observed to have the medicine, as renewed, of uniform strength; and it is best, in using a fresh sample, to return to the minimum dose.

POTASSII CYANIDUM (*Cyanide of Potassium*), (KCy), is used as a substitute for hydrocyanic acid, and has the advantage of being a more uniform chemical product, and less liable to undergo decomposition. It is made by heating together ferrocyanide of potassium and carbonate of potassium, and occurs in white, opaque, amorphous pieces, having a sharp, somewhat alkaline and bitter-almond taste, and an alkaline reaction; its solution yields the odour of hydrocyanic acid, when exposed to the air. It is deliquescent, very soluble in water, and sparingly so in alcohol. Its medicinal and poisonous effects are the same as those of hydrocyanic acid. Dose, gr. $\frac{1}{8}$ in half an ounce of distilled water, to be repeated and increased. The addition of a few drops of some vegetable acid frees the hydrocyanic acid, and the same effect is produced by the acids of the stomach.

OLEUM AMYGDALÆ AMARÆ (*Oil of Bitter Almond*), contains hydrocyanic acid, and may be used for the same purposes. It is obtained by distillation from the kernel of the fruit of Amygdalus communis, variety *Amara* (*Nat. Ord.* Amygdaleæ), and is of a yellowish colour, with a bitter, acrid, burning taste, and the peculiar odour of the bitter almond, which is different from that of hydrocyanic acid. It is heavier than water, slightly soluble in it, and soluble in alcohol and ether. It contains hydride of benzoyl and hydrocyanic acid, which are developed from a principle termed *amygdalin*, and water, under the influence of an albuminous ferment termed *emulsin:* thus, amygdalin ($C_{20}H_{27}NO_{11}$) + water ($2H_2O$) = hydride of benzoyl (C_7H_5OH) + HCN + glucose ($2C_6H_{12}O_6$). The effects of this oil upon the system are closely analogous to those of hydrocyanic acid, and its strength is about four times that of the diluted officinal acid. Dose, for internal use, a quarter to half a drop in emulsion; as an external application, one drop to a fluidounce of menstruum. *Bitter Almond Water* (aqua amygdalæ amaræ), is used as a vehicle for narcotic medicines. Dose, half a fluidounce.

SYRUPUS AMYGDALÆ (*Syrup of Almond*), made from both the sweet and bitter almonds, is slightly impregnated with the virtues of hydrocyanic acid, and is a pleasant vehicle for cough mixtures. The following is the formula for preparing it: Rub twelve troyounces of blanched sweet almonds and four troyounces of bitter almonds to a fine paste, adding, during the trituration, three fluidounces of water and twelve troyounces of sugar. Mix the paste with two pints and thirteen fluidounces of water, strain, and dissolve in this solution, at a gentle heat, sixty troyounces of powdered sugar.

CAMPHORA—CAMPHOR.

Camphor is a peculiar CONCRETE SUBSTANCE derived from Camphora officinarum, or the Camphor-Laurel (*Nat. Ord.* Lauraceæ), a large evergreen tree of China, Japan, and Cochin-China. All parts of the tree are strongly impregnated with camphor, which is obtained from the roots and branches by sublimation. In this state it is known in commerce as *crude camphor*, and consists of dirty grayish grains, adhering in crumbling masses. *Japan* camphor (called also *Dutch* camphor), has a pinkish colour, and is purer than the *China* camphor, but is not brought to the United States. The crude camphor, as imported from Canton, is not found in the shops, until it is purified by resublimation with lime, when it is termed *refined camphor*.

This occurs in large hemispherical or convex-concave cakes, perforated in the middle. It is solid at ordinary temperatures, soft and somewhat tough, but may be readily powdered by the addition of a few drops of alcohol. It is translucent, has a strong, fragrant odour, and an aromatic, bitter, afterwards cooling taste. It is volatile, highly inflammable, lighter than water, and very slightly soluble in it, but soluble in alcohol, ether, chloroform, oils, and acids. Water, added to the spirit of camphor, precipitates the camphor.

A valuable camphor is known in the East, which is found in a concrete state in the cavities and fissures of the trunk of Dryobalanops Camphora, a tree of Borneo and Sumatra. The Borneo camphor occurs in small fragments of crystals, which are transparent, brittle, and harder than the laurel camphor. An oil, or liquid camphor, is also obtained from the Dryobalanops, which is more highly esteemed in Oriental countries than the camphor itself.

Camphor is composed of carbon, hydrogen, and oxygen ($C_{10}H_{16}O$). It has been considered to be an oxide of a hypothetical base called *camphogen* or *camphene*, which is isomeric with the oil of turpentine. When heated, it yields an oil, called *oil of camphor*. By passing hydrochloric acid into oil of turpentine, a substance is obtained called *artificial camphor*.

Physiological Effects.—The topical action of camphor is irritant. After its absorption, its effects, in small doses, are moderately stimulant, exhilarant, and anodyne, with a determination to the skin. In large doses, it causes considerable disorder of the cerebro-spinal system, and generally depression of the circulation: and in excessive quantity, it acts as a powerful acro-narcotic poison, occasioning burning heat in the stomach, violent convulsions, and maniacal delirium. It is also an anaphrodisiac. In cases of poisoning, after evacuating the stomach, opium, wine, &c., are to be administered.

Medicinal Uses.—From its combined narcotic and diaphoretic powers, camphor is a valuable remedy in the treatment of dysentery, and is much employed in this disease, either in combination with opium, or as a substitute for the latter. In the early stages of cholera, and in flatulent diarrhœa, it is also greatly prescribed. As a diaphoretic stimulant and antispasmodic, it is useful in the low stages of typhoid and typhus fevers, and in typhoid conditions of the system generally. In many forms of mental disorder, it calms irritability, relieves despondency, and induces sleep. And it has no superior among the anodynes, in allaying irritation or pain of the genito-urinary organs, as in dysmenorrhœa, uterine after-pains, strangury, nymphomania, chordee, &c. From its anodyne and sudorific properties, it is also applicable to the treatment of chronic rheumatism and gout. *Externally*, camphor is employed as an anodyne in rheumatism, and as a discutient in chronic inflammatory affections. Powdered camphor, sniffed into the nostrils, is a good remedy in coryza and influenza.

Administration.—The medium dose, in substance, is gr. v to gr. x; but it may vary from gr. j to ℈j. It is best given in emulsion, made by rubbing up the camphor with loaf sugar, gum arabic, myrrh, and water. The form of pill is objectionable from the difficulty with which it is dissolved in the gastric liquors.

AQUA CAMPHORÆ (*Camphor Water*), is made by rubbing up camphor (120 grains) with 40 minims of alcohol, and subsequently with carbonate of magnesium (half a troyounce) and distilled water (two pints). The carbonate is used to promote the solution of the camphor, and is afterwards separated by filtration. Dose, f℥j (containing about gr. iij) to f℥ij or iij. The *spirit* (four troyounces to alcohol Oij), is chiefly used as an embrocation, but it may be given internally, where the action of the alcohol is not objectionable, in the dose of gtt. v. to f℥j.

LINIMENTUM CAMPHORÆ (*Liniment of Camphor*), consists of camphor (1 part), dissolved in olive oil (4 parts): a mild embrocation.

LINIMENTUM SAPONIS (*Soap Liniment*), is made by digesting soap (four troyounces) and camphor (two troyounces) with oil of rosemary (half a fluidounce), in alcohol (two pints) and water (six fluidounces). It is a yellow oleaginous liquid, and is used as an anodyne and gently rubefacient application, in gouty and rheumatic pains, sprains, bruises, &c.

OLEUM CAMPHORÆ (*Oil of Camphor*), the volatile oil obtained from Camphora officinarum, is a light reddish-brown fluid, with the odour and taste of camphor. It has medicinal properties similar to those of camphor, but is more stimulant, and therefore especially adapted to affections of the stomach and bowels. Dose, 2 or 3 drops. It is used also externally.

PHYSOSTIGMA—CALABAR BEAN.

This is the seed of a perennial climbing plant of the western coast of Africa, which has received the name of Physostigma venenosum (*Nat. Ord.* Fabaceæ). The SEED is about the size of a large horse-bean, irregularly kidney-form in shape, with a firm, hard, brittle integument, when recently gathered of a gray colour, but gradually deepening into a dark chocolate-brown. The inner kernel is by far the more active portion; it is hard, white, pulverizable, of an edible taste, without bitterness or acridity. Alcohol, but not water, extracts its medicinal virtues. It yields an active alkaloid principle, termed *physostigmia* or *eseria*, sparingly soluble in water, but more soluble in alcohol, ether, and chloroform.

The calabar bean has long been used among the negroes of Western Africa, as an ordeal to determine the guilt or innocence of accused individuals, whence its name, the *ordeal bean of Calabar*. It has been found, in full medicinal doses, to produce giddiness, torpor, paleness and coolness of the surface, weak and irregular pulse, relaxation of the muscular system, and drowsiness, but not stupor. An interesting effect of its action is a remarkable power of contracting the pupil, whether taken internally, or applied externally; and it also contracts the ciliary muscle, which regulates the accommodating power of the eye. As a neurotic, its influence is directed rather to the spinal marrow than the brain, suspending or destroying the power of the former of conducting impressions. It is allied in its effects to woorara and conium, but differs from them in its tendency to produce muscular twitchings, and in contracting the pupil. In cases of poisoning, after emptying the stomach, the hypodermic administration of a solution of atropia is the best physiological antidote.

Calabar bean has been found highly efficacious in traumatic tetanus. It has been used also with success in chorea, and in poisoning from strychnia, and spasmodic cholera. In ophthalmic surgery, its employment is obvious, either to produce contraction of the pupil, or to increase the power of accommodating the eye to distances.

The dose of the kernel is laid down as two or three grains, to begin with, gradually increased. By exhausting the kernel with alcohol, an *extract* (alcoholic) is obtained, of which the dose is one-eighth of a grain. A good form of administration is the *tincture* (which is not officinal), which may be made from the alcoholic extract, in the proportion of twelve grains to an ounce of alcohol—dose, 10 drops; or a solution in glycerin may be used. Paper, impregnated with a concentrated tincture of the bean, and afterwards dried, has been applied locally to the eye.

COCCULUS—COCCULUS INDICUS.

This is the DRIED SEED of Anamirta Cocculus, (*Nat. Ord.* Menispermaceæ), a climbing shrub of India. The fruit is a one-celled berry, of a dark, purplish colour, with a soft pulp, and a single *seed*. This, when dried, is about the size of a pea, of a dark-grayish colour, and consists of a thin, dry, blackish, wrinkled integument, containing a whitish, oily, inodorous, very bitter kernel. The active properties reside in a peculiar white, crystallizable, bitter principle, termed *picrotoxin*, which is partially soluble in water, and very soluble in alcohol, chloroform, and ether. In the shell, an alkaloid termed *menispermia* has been found, and a neutral principle of the same composition as the alkaloid, termed *paramenispermin*.

Effects and Uses.—Cocculus Indicus is an acrid cerebro-spinant narcotic, capable in large doses, of producing death. It has not been much used internally; but, in the form of decoction or ointment, it is employed to destroy lice and other parasites, and for the cure of tinea and porrigo of the scalp. It is said to prevent the secondary fermentation of malt liquors, into which it is sometimes introduced as an adulteration. Cocculus Indicus is not officinal.

WOORARA.

This substance, termed also *woorari*, *woorali*, and *curare*, has long been known as a powerful poison, prepared by the Indians in South America, and, of late years, has been employed as a medicine. Its source is unsettled, but it is generally considered to be an extract from the bark of an unknown plant. It is brought from the shores of the Amazon, and occurs in the form of dark-brown or grayish lumps or powder, of an intensely bitter taste, and, when triturated, of a powerful odour. A principle termed *curarine* is said to have been extracted from woorara.

Effects and Uses.—Woorara is ranked with the sedative narcotics, and is considered to destroy life by more or less rapid paralysis of the respiratory muscles. A peculiarity of its action is that it is comparatively innoxious when taken by the stomach, being either not absorbed at all in this viscus, or so slowly, as to allow of its elimination by the kidneys, before dangerous accumulation in the blood. Hence, for therapeutic purposes, it must be employed either endermically to a blistered surface, or by hypodermic injection. It is very similar in its action to conium, and may be employed therapeutically to fulfil the same indications. The amount administered *endermically* is from a half to three-quarters of a grain daily.

ORDER II.—ETHEREAL ANÆSTHETICS.

The term, Anæsthetics (from *α*, *non*, and *αἴσθησις*, *sensation*), properly speaking, includes all agents which diminish sensibility and relieve pain. It has, however, been used to denominate a class of ethereal remedies, which are applied by inhalation, and produce such a condition of temporary insensibility, as to prevent pain during surgical operations and parturition.

The vapours usually employed to produce anæsthesia are those of ETHER and CHLOROFORM. Many other substances have, however, lately been introduced as anæsthetics.

ÆTHER—ETHER.

Ether is prepared by the distillation of alcohol and sulphuric acid, and is afterwards rectified by redistillation with solution of potassa. For inhalation, however, it is further purified by being shaken with water, by which it is freed from alcohol, and this, as well as acid contaminations, are afterwards removed by the agency of chloride of calcium and freshly calcined lime. Thus purified, it is designated as ÆTHER FORTIOR—STRONGER ETHER.

Although commonly termed sulphuric ether, in allusion to the sulphuric acid used in its preparation, yet ether contains no sulphuric acid. By the action of the acid upon alcohol, this substance, which is chemically a hydrated oxide of ethyl, is deprived of the elements of water, and is converted into the oxide of ethyl or ether, for which the formula is $C_4H_{10}O$, or $(C_2H_5)_2O$.

Ether is a transparent, colourless liquid, with a strong, fragrant odour, and a hot, pungent taste. It wholly evaporates in the air, so rapidly as to cause a considerable degree of cold, is very inflammable, combines with alcohol and chloroform in every proportion, and dissolves in ten times its volume of water. The sp. gr. of pure ether is 0.713, of *stronger ether*, 0.728, of ordinary *officinal ether*, 0.750. The boiling point of *stronger ether* is about 98° F.

Effects and Uses when swallowed.—When taken into the stomach, ether produces a primary stimulant and secondary narcotic effect, the stage of excitement being, however, very transient. It has long been employed as an antispasmodic and anodyne remedy in asthma, angina pectoris, hysteria, cramp of the stomach and bowels, spasm of the gall ducts, &c.; and from its combined stimulant and antispasmodic virtues, it has been found useful in the latter stages of typhus, attended by subsultus tendinum, &c. As a *topical* anodyne, ether is a very good application in nervous headache and earache; it has been also applied with advantage in aphthæ, stomatitis, diphtheria, and other affections of the mouth and throat; and, from its refrigerant effects, it has been used in the reduction of strangulated herniæ, and as a cooling lotion in cerebral affections. If evaporation be repressed, when it is applied locally, it acts as a rubefacient, and may be employed for counter-irritation.

Dose, fʒss to fʒj, to be increased when habitually used. It may be incorporated with water, by rubbing it up with spermaceti, in the proportion of two grains to a fluidrachm of ether, or it may be given in capsules of sugared gum.

Effects and Uses when inhaled.—The first effects of the inhalation of ether are a sense of strangulation and cough, from its local irritant action. When the vapour is absorbed into the system through the pulmonary surface, the nervous functions are successively and progressively affected. The mental faculties and volition become first impaired; insensibility and unconsciousness rapidly supervene, *during which susceptibility to pain is lost;* and the patient lies in a trance-like sleep, resembling death. This condition is often preceded by one of excitement, during which patients sometimes weep, laugh, moan, sing, rave, or present pugnacious manifestations. In the beginning of etherization, the circulation is accelerated, but it is afterwards depressed. The period of full ether-narcosis lasts from five to ten minutes, and the patient ordinarily recovers without serious inconvenience, although headache, nausea, drowsiness, and languor sometimes ensue for a few hours. Occasionally, congestion of the brain or lungs, cataleptic rigidity with prolonged insensibility, and, in females, hysterical phenomena ensue after etherization; but these effects are uncommon, and it is believed that death has never followed the use of ether, when care has been taken to admit atmospheric air into the lungs along with the ether. During the stage of insensibility, convulsive twitches or muscular rigidity are occasionally noticed; the breathing is sometimes stertorous; the iris becomes fixed; the pupils are dilated; the eyeballs are upturned; and the orbicularis palpebrarum does not contract when touched. Insensibility to pain in some cases takes place before unconsciousness; and, when patients are recovering from the latter state, the mental faculties are often completely restored, while insensibility to pain continues.

Since the year 1846, the inhalation of ether, first resorted to in our own country, has been practised very generally in all parts of the world, with the greatest success, for the prevention of pain in surgical operations; and its use has been also extended with the happiest results to the relief of pain in labour.

It should not be exhibited where disease of the heart or brain, or serious obstruction of the lungs exists, or when from any cause there is unusual tendency to syncope, and precaution should be taken to guard against asphyxia; but, when administered with proper care and discrimination, it is attended with little or no danger or unpleasant results of any kind.

The quantity of ether necessary to effect etherization is about two ounces; and it may be conveniently applied by means of a cone of stiff paper, shaped so that its base will fit over the nose and mouth of the patient, and into which a napkin, or small towel, or hollowed-out sponge is placed; the sponge should be first soaked in warm water, squeezed dry, and saturated with pure ether. It is then applied to the mouth and nostrils, the mouth being permitted occasionally to receive atmospheric air; and, if irritability of the air-passages occur, this is to be gradually overcome. From three to five minutes are required to produce anæsthezation, and its occurrence is known by closure of the eyelids (if they have been previously open), failure to respond to questions, and muscular relaxation. The sponge is then to be removed, and may be reapplied from time to time if necessary.

Etherization is less apt to produce nausea, if practised upon an empty stomach, and the administration of a little brandy and laudanum promotes its action.

Etherization has been also resorted to in a variety of morbid conditions, in which the administration of narcotics and antispasmodics has been found useful. It exerts a powerful control over the violent types of spasmodic disease, and has been prescribed with the greatest advantage in hysteria, tetanus, poisoning from strychnia, asthma, chorea, convulsions, puerperal eclampsia, whooping-cough, dysmenorrhœa, and almost every description of spasm; and as a relaxant in the reduction of dislocations.

Local anæsthesia and congelation may be produced through the agency of the ether spray applied to a part by the atomizer, (see p. 44).

CHLOROFORMUM—CHLOROFORM.

Chloroform is usually obtained from the distillation of alcohol with chlorinated lime, and, for medicinal use,

COMMERCIAL CHLOROFORM (*chloroformum venale*), is purified by agitation with one-fifth its weight of sulphuric acid, which destroys the contamination of chlorinated pyrogenous oil; and the sulphurous acid formed and the water present are afterwards removed by means of a watery solution of carbonate of sodium, and of stronger alcohol and lime. The purest chloroform, for internal use, is now made from the hydrate of chloral.

PURIFIED CHLOROFORM (*Chloroformum Purificatum*) is a colourless, volatile liquid, of a bland, ethereal odour, and a hot, aromatic, saccharine taste. It is not inflammable, is slightly soluble in water, and freely soluble in alcohol and ether. It has extensive solvent powers, dissolving camphor, the fixed and volatile oils, most resins and fats, iodine, bromine, the organic alkalies, &c. The purest chloroform has a sp. gr. of 1.5022. Officinal chloroform has a sp. gr. of 1.480, when it contains a little alcohol; and, as usually found, its sp. gr. is about 1.475, when it contains more alcohol, and is less apt to become acid. The boiling point of pure chloroform is 142° F. It is, chemically, a terchloride of formyl, $CHCl_3$. Chloroform is sometimes contaminated with chlorinated pyrogenous oil (a very injurious impurity); this may be detected and removed by strong sulphuric acid, which gives the chloroform a colour varying from yellowish to reddish-brown, according to the amount of impurity. The most delicate test for the presence of alcohol is the binitrosulphuret of iron, which, when agitated with chloroform, will produce a brown tint if alcohol be present.

Physiological Effects.—The effects of chloroform on the system are analogous to those of ether, but much more rapid and powerful. When inhaled, in the dose of a fluidrachm or more, it rapidly induces anæsthetic sleep, with great relaxation of the muscles, and the most complete insensibility to painful agents. The period at which insensibility occurs varies from fifteen seconds to two minutes; and it continues usually between five and ten minutes, and may be prolonged considerably, by renewals of the inhalation. The patient usually recovers without recollection of what has occurred during the state of insensibility, and with few or no uncomfortable sequelæ. Sensibility to pain is often very much obliterated, even before consciousness is lost.

The administration of chloroform has, in some cases, been attended with fatal syncope, due to heart-paralysis. This has ordinarily occurred with such rapidity as to render remedial interference unavailable; but, at the slightest approach of symptoms of the kind, the patient should be placed in a recumbent position, cold affusions should be applied, and, above all, electro-magnetism should be resorted to. It would be proper always to have an eletro-magnetic machine ready for use, when chloroform is inhaled.

Topically applied, and when its evaporation is prevented, chloroform acts as an irritant, and soon vesicates the skin—powerfully diminishing painful impressions during its application.

Medicinal Uses.—Chloroform is prescribed by the stomach as an anodyne and antispasmodic, in all the cases to which ether is applicable, and has the advantage of a more agreeable taste. It has been found particularly useful to relieve the pain and vomiting of cancer of the stomach, and also in colic and cholera. It has been also extolled as an antiperiodic in the treatment of intermittent fevers. Externally, it is used as a topical anodyne, and also as a stimulating application to foul and indolent ulcers, and occasionally for its constitutional effects.

Dose, from f℈ss to f℈j, in sweetened water or mucilage; to be repeated. As an anti-neuralgic liniment, f℈j to f℥ij of camphor liniment; or as a rubefacient and anodyne, undiluted, on linen, covered with oiled silk, to prevent evaporation. As a wash or gargle, f℥j or ij to water Oj.

The introduction of chloroform, as an anæsthetic, took place shortly after that of ether; and, from its greater intensity of action, its freedom from irritating effects on the bronchial mucous membrane, its more agreeable odour, and its non-inflammability, it has been extensively used, particularly in Great Britain, to the exclusion of ether. A very considerable number of fatal cases have, however, occurred from the inhalation of this agent, where its administration did not appear in any way counter-indicated; and it can scarcely be considered a perfectly safe remedy. It is employed as an anæsthetic, anodyne, and antispasmodic, to fulfil the indications to which ether is applicable. It is also used hypodermically.

The *dose* for inhalation is a fluidrachm, to be repeated in two minutes, if anæsthesia be not produced; and its effects may be renewed from time to time, without injury. It may be applied on a handkerchief, held near the nose or mouth, care being taken to allow a proper admixture of atmospheric air.

A solution of chloroform in ether has been used in the United States, but, from the unequal volatilization of the two liquids, it must be difficult to modify their effects by combination.

SPIRITUS CHLOROFORMI (*Spirit of Chloroform*), is a solution of a troyounce of chloroform in twelve fluidounces of diluted alcohol; a convenient form for internal exhibition. *Dose*, f℥j.

Linimentum Chloroformi (*Liniment of Chloroform*), is made by mixing three parts of chloroform with four parts of olive oil.

Mistura Chloroformi (*Mixture of Chloroform*), is made by mixing chloroform, in which camphor is dissolved (*sixty grains* in *half a troyounce* of chloroform), with six fluidounces of water, by the intervention of the yolk of an egg. *Dose*, f℥ss–f℥j.*

*Under the name of *chlorodyne*, a combination containing chloroform is much used, for which the following is a formula: Muriate of morphia, 8

Since the discovery of the anæsthetic properties of ether and chloroform, many other substances have been employed for the purpose of anæsthesia. Of these may be mentioned:

I. RHIGOLENE, a petroleum naphtha, obtained by the distillation of petroleum. It is the lightest of all known liquids, having a sp. gr. 0.625, is highly volatile and inflammable, boils at 70° F., and in its composition is a hydrocarbon, containing no oxygen. It is nearly odourless, and has been employed to produce local anæsthesia through the agency of the atomizer, and is the most convenient, most rapid, and most easily controlled freezing liquid that can be used. Its name is derived from ριγος, *extreme cold.*

II. BICHLORIDE OF METHYLENE.—This liquid is most easily procured by the action of nascent hydrogen (developed from zinc, water, and sulphuric acid), upon chloroform. Its composition is CH_2Cl_2. It is a colourless fluid, having a pleasant ethereal odour like that of chloroform, boils at 88° F., has sp. gr. 1.34, and mixes with ether and chloroform in all proportions. It is said nearly to equal chloroform in efficacy, with less danger to life, while its effects are much more rapid. It is used in about the same dose as chloroform, but has not been employed in the United States.

III. METHYLIC ETHER, made by digesting methylic alcohol with strong sulphuric acid, is a gaseous substance, lately employed. Under the name of *methyl-ethylic ether*, it has been used, dissolved in ethylic ether, and is said to produce rapid anæsthesia, without spasm, syncope, or asphyxia, during inhalation, or subsequent nausea. One or two drachms may be introduced into a bag inhaler, and the gas is volatilized by means of a hand bellows.

IV. COMPOUNDS OF AMYL.—Various compounds of amyl

grains; oil of peppermint, 16 minims; stronger ether, a fluidounce; extract of liquorice, 2½ troyounces; pure chloroform, stronger alcohol, and molasses, each, 4 fluidounces; diluted hydrocyanic acid, 2 fluidounces; syrup, 17½ fluidounces: dissolve the morphia and oil in the alcohol, and add the chloroform and ether, mix the liquorice, syrup, and molasses, shake the two mixtures, and add the hydrocyanic acid—dose, 5 to 10 minims, the vial to be well shaken.

(C_5H_{11}), products derivable from the oxidation of starchy matter, have been proposed as anæsthetics. *Amylic alcohol*, or fusel oil (the hydrated oxide of amyl, $C_5H_{11}HO$), is one of the products of the alcoholic fermentation. It is a colourless, oily liquid, of a strong, offensive odour, and an acrid, burning taste. When inhaled by animals, it has been found to produce muscular paralysis and convulsions. *Amylene* (C_5H_{10}) is prepared by distilling amylic alcohol with a concentrated solution of chloride of zinc. It is a colourless, mobile liquid, having a peculiar disagreeable smell. Of the amyl series, *amylene* alone can be considered as a true anæsthetic, that will produce complete insensibility to pain. An extreme dose is, however, required for this purpose, and its operation is dangerous to life. The *hydruret*, *iodide*, *acetate*, and *nitrite* of amyl have also been employed. Of these compounds, however, the NITRITE alone appears likely to come into use as a therapeutic agent. The NITRITE OF AMYL is prepared by heating one part of strong nitric acid with two parts of rectified fusel oil until reaction just commences, when the fire is withdrawn. After the violent reaction has subsided, heat is again carefully applied. The distillate obtained below 212° F., is rectified over carbonate of potassium, with the precaution to collect only that portion distilling between 202° and 206° F. It is a nitrite of the oxide of amyl, and is an amber-coloured, volatile, inflammable liquid, of sp. gr. 0.913, boiling at 182° F., with an odour and taste like that of ripe pears. Its composition is $C_5H_{11}NO_2$. It is not a true anæsthetic, as it does not destroy consciousness, unless a condition approaching to death is produced. It exercises, however, a rapid and powerful influence on the heart and circulation, and as an excitant of vascular action may be considered the most energetic agent as yet physiologically discovered. In has been employed to rouse the system in cases of syncope and prostration, and has been also found efficacious in relieving the pain of angina pectoris, in asthma, and as a general relaxer of muscular spasm. Experiments upon animals show it to be also a physiological antidote in cases of poisoning from strychnia, and it would probably prove efficacious in tetanus. *Dose*, 5 to 6 drops.

V. Tetrachloride of Carbon.—This substance, termed also bichloride of carbon and chlorocarbon (CCl_4), is made by passing the vapour of bisulphuret of carbon, together with chlorine, through a red-hot porcelain tube; and is purified by agitation with an alcoholic solution of potash, afterwards washing with water, and subsequently redistilling, It is a transparent, colourless fluid, having an ethereal and sweetish odour, not unlike that of chloroform. Its sp. gr. is high, 1.56, and its boiling point, 170° F. It is miscible in all proportions with ether and chloroform. Chlorocarbon has been employed by inhalation as an antispasmodic, anodyne, and anæsthetic, and has the advantage of a pleasant smell and freedom from nauseating effect. For full and prolonged anæsthesia, however, there are objections to its use in the heaviness of its vapour, its insufficient volatility, and the consequent difficulty of its elimination from the system. It may be inhaled to the extent of f℥i. A mixture of one part of chlorocarbon and six parts of chloroform is recommended as a safe and agreeable anæsthetic. The Tetrabromide of Carbon (CBr_4) has very recently been added to our list of anæsthetics. It may be made by heating bisulphuret of carbon in a sealed tube with bromide of iodine. It is a white substance, crystallizing in plates, of an ethereal odour, somewhat resembling that of tetrachloride of carbon, and sweetish taste. It is insoluble in water, but dissolves in ether, alcohol, bisulphuret of carbon, chloroform, bromoform, benzole, and petroleum.

VI. Nitrous Oxide Gas was the substance by which anæsthesia was in the first instance produced, in the hands of Mr. Horace Wells, a dentist of Hartford, Connecticut. It is made by the decomposition of nitrate of ammonium by heat. Its composition is N_2O. It is a colourless, respirable gas, absorbable by water, and the solution, like the gas itself, has a faint, agreeable odour and sweet taste. This gas is both a pleasant and efficient anæsthetic, more rapid, and at the same time more transitory in its action than either ether or chloroform, and free from disagreeable or serious consequences. It is well adapted to employment in the extraction of teeth, or in short, minor surgical operations, but its effects are too transient for the anæsthesia required in protracted operations. The amount necessary to produce anæsthesia (one or two gallons), as well as the complicated apparatus required for its administration, constitute also an objection to its general use. It is best administered from an India-rubber bag, containing about eight gallons of the gas, furnished with a mouth-piece with two valves, one of which is designed for the throwing out of the respired gas. Water, impregnated with about five times its volume of nitrous oxide, has been used internally as a stimulant, in the dose of half a pint to a pint and a half, during the course of the day. In experiments upon dogs, nitrous oxide water injected into the bowels has been found to act as a physiological antidote in cases of poisoning from chloroform, carbonic acid, hydrocyanic acid, and other agents.

ORDER III.—ANTISPASMODICS.

Antispasmodics are medicines that allay irregular nervous action. Their effects upon the economy in a state of health are not very decided, and are limited to a slight stimulation of the circulation, and exhilaration of the mental faculties. Their influence is, however, strikingly shown in certain deranged conditions of the nervous system, particularly in those forms of spasm, which depend upon idiopathic or primary nervous disorder, and are known under the designation of *hysteria*. They are also useful in many varieties of mental disturbance, as wakefulness, hypochondriasis, and even insanity, and are often preferable to narcotics in the treatment of these cases, from their comparative freedom of action on the brain. They are all distinguished by a powerful odour.

ASSAFŒTIDA—ASSAFETIDA.

Assafetida is a GUM-RESINOUS EXUDATION, obtained from the ROOT of Narthex Assafœtida (*Nat. Ord.* Apiaceæ). This plant is a native of Persia, and has a large, tapering root, the size of a man's leg, with long, lanceolate leaves, springing directly from the root, and an erect stem, from six to nine feet in height, rising from the midst of the leaves. The drug is obtained from incisions made into the root, or by taking successive slices of it. The exuded juice is scraped off, hardened in the sun, and afterwards packed for exportation. It occurs in masses of varying size, consistence, and colour, but is usually whitish, intermixed with darker spots, and becomes reddish, and finally brown, by exposure to the air. It is sometimes soft and adhesive, at other times hard and brittle, and is not readily powdered, except at a low temperature. It breaks with a waxy lustre, and the best samples appear to be composed of irregularly-shaped tears. Its taste is unpleasant, bitter, and acrid; its odour powerful, alliaceous, and fetid.

Assafetida is a gum-resin, united to a volatile oil. The gum is dissolved by water; and the mucilage thus formed suspends the resin and volatile oil. The resin and volatile oil are soluble in alcohol; but the tincture becomes milky on the addition of water, owing to the separation of the resin.

Physiological Effects.—Assafetida, when taken into the stomach, produces a local stimulant and carminative effect. After absorption, it proves a moderate excitant and exhilarant, and exerts a marked influence upon morbid conditions of the nervous system. It also stimulates the mucous secretions generally, and increases the peristaltic action of the bowels. Its volatile oil is absorbed, and the odorous principle is recognised in the secretions, especially in the perspiration.

Medicinal Uses.—No medicine is more highly esteemed as a direct antispasmodic than assafetida. It is much resorted to in the various forms of hysteria, and is particularly valuable in relieving the mental depression, which constitutes one of the protean types of this disorder. In other spasmodic diseases, as chorea, asthma, whooping-cough, &c., it is a favorite remedy with many practitioners; and, from its combined expectorant and antispasmodic properties, it is particularly adapted to spasmodic pectoral affections. In certain diseases of the abdominal viscera, as flatulent colic and costiveness, assafetida is often useful as an antispasmodic and laxative enema. It is also prescribed as a stimulating emmenagogue, when the uterine disorder is attended with a disturbance of the nervous functions.

Notwithstanding its disagreeable odour, this drug is largely used as a condiment in Asia; and, even in the refined cookery of Europe, its flavour is admired. Many persons take it habitually for its exhilarant effects; and, when used as a medicine, it generally becomes acceptable.

Administration.—Dose, gr. v to ℈j, in pill. It is most frequently given in the form of *mixture* (*Mistura Assafœtidæ*,—ʒij, rubbed gradually with water Oss),—dose, f℥ss to f℥j, repeated, or as an enema, f℥ij to f℥iv. This mixture, from its whiteness and opacity, is sometimes called *lac assafœtidæ*, or *milk of assafetida*. *Pills of assafetida*, made by beating up three parts of assafetida with one part of soap and a little water, are officinal, each pill containing 3 grains of the gum-resin. The *tincture* (four troyounces to alcohol Oij—dose fʒj), is a good preparation, where the alcohol is not objectionable. A *plaster* is used externally in whooping-cough and catarrh; it is made by dissolving *twelve troyounces* of assafetida and *six troyounces* of galbanum in three pints of alcohol, evaporating to the consistence of honey, and to this adding *twelve troyounces* of lead-plaster and *six troyounces* of yellow wax, previously melted together. *Suppositories of Assafetida* are made by mixing a fluidounce of the tincture, evaporated to the consistence of a thick syrup, with 320 grains of oil of theobroma.

GALBANUM.

Galbanum is a GUM-RESIN obtained from an undetermined Eastern plant. It is met with in the form of tears, or more commonly in lumps, of a brownish colour, and has a peculiar balsamic odour, and a hot, bitter, acrid taste. It is a gum-resin united to a volatile oil. Its effects are similar to those of assafetida, but less active; and it is chiefly employed externally, as a stimulant and resolvent to indolent swellings.

The *compound pills of galbanum* are used as antispasmodic and emmenagogue; they are made by beating into a pilular mass *thirty-six grains* of galbanum and myrrh, each, and *twelve grains* of assafetida, with a little syrup, the mass to be divided into 24 pills,—dose, 3 to 5 pills. Galbanum forms the basis of the *compound galbanum plaster*, which contains eight parts of galbanum, one part of turpentine, three parts of Burgundy pitch, and thirty-six parts of plaster of lead.

AMMONIACUM—AMMONIAC.

This is a GUM-RESINOUS EXUDATION obtained from Dorema Ammoniacum (*Nat. Ord.* Apiaceæ), a plant of Persia. It comes in tears or lumps, of an irregular shape, yellowish on the outside, whitish within, is moderately hard and brittle, and has an unpleasant, bitter, and rather acrid taste, with a peculiar smell, somewhat like that of galbanum. It is a gum-resin, with a little volatile oil. Its effects are similar to those of assafetida; but it is seldom used, except as an antispasmodic expectorant in chronic catarrh. Dose, gr. x to xxx. A *mixture* and *plaster* are officinal. The *mixture* has the same formula as *mixture of assafetida;* the plaster is made by dissolving *five troyounces* of ammoniac in half a pint of diluted acetic acid, straining, and evaporating to a proper consistence. A *plaster of ammoniac with mercury* is also officinal.

VALERIANA—VALERIAN.

Valeriana officinalis, or Wild Valerian (*Nat. Ord.* Valerianaceæ), is a perennial European plant, growing to the height of three or four feet, with serrated leaves, and small, reddish-white fragrant flowers. The ROOT is the portion used, and consists of numerous long, slender, cylindrical fibres, attached to a rough, tuberculated head. The colour of the dried root externally is yellowish or brown, and internally white; when powdered, it is yellowish-gray. It has a peculiar, powerful odour, of which cats are fond, and a bitterish, subacrid, aromatic taste. Water and alcohol extract its virtues, which depend on the presence of a *volatile oil*, from which a peculiar colourless, volatile acid, called *valerianic*, may be separated.

Effects and Uses.—Valerian generally acts as an energetic excitant and antispasmodic, although at times it makes but a feeble impression on the system. It is much used as a nervous excitant and antispasmodic in the various forms of hysteria, and occasionally, also, in epilepsy, chorea, hemicrania, hypochondriasis, delirium tremens, &c.

Dose of the *powder*, from ʒss to ʒjss, three or four times a day; of the *infusion* (half a troyounce to Oj of water), f℥j to ij; of the *tincture* (four troyounces to diluted alcohol Oij), fʒj; of the *ammoniated tincture* (four troyounces to aromatic spirit of ammonia Oij—an excellent preparation), fʒj to ij; of the *fluid extract*, fʒj; of the *extract* (*alcoholic*) gr. x to xxx; of the *oil*, 4 or 5 drops.

ACIDUM VALERIANICUM (*Valerianic Acid*). ($HC_5H_9O_2$), which is found in valerian-root, is usually prepared artificially by the action of bichromate of potassium and sulphuric acid upon amylic alcohol, and occurs as an oily, colourless liquid, of a caustic taste, and strong odour, resembling, but different from that of valerian. It is used for the manufacture of

AMMONII VALERIANAS (*Valerianate of Ammonium*).—This salt, made by combining valerianic acid with ammonia (obtained by the reaction of lime upon chloride of ammonium), occurs in snow-white, quadrangular plates, of an offensive odour like that of valerianic acid, and a sharp, sweetish taste. It deliquesces in a moist air, effloresces in a dry one, and is very soluble both in water and alcohol. Potassa and the mineral acids decompose it. It is much employed in neuralgia, nervous headache, hysteria, chorea, epilepsy, &c. *Dose*, gr. ij–viij, given in coated pills; or an elixir, prepared with aromatics* may be used.

* Take of valerianate of ammonium, ʒi; fluid extract of vanilla, f℥ss; cd. tinct. of cardamom, fʒvi; curaçoa, fʒij; water, f℥iv; mix. Dose, a teaspoonful three times a day.

CYPRIPEDIUM.

The ROOT of Cypripedium pubescens and of Cypripedium parviflorum (*Nat. Ord.* Orchidaceæ), common indigenous plants, known under the numes of *ladies' slipper*, and *moccasin plant*, are recognized in the secondary list of the U. S. Pharmacopæia. They grow to the height of one or two feet, with large many-nerved, plaited leaves, and large handsome flowers resembling the Indian moccasin; C. pubescens (*yellow ladies' slipper*), has yellow flowers. The *dried root* is several inches long, bent, with a small knotted dark head, and numerous fibres, of a yellowish-brown colour, of an aromatic odour, and a bitter, sweetish; somewhat pungent taste. It contains a volatile oil and bitter principle, and has been used as a substitute for valerian. Dose of the *powdered root*, gr. xv, three times a day. An infusion and tincture are also used; by precipitating the tincture, an oleoresin is obtained, of which the dose is half a grain to three grains.

SCUTELLARIA—SKULLCAP.

The HERB of Scutellaria lateriflora (*Nat. Ord.* Labiatæ), an indigenous perennial herb, found in moist localitics, growing to the height of one or two feet, with ovate, acute, dentate, petiolate, opposite leaves, and small pale-blue flowers in leafy racemes, is considered by many American practitioners to possess valuable antispasmodic properties. An *infusion* (two troy-ounces to boiling water Oj) may be taken ad libitum; and a *fluid extract* is also used. S. pilosa and integrifolia have a more bitter taste, and have been used as tonics.

DRACONTIUM—SKUNK-CABBAGE.

Dracontium fœtidum, Ictodes fœtidus, Symplocarpus fœtidus, or Skunk-Cabbage (*Nat. Ord.* Araceæ), is an indigenous plant, growing in moist situations, which flowers in April and May, and afterwards sends up numerous large and luxuriant leaves. The fresh ROOT has a strong, fetid odour, and an acrid taste, but loses these properties by being kept. It is stimulant, anti-spasmodic, and narcotic, and is employed in hysteria, asthma, chronic catarrh, &c. Dose, gr. x to xx, gradually increased. It is also given in the form of *infusion.* The leaves are used in the country to keep up the discharge from blistered surfaces, and to stimulate indolent ulcers.

The following vegetable substances, used as articles of diet, may be ranked also with antispasmodics.

I. THEA—TEA, the *dried leaves* of Thea Chinensis (*Nat. Ord.* Ternstromiaceæ), an evergreen shrub, of China and Japan, whence the markets of the world are supplied. The most important constituents of tea are essential oil (upon which the flavour depends), tannic acid, and a crystalline, volatilizable, nitrogenous alkaloid principle, termed *theina.*

II. CAFFEA—COFFEE, the SEED of Coffea Arabica (*Nat. Ord.* Cinchonaceæ), a small tree, which is a native of Southern Arabia and Abyssinia, and is cultivated in various tropical and semi-tropical countries. Coffee contains a nitrogenous principle, *caffeina* ($C_8H_{10}N_4O_2 + H_2O$), which is considered to be identical with *theina*, and two peculiar principles, one resembling tannin, termed *caffeo-tannic acid,* and the other termed *caffeic acid.* The volatile oil, upon which the flavour depends, is developed by roasting. Coffee may be used for the general indications of antispasmodics, and is besides especially efficacious in relieving the sopor produced by opium poisoning. Both tea and coffee lessen the uric acid and increase the urea in the urine.

III. THEOBROMA—CHOCOLATE (noticed more at length under the head of demulcents—see *Oil of Theobroma*) contains a nitrogenous principle, *theobromia*, nearly identical in composition with caffeina ($C_7H_8N_4O_2 + H_2O$).

IV. ERYTHROXYLON COCA—COCA.—The leaves of this plant, a shrub, about six feet in height, have long been used as a masticatory by the Indians in Peru, for the purpose of enabling them to undergo fatigue, hunger, and thirst. Statements have been recently made, of the medicinal efficacy of this substance as a nervous stimulant, in doses of half an ounce, in infusion. An alkaloid principle, termed *cocaina*, has been found in coca.

V. PAULLINIA—GUARANA.—This occurs in chocolate-coloured cylinders, which are worked up from the fruit of Paullinia Sorbilis (*Nat. Ord.* Sapindaceæ), a plant of Brazil, where it is used to make a common and highly esteemed beverage. It is said to contain twice as much *theina* as the best tea. It is recommended medicinally, as a tonic, astringent, and antispasmodic and has been found especially useful in sick-headache; dose, one or two drachms, or an alcoholic extract may be given in doses of ten or twenty grains.

VI. MATE.—Under this name, the dried leaves of Ilex Paraguaiensis, a small tree or shrub of Paraguay, cultivated also in other parts of South America, are extensively used as a beverage throughout the Atlantic region of that continent. *Paraguay tea*, as it is termed, has a balsamic odour and bitter taste, and contains a principle identical with *caffeina* and *theina*, and also tannic acid.

MOSCHUS—MUSK.

Musk is a peculiar CONCRETE SECRETION obtained from Moschus moschiferus, the Musk Deer, an animal rather larger than the goat and resembling the deer in its characters, which inhabits the mountainous portions of Central Asia. The musk-bag is found only in the male, and lies between the umbilicus and prepuce. It is an oval pod, about two and a half inches long, and one and a half broad, flat on one side, and convex and hairy on the other, and in a full-grown animal contains from ℥jss to ℥vj, of a liquid secretion, which, when dried, is musk. Two kinds are known in commerce, the China and the Russia Musk, the former of which is much the stronger.

Musk occurs in grains or lumps concreted together, of a reddish-brown colour, and has usually some hairs of the pod mixed with it. It has a powerful diffusive, aromatic odour and a bitterish taste. It is inflammable, leaving a light spongy charcoal. On analysis, it yields ammonia and a variety of other constituents, but the odorous principle has not been isolated. It is partially soluble in water and alcohol, and completely so in ether.

Owing to its high price, musk is greatly sophisticated. Sometimes artificial pods are met with, which may be distinguished from the genuine, by the absence of the remains of the penis and of an aperture in the middle of the hairy coat. The musk itself is more frequently adulterated, by mixture with dried blood, and a variety of substances. Indeed, little if any genuine musk is found in the shops.

Effects and Uses.—Musk is a powerful excitant and antispasmodic, without much effect on the cerebral functions. If a pure article could be obtained, it would have no superior as a direct antispasmodic in the treatment of essential nervous disorders—hysteria, epilepsy, chorea, and hiccough, and as a combined excitant and antispasmodic in the latter stages of typhus, and in typhoid pneumonia. But it is now little prescribed, owing to the difficulty of procuring it good.

Administration.—It may be given in the form of bolus or emulsion. Dose, gr. x, to be repeated every two or three hours.

An article, termed ARTIFICIAL MUSK, is made by the addition of one part of rectified oil of amber to three parts of nitric acid. It resembles musk both in sensible and medicinal properties, and it has been prescribed in its stead, in the same dose.

CASTOREUM—CASTOR.

This is a peculiar CONCRETE SUBSTANCE, found in membraneous follicles, which exist between the anus and external genitals of the Castor fiber, or Beaver. It occurs in the form of solid unctuous masses, contained in pairs of sacks about two inches in length, of a brownish-black colour externally, and of a reddish-brown colour internally. It has a peculiar, penetrating, disagreeable smell, and a bitter, acrid, nauseous taste. It is soluble in alcohol and ether. Castor contains, with other matters, a *volatile oil*, a peculiar neutral crystalline substance, termed *castorin*, and *salicin*, the bitter principle of the willow. According to many authorities, the *oil* is a derivative of salicin.

Effects and Uses.—Castor is moderately excitant and antispasmodic, and is very analogous in its effects to musk. It is not much used. Dose of castor in substance, gr. x to gr. xx; of the *tincture* (two troyounces to alcohol Oij), f℥j to f℥ij.

OLEUM SUCCINI RECTIFICATUM—RECTIFIED OIL OF AMBER.

Amber, Succinum, is a sort of fossil resin found in various parts of the world, and comes to this country from the shores of the Baltic. It is a hard, brittle substance, usually translucent, and of a pale golden-yellow colour, insipid, and inodorous, except when heated. By distillation, it yields an *oil*, OIL OF AMBER (*oleum succini*), which when rectified (by the distillation of one part of the *oil* with six parts of water), is employed medicinally. The oil is nearly colourless at first, but gradually becomes brown, has a strong, peculiar odour, and a pungent, acrid taste. It is soluble in alcohol. An acid called *succinic* is also obtained from amber.

Effects and Uses.—Oil of amber is excitant and antispasmodic, and has been used in hysteria, epilepsy, tetanus, pertussis, hiccough, and amenorrhœa. It is chiefly employed as an external application, and is a good remedy in pertussis and convulsions of children. Dose of the oil, gtt. v to gtt. xv, given in emulsion. For external use, it may be mixed with three or four parts of olive oil and brandy, with one part of laudanum added.

OLEUM ÆTHEREUM—ETHEREAL OIL.

This substance, known also as *oil of wine*, is a result of the distillation of alcohol with a large excess of sulphuric acid; it is afterwards mixed with an equal volume of stronger ether.

It is a transparent, nearly colourless, volatile liquid, of a peculiar, aromatic, ethereal odour, and sharp, bitter taste, sparingly soluble in water, but readily dissolved by alcohol or ether. Sp. gr. 0.91. It has antispasmodic properties, but is used in medicine only as an ingredient of the Compound Spirit of Ether.

SPIRITUS ÆTHERIS COMPOSITUS—COMPOUND SPIRIT OF ETHER.

This preparation, known as *Hoffman's Anodyne*, is a solution of ethereal oil (f℥vj), in ether (Oss), and alcohol (Oj). It is a colourless, volatile, inflammable liquid, having an aromatic, ethereal odour, and a burning, slightly sweetish taste. It becomes milky on being mixed with water, owing to the precipitation of the ethereal oil.

Effects and Uses.—Hoffman's Anodyne has the antispasmodic and stimulant effects of ether, and derives additional tranquillizing and anodyne properties from the ethereal oil present; it is also an efficient carminative. It is much used in hysteria, and is often added to laudanum, to prevent the nausea which the latter sometimes excites. Dose, f℥j to f℥ij, in sweetened water.

ORDER IV.—TONICS.

Tonics, called also corroborants, are medicines which produce a gradual and permanent increase of nervous vigour. It is only, however, in certain conditions of disease that they manifest this invigorating influence; as, in a state of health, they often act as irritants, or even nauseants. Their local effects are similar to their general effects. They exalt the nervous functions of the parts to which they are applied, and increase their firmness and density. When taken into the stomach, they produce a twofold corroborant effect, improving the digestive powers by their local action, and strengthening the system generally by their cerebro-spinal influence.

Tonics differ from stimulants only in the more permanent character of their effects. The more powerful tonics are closely allied to the narcotics in their action, producing, in overdoses, giddiness, loss of sight and of hearing, convulsions, delirium, and even death. And this analogy is further illustrated by the curative power of tonics in the relief of painful and spasmodic diseases, as neuralgia, rheumatism, chorea, and epilepsy.

The articles of this class may be divided into *vegetable* and *mineral* tonics. The vegetable tonics are characterized by *bitterness;* and it is said that they owe their bitterness and medicinal activity to a principle which has been termed bitter extractive. It is doubtful, however, whether any such proximate principle has really been obtained. The mineral tonics unite astringent with tonic properties; and the preparations of iron produce a further corroborant effect, by increasing the red colouring matter of the blood.

The therapeutic application of tonics comprises a diversified range of diseases. They are employed as stomachics in dyspepsia, and as general corroborants in convalescence from acute diseases, in chronic affections accompanied by marasmus and cachexia, in exhaustion and debility, in typhus and gangrene, and in typhoid conditions of the system generally. But their most striking and valuable powers are shown in their febrifuge influence upon miasmatic diseases. The modus medendi here is obscure, but the curative agency is undoubtedly due to a powerful impression upon the central organs of the nervous system. The antineuralgic and antispasmodic properties of tonics have already been alluded to. They also enjoy considerable reputation in the treatment of chronic bowel-complaints, where they act by restoring tone to the debilitated intestinal tube; and, on the other hand, they are often useful as laxatives in torpid conditions of the alimentary canal.

VEGETABLE TONICS.

The vegetable tonics may be arranged into three sections, viz.: 1. The pure bitters. 2. The aromatic bitters, which contain a stimulant volatile oil, and are aromatic as well as tonic. 3. The astringent bitters, which contain tannic and gallic acids, and are both astringent and tonic: this group contains cinchona, the most powerful and important of the vegetable tonics. The bitter principle is found also in many medicines belonging to other classes, as rhubarb, aloes, taraxacum, &c., and gives them tonic properties.

SIMPLE BITTERS.

QUASSIA.

Quassia is the WOOD of Simaruba excelsa (*Nat. Ord.* Simarubaceæ), a lofty tree of Jamaica and other West Indian islands. It is imported from the West Indies in billets of various sizes, which are found in the shops in the form of chips or raspings. Externally, it is covered with a smooth, brittle bark; the wood is white, but becomes yellowish by exposure. It has no odour, but an intensely permanently bitter taste. Water and alcohol extract its virtues, which are said to depend on a neutral principle termed *quassin* ($C_{10}H_{12}O_2$).

The article originally known as Quassia was the root and wood of Quassia amara, a shrub of Surinam, but this does not now reach our markets. It is thought to have possessed much more decided tonic properties than the drug now found in commerce.

Effects and Uses.—Quassia is a mild tonic, free from stimulant or astringent effects, and is employed principally in dyspepsia, want of appetite, and other stomachic affections. It is much used to give additional bitterness to malt liquors. Dose, in *powder*, ℈j to ʒj, three or four times a day; but the best form of administration is that of *infusion* (ʒij in water Oj), in doses of f℥ss to f℥iij; the infusion is a good remedy for ascarides, given by injection. An *extract* (aqueous) is given in the dose of gr. v, but it is principally used as an excipient for the administration of the mineral tonics. Of the *tincture* (two troyounces to diluted alcohol Oij), the dose is f℥j to f℥ij.

SIMARUBA.

Simaruba is the BARK of the ROOT of Simaruba officinalis (*Nat. Ord.* Simarubaceæ), a tall tree of Jamaica and many parts of South America. It occurs in long pieces of various sizes, which are much rolled or quilled, of a brownish-yellow colour externally, and yellow internally. It contains a bitter principle, analogous to quassin, and resembles quassia in its medicinal effects.

COPTIS—GOLDTHREAD.

Fig. 10.

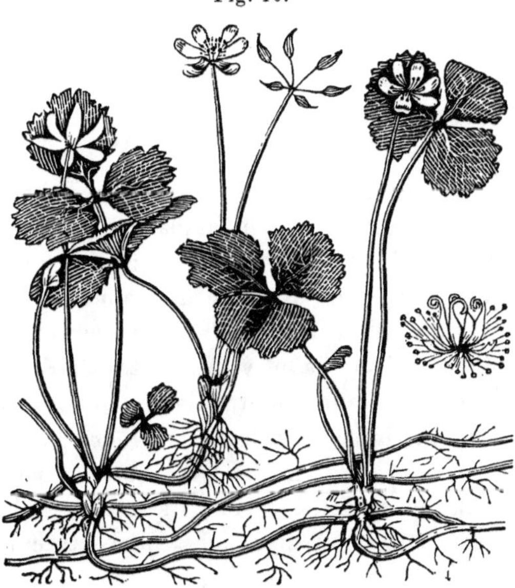

Coptis trifolia, or Goldthread (*Nat. Ord.* Ranunculaceæ), is a small, evergreen, herbaceous plant, resembling the strawberry-vine, with perennial creeping roots, slender stems, round ternate leaves, and a single small white flower, which appears through the spring till midsummer. It belongs to the northern regions of America and Asia, and abounds in swampy places in Canada and New England. The parts used are the ROOTS, which should be gathered in autumn, and carefully dried. They are of a bright-golden colour, and give the name by which the plant is commonly known. They contain the alkaloid *berberina.* The roots of a variety of coptis, derived from Assam in Asia, *Coptis teeta,* have been introduced into Europe; they possess analogous properties to those of *C. trifolia.*

Effects and Uses.—Goldthread is a pure and powerful bitter, similar in its effects to quassia, but much more palatable, and is a very good stomachic tonic. It is also employed in New England as a topical application in aphthous and other ulcerations of the mouth. It is usually given in the form of *tincture* (a troyounce to diluted alcohol Oj), in the dose of f℥j, and of *infusion* (half a troyounce to water Oj); these preparations are not, however, officinal.

GENTIANA—GENTIAN.

Gentian is the ROOT of Gentiana lutea or Yellow Gentian (*Nat. Ord.* Gentianaceæ), a perennial plant of the mountainous parts of Central and Southern Europe, growing to the height of two or three feet, with broad, ovate, opposite leaves, and handsome whorled, yellow flowers. It is imported in cylindrical, branched, twisted pieces, of various sizes, marked by transverse annular wrinkles and longitudinal furrows. Externally, it is grayish-brown, internally, brownish-yellow, and of a soft spongy texture. Its odour in the fresh state is peculiar and disagreeable, but, when dried, feeble; its taste is slightly sweetish and intensely bitter. Water and alcohol extract its virtues. It contains a peculiar oil and acid, pectin, grape sugar, and a bitter principle, termed *gentiopicrin* or *gentianin,* ($C_{40}H_{30}O_{24}$), which is crystallizable, soluble in water and alcohol, and ranks with the glucosides. Other species of gentian are employed as substitutes for the yellow gentian.

Effects and Uses.—Gentian is a pure bitter, without either astringency or much aroma. In full doses it is more disposed to relax the bowels than the other simple bitters; and, like others of the vegetable tonics, in excessive doses, it is capable of producing narcotic effects. It is an admirable stomachic in dyspepsia and gastric disorders, and is also used in the various forms of constitutional debility.

Administration.—In the form of *powder*, the dose is gr. x to ℨss. But it is usually given in the form of *compound infusion* (half a troyounce to water f℥xiv, with alcohol f℥ij, and bitter orange-peel and coriander, each ℨj), dose f℥i, 3 or 4 times a day; *compound tincture* (tinctura Gentianæ composita, gentian, two troyounces, bitter orange-peel, a troyounce, cardamom, half a troyounce, to diluted alcohol Oij), in the dose of fℨj to fℨij; *extract* (*aqueous*), in the dose of gr. x to ℨss; and *fluid extract*, in the dose of fℨss–j.

FRASERA—AMERICAN COLUMBO.

The ROOT of Frasera Walteri (*Nat. Ord.* Gentianaceæ), an elegant plant of our Southern and Western States, may be used as a substitute for gentian and columbo. Dose, ℨss–ℨj; or an *infusion* (a troyounce to boiling water Oj), may be given.

SABBATIA.

Sabbatia angularis, American Centaury, or Centaury (*Nat. Ord.* Gentianaceæ), is a very common annual indigenous plant, with an erect stem, one or two feet high, opposite ovate leaves, and numerous terminal flowers of a rich rose-colour, nearly white in the centre. It is found in low meadow-grounds or neglected fields in most parts of the United States, and flowers in August and September. The HERB is officinal, and should be gathered while in flower. It has a very bitter taste, and yields its virtues to both water and alcohol.

Effects and Uses.—Centaury is a pure bitter, with no astringency, and very little aroma. It is an excellent stomachic,

Fig. 11.

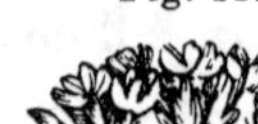

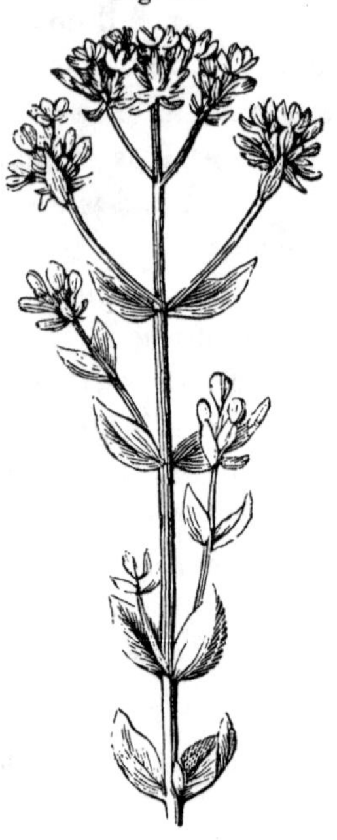

and may be used also as a general corroborant. It is said to act as an emmenagogue when given in warm infusion, and, like the bitters generally, has had anthelmintic properties ascribed to it. The best form of exhibiting it is *infusion* (a troyounce, to boiling water Oj), of which the dose is a wineglassful when cool; of the *powder* ʒss to ʒj may be given.

CALUMBA—COLUMBO.

Columbo is now generally ascribed by botanists to two species of plants known as Jateorrhiza palmata and Jateorrhiza Calumba (*Nat. Ord.* Menispermaceæ), designated by some writers still under the old name of cocculus palmatus, climbing plants of Mozambique, on the south-eastern coast of Africa. The ROOT is the officinal portion, and is known in Africa under the name of *Calumb*. It consists of fleshy tubers, with numerous offsets, which are the portions used, the main root being too fibrous. They are sliced, strung on cords, and dried in the sun; and are found in the shops in round pieces about a quarter of an inch thick, externally of a brown, wrinkled appearance, and internally yellow. The odour is slightly aromatic, and the taste very bitter. Owing to the starch which is found in columbo, it is liable to be worm-eaten. It contains, besides a large proportion of starch, a peculiar azotized substance, and two bitter principles, *colombin* and *berberina*. Water and alcohol take up its virtues; and, from its liability to attract moisture from the air, it should not be kept in the form of powder.

Effects and Uses.—Columbo is a very agreeable demulcent tonic, particularly acceptable to the stomach, and hence well adapted to the convalescent stages of acute disorders of the bowels and of fevers. It is also a good preparation in the sickness of pregnant women, and is one of the best of the stomachics in all cases where there is unusual delicacy of the stomach. In its native country, it is much employed in the treatment of dysentery.

Administration.—The dose of the *powder* is gr. x to gr. xxx. It is best given in the form of *infusion* (half a troy-ounce to boiling water Oj, dose, f℥j to f℥ij), which should be used at once, as it is liable to spoil. Of the *tincture* (four troy-ounces to diluted alcohol Oiij), f℥j to f℥iv may be given. Columbo is often combined with aromatics, iron, and alkalies, and is sometimes added to purgative mixtures.

Berberina ($C_{20}H_{17}NO_4$), the alkaloid found in Columbo, is widely diffused in the vegetable kingdom, and is obtained from numerous plants of the natural orders *Berberaceæ*, *Menispermaceæ*, and *Ranunculaceæ*, as barberry, yellow-root, hydrastis, goldthread, and others. It has been employed, in the form of muriate and sulphate, as a tonic and febrifuge, in doses of from one to ten grains.

CHIRETTA.

The HERB and ROOT of Agathotes Chirayta (*Nat. Ord.* Gentianaceæ), an East Indian plant, found in the northern mountainous parts of India, have been introduced into Europe, under the name of Chiretta or Chirayta, where it now ranks among the best simple bitters. It contains a peculiar bitter neutral substance, termed *chiratin;* in medicinal properties, it resembles gentian, and may be used in the same way.

XANTHORRIZA—YELLOW-ROOT.

The ROOT of Xanthorriza Apiifolia (*Nat. Ord.* Ranunculaceæ), an indigenous shrub, of our Southern and Western States, is a good simple bitter, which agrees very well with the stomach.

AROMATIC BITTERS.

SERPENTARIA.

The ROOTS of several species of Aristolochia are known under the name of Virginia Snakeroot. The most familiar is A. serpentaria (*Nat. Ord.* Aristolochiaceæ), an herbaceous indigenous plant, with a perennial root, composed of numerous slender fibres, arising from a knotty, brown head, one or more stems, eight or ten inches in height, heart-shaped, pointed, yellowish-green leaves, and purple, tubular flowers, springing up close to the root. It grows in our Southern and Southeastern states, in shady woods and on hill-sides, flowering in May and June; but from the great demand for the roots it has become scarce. A. reticulata is a variety found in the Southwestern States.

Virginia Snakeroot is found in the shops, in tufts of long, slender, matted fibres, attached to a knotty, rugged head. They are brittle, and of a yellowish-brown colour. The odour is aromatic and agreeable; the taste somewhat pungent, bitter, and aromatic. Water and alcohol extract its virtues, which depend on the presence of a volatile oil and a bitter principle.

Fig. 12.

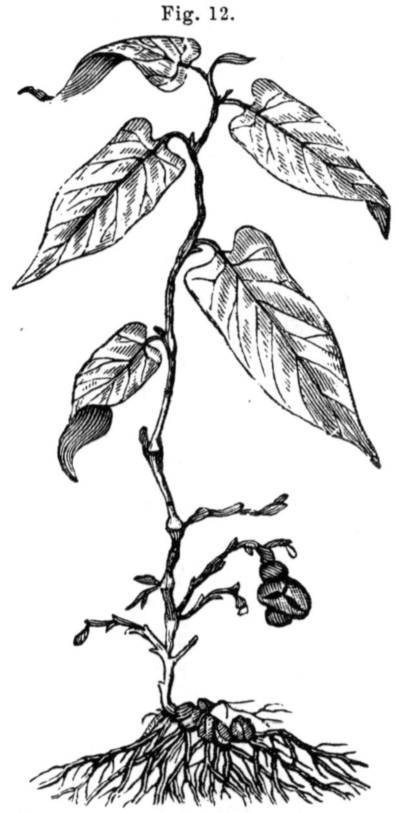

The roots of A. reticulata are very commonly substituted for those of A. serpentaria, from which they differ only in the larger size of their fibres. They are quite equal to the latter, and are even thought to contain a larger proportion of volatile oil.

Effects and Uses.—Virginia Snakeroot is a combined stimulant and tonic, with diuretic or diaphoretic properties, according to the mode of its administration. It is much used in the latter stages of fevers, and in other acute diseases, and is frequently combined with Peruvian bark, in the treatment of intermittents. The proper form of administration is that of *infusion* (half a troyounce to boiling water Oj), in doses of f℥j to f℥ij, repeated. Of the *tincture* (four troyounces to diluted alcohol Oij), the dose is f℥j to f℥ij; of the *fluid extract*, f℥ss–f℥j. *Huxham's Tincture* contains serpentaria.

ANTHEMIS—CHAMOMILE.

Anthemis nobilis, or Chamomile (*Nat. Ord.* Asteraceæ), is a small, herbaceous, trailing European plant, cultivated extensively both in Europe and this country. The FLOWERS are described by the U. S. Pharmacopœia as the portion used, but the ENTIRE HEADS are really the commercial article. The flowers consist of small spheroids, with convex, yellow disks, and numerous white, spreading rays. By cultivation they become double. In Europe the single heads are preferred, as the aromatic properties reside in the disks, which are larger in the single-flowered wild plants; but in this country, the cultivated, double heads, which are not inferior in tonic virtues, are used. Chamomile flowers have a bitter, aromatic taste, and a strong, peculiar odour, both of which are imparted to water and alcohol. They contain a volatile oil, bitter extractive, and a little tannic acid.

Effects and Uses.—Chamomile, in small doses, is a mild, agreeable aromatic tonic, and, in large doses, acts as an emetic. The cold infusion is much employed as a stomachic, and the hot infusion is given to aid the operation of emetics. The flowers, boiled in water, form a good fomentation to inflamed parts. The usual form of administration is the *infusion* (half a troyounce to water Oj). Dose, as a stomachic, f℥ij, two or three times a day, cold; as an emetic, hot, ad libitum.

COTULA (*Mayweed*). Anthemis (or Maruta) cotula, Wild chamomile, or Mayweed (*Nat. Ord.* Asteraceæ), an herbaceous plant, indigenous in Europe, but extensively naturalized in the United States, resembles chamomile very closely, both in botanical characters and in properties, and is used as a substitute for it in domestic practice.

MATRICARIA (*German Chamomile*). The FLOWERS of Matricaria chamomilla (*Nat. Ord.* Asteraceæ), an annual European plant, possess properties very similar to those of chamomile. They are considerably smaller than common chamomile, and have a larger proportion of disk florets compared with those of the ray. They are not much employed in this country.

EUPATORIUM—THOROUGHWORT.

Eupatorium perfoliatum, Boneset, or Thoroughwort (*Nat. Ord.* Asteraceæ), is a very common indigenous plant, growing

Fig. 13.

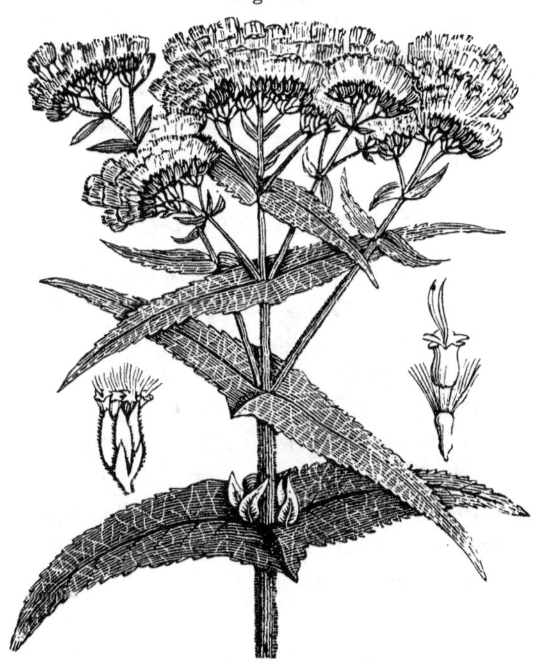

in wet grounds in every part of the United States. It has a perennial root, with numerous herbaceous stems, from two to five feet high, long, narrow leaves, perforated by the stems, and numerous white flowers, forming a flattened summit to the plant, which appear in August, continuing in bloom till October. The LEAVES and TOPS are the officinal portion. They have a faint odour, a strongly bitter taste, are soluble in water or alcohol, and contain a peculiar bitter principle, gum, tannic acid, resin, salts, and other matters. E. teucrifolium, E. aromaticum, and other native species, are almost identical in their properties with E. perfoliatum.

Effects and Uses.—Thoroughwort is a stimulant tonic, diaphoretic, and expectorant, and in large does proves emetic and laxative. It is a good stomachic in dyspepsia, and, from its combined corroborant, expectorant, and diaphoretic properties, is an excellent remedy in epidemic influenza, and in the later stages of pneumonia and bronchitis. It is also used with good effect in rheumatism, and in intermittent, remittent, and typhoid fevers. It should be given in *infusion* (a troyounce to boiling water Oj), f℥ij of which may be taken cold, as a stomachic, three or four times a day, and in freer warm draughts as a diaphoretic.

ABSINTHIUM—WORMWOOD.

The TOPS and LEAVES of Artemisia Absinthium, or Wormwood (*Nat. Ord.* Asteraceæ), a European plant, naturalized in New England, are ranked among the aromatic bitters, but are not now much employed. They may be given in *infusion* (a troyounce to boiling water Oj)—not officinal.

Wormwood contains an essential oil, which possesses narcotic properties, producing epileptiform convulsions, and, in large doses, is capable of causing fatal results. A *liqueur*, termed *absinthe*, containing the oil in question, is much used in France, with highly pernicious effects.

MAGNOLIA.

The BARKS of Magnolia glauca, Magnolia acuminata, and Magnolia tripetala (*Nat. Ord.* Magnoliaceæ), indigenous trees, remarkable for the beauty of their foliage, and the size and fragrance of their flowers, are officinal, and rank with the aromatic bitters. The barks of the trunk, branches, and root, are alike officinal; but those of the last are the most active. They contain a volatile oil, a green resin, and a peculiar crystallizable bitter principle. The aromatic property is impaired by drying, and is lost when the barks are long kept.

They are used as gentle stimulant tonics and diaphoretics, in the low stages of fever, rheumatism, &c. An *infusion* may be given, but the best solvent is diluted *alcohol.*

LIRIODENDRON—TULIP-TREE BARK.

The BARK of Liriodendron tulipifera, the Tulip-tree, or American Poplar (*Nat. Ord.* Magnoliaceæ), the well-known pride of the American forest, remarkable for its size, foliage, and beautiful tulip-shaped flowers, closely resembles those of magnolia in its medicinal properties, but is less aromatic and more stimulant. It is said to contain a peculiar principle, termed *liriodendrin.* It may be given in *powder*, in the dose of ℈j to ʒij; and in *infusion*, *decoction*, and *tincture.*

ANGUSTURA.

Angustura BARK is derived from Galipea officinalis (*Nat. Ord.* Rutaceæ), a small tree of the district of country bordering on the Orinoco river, in South America. It occurs in pieces of various lengths and sizes; sometimes flat, sometimes slightly curved, but rarely entirely quilled. Externally, it is of a light-gray colour, and is covered with lichens, with a soft, spongy epidermis, which is readily scraped off; internally, the colour is yellowish-brown. It has a disagreeable smell, and a bitter, aromatic, somewhat pungent taste. It imparts its virtues to water and alcohol, and contains a volatile oil and a bitter principle, termed *cusparin.* The bark of Strychnos nux vomica has been sometimes mixed with Angustura bark, and is thence known as *false angustura bark.*

Effects and Uses.—Angustura bark is a stimulant tonic, and in large doses acts on the stomach and bowels. From its liability to adulteration with the bark of strychnos nux vomica, it has fallen into disuse, and it has no superiority over serpentaria, and others of the indigenous aromatic bitters. Dose, in *powder*, gr. x to ʒss; of the *infusion* (half a troyounce to boiling water Oj), f℥ij, repeated.

CASCARILLA.

This is the BARK of Croton Eluteria (*Nat. Ord.* Euphorbiaceæ), a small tree of the Bahamas and other West India islands. It occurs sometimes in the form of small thin fragments—sometimes in that of rolled pieces, one or two inches long, occasionally longer, and varying in size from that of a quill to that of the little finger. It is usually covered with a grayish-white rugous epidermis, and is of a brown colour beneath. It has a warm, spicy, and bitter taste, and an aromatic, agreeable odour, which is particularly fragrant when it is burned. It yields its properties to alcohol, and partially to water; and contains volatile oil, resin, and a bitter principle, called *cascarillin.*

Effects and Uses.—Cascarilla is a very pleasant aromatic bitter, causing neither vomiting nor purging, and hence agreeing very well with the stomach. It may be given in *powder*, in the dose of ℈j to ʒss; but this is a less agreeable form than the *infusion* (a troyounce to boiling water Oj), of which the dose is f℥ij.

CANELLA.

This is the BARK of Canella alba (*Nat. Ord.* Meliaceæ), a large tree of the West Indies and South America. It comes in quilled pieces of a whitish-yellow colour, or in flat fragments, which are thicker and darker. It has an aromatic odour, and a warm, pungent, aromatic, and somewhat bitter taste. It imparts its virtues to alcohol, and partially to water; and contains volatile oil, resin, bitter extractive, gum, &c.

Effects and Uses.—An aromatic tonic, little employed except in combination. *Pulvis Alöes et Canellæ* (*Powder of Aloes and Canella*) popularly known as *hiera picra*, consists of aloes *four parts*, canella *one part;* dose, gr. x. to ℈j.

ACHILLEA—YARROW.

Achillea Millefolium, Milfoil, or Yarrow (*Nat. Ord.* Compositæ Senecionideæ), a perennial herb, common to the old and new continents, growing to the height of twelve or eighteen inches, with doubly pinnate, minutely divided leaves, and whitish flowers, possesses mild stimulant tonic properties, with some astringency. The LEAVES and FLOWERING TOPS are the portion to be employed. Of the *infusion*, made in the proportion of an ounce to the pint, a wine-glassful or more may be given. It yields a *volatile oil*, which has been used in the dose of 20 or 30 drops.

ASTRINGENT BITTERS.

CINCHONA.

The name Cinchona (derived from the Countess del Cinchon, wife of a viceroy of Peru) is applied to the BARK of different species of Cinchona (*Nat. Ord.* Cinchonaceæ), large trees which grow in the mountainous regions of the western portions of South America, from the nineteenth degree of south latitude to about the tenth degree of north latitude. Three principal varieties of cinchona are known in commerce: CINCHONA FLAVA (*Yellow Bark*), called in commerce *Calisaya Bark*, derived from Cinchona Calisaya; CINCHONA PALLIDA (*Pale Bark*), called in commerce *Loxa* and *Lima Bark*, derived from Cinchona Condaminca and Cinchona Micrantha; and CINCHONA RUBRA (*Red Bark*), derived from Cinchona Succiruba. The Pharmacopœia now recognizes, however, as officinal the BARKS of all species of the genus Cinchona, which contain at least two per cent. of the proper cinchona alkaloids.

Peruvian Bark is brought to the United States from the Pacific ports of South America. It is obtained by stripping the trunks and branches of the Cinchona trees during the dry season, and is dried by exposure to the sun, during which process the smaller pieces usually become quilled.

1. The *Yellow* or *Calisaya Bark* comes both in quilled and flat pieces. The former are from three or four inches to a foot and a half long, from a quarter of an inch to two or three inches in diameter, and of variable thickness. They have a brownish epidermis (with longitudinal wrinkles and transverse fissures), which possesses none of the virtues of the bark. The bark itself is one or two lines thick, compact, of a short, fibrous texture, and when broken presents shining points. The flat pieces, which are derived from the larger branches and trunk, are usually destitute of epidermis, are more roughly marked externally, and are of a browner hue than the quilled pieces. They are also less compact, less bitter, and of less medicinal virtue. The yellow bark is distinguished from the other barks by its much more bitter taste; its comparative freedom from astringency; its brownish-yellow, somewhat orange colour, which is still brighter in the powder; and by *containing a large proportion of quinia with very little cinchonia.*

2. The *Pale Bark* comes in cylindrical pieces of variable length, sometimes singly, sometimes doubly quilled, from two lines to an inch in diameter, and from half a line to two or three lines in thickness—the best kinds being about the size of a goose-quill. Their exterior surface is rough, marked with fissures, and of a grayish colour, owing to adhering lichens. Their interior surface is of a cinnamon colour, and, in the finer sorts, smooth. The colour of the powder is a pale fawn. The taste is moderately bitter, and somewhat astringent; the odour feeble, but rather aromatic in the powder and decoction. The pale barks, of which there are two varieites, Loxa Bark and Huanuco or Lima Bark, *contain a much larger proportion of cinchonia than of quinia;* and, from their yielding little quinia, have fallen into disuse in the United States.

3. The *Red Bark* usually comes in large, thick, flat pieces; sometimes also in quills from half an inch to two inches in diameter. They are covered with a reddish-brown, rugged epidermis, beneath which is a dark-red, brittle, and compact layer, the interior parts being woody and fibrous, and of a lively brownish-red colour. The taste of red bark is bitter and astringent; its odour not different from that of the other barks; its powder is reddish. It *contains considerable quantities both of quinia and cinchonia.*

Under the name of CARTHAGENA BARKS, several common varieties of cinchona were long brought to this country from the northern Atlantic ports of South America. They were of inferior quality, and were therefore not recognized by the Pharmacopœias; but, since the reduced supply and consequent high price of the Calisaya bark, large quantities of very good bark have been imported from New Granada, and are now used in the manufacture of quinia, under the name of Colombian barks.

Within a few years, the cultivation of several varieties of Cinchona trees has been successfully introduced into Southern India, and valuable specimens of red bark (the product of C. succirubra), equal to that of South America, have been sent to Europe; and, lately, a new variety, C. officinalis, of rapid growth, has been successfully cultivated.

Chemical Constituents.—The most important constituents of cinchona are two alkaloid principles, termed *quinia* and *cinchonia*, which exist chiefly in combination with an acid called *kinic*. These alkaloids are found in different proportions in the different barks, quinia being obtained from the *yellow* bark most abundantly, cinchonia from the *pale* bark, and the two principles in about equal proportion from the *red* bark. Two other valuable alkaloids, *quinidia* and *cinchonidia*, are found (also as *kinates*), most abundantly in the *pale* and *Carthagena* barks; but, to a certain extent in all. Other principles found in cinchona are cincho-tannic acid, colouring matter, kinovic acid, starch, fatty matter, kinate of lime, lignin, &c. Gum is found in the pale bark, but not in the yellow or red bark.

Quinia is obtained by heating the sulphate with an alkaline solution. QUINIÆ SULPHAS (*Sulphate of Quinia*), is prepared in the following manner: Powdered yellow bark is boiled in water acidulated with muriatic acid, by which the alkaloid is separated from its combination with kinic and other acids, to form a soluble muriate. By the addition of lime, this salt is decomposed, and quinia precipitated. The precipitate is washed with distilled water, and is separated from insoluble impurities by digestion in boiling alcohol, which is afterwards distilled off. To the residual brown viscid mass, dissolved in distilled water, and heated to the boiling point, sulphuric acid is added, in quantity sufficient to dissolve the quinia. The liquor is then boiled with animal charcoal, filtered, and set aside to crystallize. The alkaloid quinia may be obtained in the form of fine crystalline needles of a silky lustre, but usually occurs as a loose white powder; it is inodorous, very bitter, sparingly soluble in cold water, but somewhat more readily so in hot water, readily soluble in alcohol, ether, chloroform, and the fixed and volatile oils. It unites with acids to form salts, the most important of which is the officinal salt, the sulphate. Its composition is $C_{20}H_{24}N_2O_2,3H_2O$. Quinia and its salts may be distinguished from all other vegetable alkalies and their salts (excepting quinidia), by striking an emerald-green colour, when treated first with fresh chlorine-water and then with ammonia. *Herapath's* test is by adding to sulphate of quinia (gr. v.), diluted acetic acid (fʒi), with alcohol (fʒss), and tincture of iodine (8 drops), heating gently over a spirit lamp till it forms a clear light-brown solution, when, as the liquor cools, right-angled, quadrate, rhombic crystals are deposited, which by reflected light appear of a copper-green colour, resembling the elytra of Spanish flies. *Cinchonia* is a white crystalline substance, less bitter than quinia, almost insoluble in cold water, very soluble in boiling alcohol, and slightly soluble in ether and the fixed and volatile oils. Its composition is $C_{20}H_{24}N_2O$. It is distinguishable from quinia by striking a white precipitate, when chlorine-water and afterwards ammonia are added; with ferrocyanine of potassium, a yellowish-white precipitate ensues.

Cinchonia being insoluble in ether, while quinia is soluble in that menstruum, the latter may by this means be readily separated from the former alkaloid. The medicinal properties of quinia and cinchonia are analogous, and the sulphate of cinchonia is now officinal. *Quinidia* is isomeric with quinia, but more crystallizable and less soluble in ether; its salts strike a white precipitate with solution of iodide of potassium. *Cinchonidia* is isomeric with cinchonia. It is usually found mixed with quinidia, the mixture being known as *commercial quinidia.* The commercial sulphate of quinidia (which is more soluble in water and alcohol than the sulphate of quinia), may be used as a substitute for the latter salt.

Incompatibles.—The alkalies and alkaline earths precipitate the alkaline principles of cinchona; tannic acid, and the tincture and compound solution of iodine, form with them insoluble compounds; the ferric salts precipitate cincho-tannic acid; solution of arsenite of potassium is also incompatible with infusions and decoctions of cinchona.

Physiological Effects.—Locally, cinchona and its alkaloids act as irritants, and have, besides, a marked antiseptic effect, arresting putrefaction and fermentation by a destructive influence upon fungi and infusoria. Cinchona produces upon the stomach a stimulant effect to the appetite and digestion, and, from the tannic acid which it contains, a slightly astringent action, not belonging to the salts of its alkaloids. If given too long, or if the stomach or bowels are in an irritable condition, it is apt soon to produce nausea, vomiting, and even diarrhœa. The constitutional effects of the cinchona preparations, within toxic limits, are powerfully tonic, marked by increased fulness with diminished irritability of the pulse, improved tonicity of the capillary vessels, and augmentation of the general vigour. Large doses produce depression, the first indications of which are upon the special senses, especially that of hearing, which undergoes subjective noises, as ringing and roaring in the ears, with partial deafness; dimness of vision is an accompaniment, though less common; the face is flushed, the eyes are suffused, with often severe headache; very large doses produce a marked sedative influence upon the pulse and temperature of the body, with sometimes dilatation of the pupils, delirium, and even convulsions; death is said in rare cases to have followed cinchona-poisoning, though immense doses of the sulphate of quinia have been taken with impunity. The cinchona alkaloids are eliminated almost exclusively by the kidneys, acting as diuretics, though they diminish the production of uric acid. They are said to arrest the amœboid movements of the white blood-corpuscles.

Medicinal Uses.—The most important therapeutic employment of cinchona is as a febrifuge in the treatment of fevers of a miasmatic origin. Its efficacy in these diseases was first made known to the world by the Jesuit missionaries in Peru, from whom it was called *Jesuit's powder.* The type of miasmatic fever in which the powers of bark are most strikingly displayed, is *intermittent;* the non-pernicious and uncomplicated forms of which it rarely if ever fails to control. It may be given in these cases from the very onset of the attack; and if, owing to gastric irritability, it is rejected by the stomach, it should be introduced by the rectum. In *remittent fevers*, cinchona is scarcely less useful than in *intermittents;* and most physicians, who practice in miasmatic districts, now concur in recommending its early exhibition in these fevers, without waiting for a remission. In the *pernicious* or *congestive* forms of intermittent and remittent fevers, the early administration of large doses of cinchona or the salts of quinia or cinchonia, in combination with stimulants, is imperatively demanded; and the hypodermic injection of the sulphate of quinia may here be necessary. As a prophylactic against miasmatic fever, the use of the preparations of cinchona is very efficacious. In the varieties of typhus, including that termed cerebro-spinal meningitis, the salts of quinia, in full doses, are generally resorted to, in conjunction with abundant alcoholic stimulation and nourishment. In yellow fever, the declining stages of typhoid fever, the malignant exanthemata, gangrene, erysipelas, carbuncle, extensive suppurations, the typhoid forms of diseases generally, the hectic of phthisis, acute rheumatism, diarrhœa, dysentery and cholera, and various disorders of the nervous system, as neuralgia, tetanus, and chorea, cinchona and its preparations are constantly employed; and, as they have been found to lessen the amount of uric acid and urea in the urine, they have been prescribed also in gout. Cinchona is also much used as a stomachic and general tonic, but, where gastric susceptibility exists, as in convalescence from acute diseases, some of the simple bitters are preferable. *Topically*, cinchona is employed as an astringent and antiseptic.

Administration.—The use of cinchona in *powder*, since the discovery of sulphate of quinia, has been very much abandoned, owing to its bulk and disagreeable taste. When exhibited in this form, half a troyounce to an ounce is the dose as a *febrifuge*, given usually in divided amounts; as a tonic, ʒj. The following officinal preparations are employed: *decoction* (a troyounce of yellow or red bark to Oj of water, to be boiled for ten minutes, and water enough added to make the decoction measure a pint; aromatic sulphuric acid fʒj may be afterwards added), dose, f℥ij, repeated; *infusion* (a troyounce of yellow or red bark to water Oj, to which aromatic sulphuric acid fʒj may be added), dose f℥ij repeated; *extract* (of yellow bark), dose gr. x to gr. xxx, equivalent to ʒj of bark; *fluid extract* (yellow), dose, fʒi, equal to ʒj of bark; *tincture* (six troyounces of yellow bark to a mixture of three measures of alcohol with one of water, Oij), dose, fʒj to fʒiv; *compound tincture* or *Huxham's tincture* (containing red bark four troyounces, bitter orange-peel three troyounces, serpentaria three hundred and sixty grains, to a mixture of three measures of alcohol with one of water, Oijss), dose, fʒj to fʒiv. In prescribing bark, opium or port wine is often given with it, when it acts on the bowels. It is also occasionally combined with serpentaria. And, when the stomach will not retain it, it has been used externally in the form of *cataplasmata*, *pediluvia*, *bark jackets*, &c., though, in such cases, it may be administered by the rectum, and the endermic or even the hypodermic exhibition of the sulphate of quinia may be resorted to.

Quiniæ Sulphas (*Sulphate of Quinia*). This salt is prepared by the process described at p. 128. It occurs in fine, silky, rather flexible, needle-shaped crystals (interlaced among one another, or grouped in small starlike tufts), which are odourless, very bitter, and slightly efflorescent. It is soluble in 740 parts of cold and 30 parts of boiling water, readily soluble in alcohol, but insoluble in ether, and by the addition of sulphuric acid is converted into a salt, which is soluble in 11 parts of cold water; its cold solution is opalescent. The officinal sulphate consists of one eq. of base to one-half of acid, and eight eqs. of water; the more soluble salt is regarded as a neutral sulphate. Sulphate of quinia is decomposed by the alkalies and their carbonates, the alkaline earths, astringent infusions, the soluble salts of lead, acetates and tartrates generally, and the compound solution of iodine. Various substances are mixed as adulterations with the sulphate of quinia. They may be detected by adverting to their relative solubility in different menstrua, as compared with the sulphate, or by chemical tests. Thus, gum and starch are left behind by alcohol; salicin becomes red on contact with sulphuric acid, &c.

Effects and Uses.—The effects of sulphate of quinia on the system are the same as those of cinchona, and, from its being less apt to disagree with the stomach, it has to a great extent superseded the use of the latter. In large doses it produces headache, ringing of the ears, and sometimes vertigo, amaurosis, deafness, delirium, dilatation of the pupils, and other evidences of a powerful action on the cerebro-spinal system; see p. 129.

Administration.—The ordinary dose of the sulphate of quinia, as a febrifuge, is gr. xvi, equal to about ℥j of bark, but as much as twenty grains, and even more, are often required; as a general tonic, gr. j to gr. vj. It may be given dissolved in some aromatic water, by the aid of aromatic sulphuric acid, also as an enema, or hypodermically. Pills of Sulphate of Quinia (*Pilulæ Quiniæ Sulphatis*), are made by beating together 24 grains of sulphate of quinia with 14 grains of clarified honey into a pilular mass, and dividing into 24 pills. Many other salts of quinia than the sulphate have been introduced into practice, but they possess no advantage over the officinal salt.

Quiniæ Valerianas (*Valerianate of Quinia*), is obtained by dissolving freshly precipitated quinia in diluted valerianic acid. It occurs in transparent or white rhomboidal tables, of the peculiar repulsive odour of valerianic acid, and an acrid, bitter taste. Soluble in alcohol and ether, and partially soluble in water. It fulfils the indications of quinia and valerianic acid, and is therefore especially useful in nervous disorders.

Crude Quinia is the impure quinia obtained from the manufacturer, before separation from the insoluble impurities. It is a soft solid of resinous aspect, nearly free from bitterness, and may be given to children in the same doses as the sulphate.

Quinoidia, quinoidine, or *amorphous quinia*, is a substance obtained by precipitation, with an alkaline carbonate, from the mother liquor left after the preparation of sulphate of quinia. When moderately heated, it appears as a resinous mass, of a yellowish-white or brownish colour, which, according to Liebig, bears the same relation to ordinary quinia that uncrystallizable sugar bears to the crystallizable. The quinia in this preparation is thought to be converted, by the action of heat, into an isomeric alkaloid, termed *quinicia;* and, by the same action, cinchonia is converted into an isomeric alkaloid, termed *cinchonicia.* It is considered equally efficacious with quinia, but requires doses rather larger than the sulphate of quinia, than which it is much more economical.

Cinchoniæ Sulphas (*Sulphate of Cinchonia*), is made from the mother-water remaining after the crystallization of sulphate of quinia. Being the most soluble of the sulphates of the four alkaloids found in bark, it remains in solution after the sulphate of quinia, and the mixed sulphate of cinchonidia and quinidia, have crystallized out. From the mother-water, it is precipitated by solution of soda, then washed with alcohol, next reconverted into a sulphate, and boiled with animal charcoal to decolorize it. It occurs in short, oblique, shining prisms with dihedral summits, of a very bitter taste, more soluble in water than the sulphate of quinia, readily soluble by alcohol, and sparingly so by ether. By the addition of sulphuric acid, it is converted into the more soluble neutral sulphate. It is now admitted to have the same remedial properties as the sulphate of quinia, but requires about one-third larger doses.

EUCALYPTUS GLOBULUS.

The LEAVES of Eucalyptus Globulus (*Nat. Ord.* Myrtaceæ), a lofty tree of Australia, have within the last few years come into notice as a febrifuge tonic. Two varieties, *latifolius* and *longifolius*, exist, the latter only of which has decided medicinal virtues; the leaves of this are ensiform, parchment-like, of a grayish-green colour, from 4 to 14 inches in length, an inch or two in breadth, of a pleasant aromatic smell, and a bitterish, rather pungent taste; the fresh leaves are more active than the dried; they owe their activity to a volatile oil, the more volatile and chief portion of which is termed eucalyptol ($C_{12}H_{20}O$). This, like quinia, has a powerful antiseptic action, and depresses the temperature of the body even more than quinia.

Eucalyptus has been given with excellent results in miasmatic fevers, in doses of from 60 grains to half an ounce of the dried leaves, or less of the fresh; a tincture is the best form (a troy-ounce to 2 fluidounces of alcohol), dose f℥ij, in some aromatic water. *Eucalyptol*, in alcoholic solution, may be given in the dose of 20 drops, repeated 2 or 3 times. It has been found efficient in whooping-cough.

CORNUS FLORIDA—DOGWOOD.

Cornus Florida, or Dogwood (*Nat. Ord.* Cornaceæ), is an indigenous tree found in most parts of the United States, and growing in the Middle States to the height of from fifteen to twenty feet. Its flowers are remarkable for large four-leaved white or pinkish involucres, which appear with us in May. The officinal portion is the BARK, that of the root being preferred. It occurs in pieces of various sizes, more or less rolled, of a reddish-gray colour, with occasionally a fawn-coloured epidermis. Its odour is slight; its taste bitter, astringent, and slightly aromatic. It yields its virtues to water and alcohol, and contains resin, bitter extractive, tannic and gallic acids, &c. The BARKS of Cornus Sericea, or Swamp Dogwood, and of

Fig. 14.

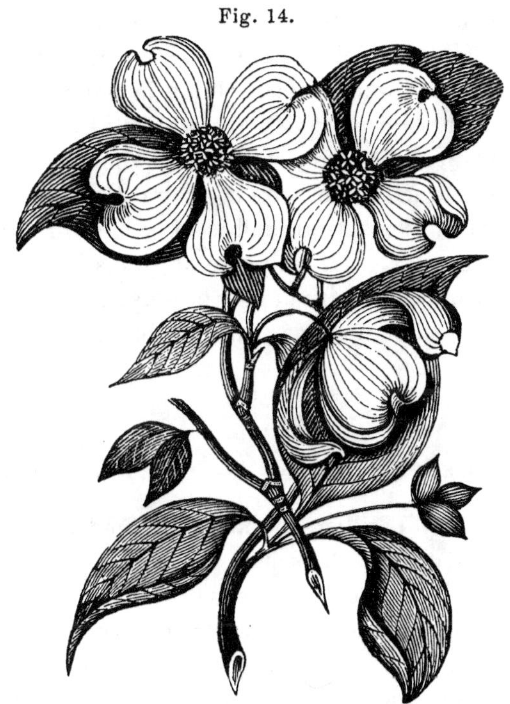

Cornus Circinata, or Round-leaved Dogwood, possess analogous properties.

Effects and Uses.—Dogwood is deservedly esteemed the best substitute for cinchona among the native astringent bitters. It is somewhat stimulant, and not unfrequently disorders the stomach. Dose, in *powder*, ℈j to ʒj; of the *decoction* (a troy-ounce to water Oj), f℥ij may be given; the *fluid extract* contains ℥i in f℥i.

SALIX—WILLOW.

The BARK of Salix alba, or the White Willow (*Nat. Ord.* Salicaceæ), is ranked among the astringent bitters. It is little employed, however, except in the form of *salicin*, its active principle ($C_{13}H_{18}O_7$) which consists of white, slender, silky crystals, inodorous, but very bitter, soluble in water and alcohol, but not in ether; it ranks with the glucosides. It has been used as a substitute for the sulphate of quinia, but it is very inferior to it as a febrifuge. As a general tonic, however, and also in diarrhœa, it is useful, and is to be given in the dose of from gr. x to gr. xxx. The sulphate of quinia is often adulterated with salicin, but the fraud may be detected by the addition of concentrated sulphuric acid, which strike a blood-red colour with salicin.

PRUNUS VIRGINIANA—WILD-CHERRY.

The wild-cherry has long been known under the name of Prunus Virginiana, which is still retained by the Pharmacopœia. This name, however, belongs to another tree, the choke-cherry; and the wild-cherry is now properly distinguished as Cerasus serotina (*Nat. Ord.* Drupaceæ). It is a large indigenous tree, attaining a great height and size in the Southwestern States, but usually with us about twenty-five to thirty feet high. The trunk is covered with a rough, blackish bark, which detaches itself semicircularly; the leaves are ovate, oblong, and acuminate; the flowers, which appear in May, are white, and are followed by fruit about the size of a pea, of a purplish-black colour, and a not unpleasant, prussic, bitterish taste. The medicinal portion is the BARK of the root and trunk, the former of which is the more active. It is found in the shops, in pieces of various lengths and sizes, deprived of the epidermis and slightly curved, of a reddish-brown colour, and a bitter, slightly astringent, aromatic taste.

It contains a bitter principle, resin, starch, and tannic and gallic acids, and yields on distillation a volatile oil, nearly identical with the oil of bitter almond, which does not pre-exist in the bark, but is formed by the action of water on amygdalin, through the agency of an albuminous principle termed emulsin, as in the bitter almond. The leaves also yield this oil. Boiling water impairs the virtues of the bark.

Effects and Uses.—Wild-cherry bark is tonic, with some astringency, and at the same time exercises a sedative influence on the nervous and circulatory systems, owing to the hydrocyanic acid, which is developed in it. It is used with excellent effect as a sedative corroborant in various forms of pulmonary irritation, particularly in the latter stages of pneumonia, and in the hectic of phthisis. It is also a useful stomachic and tonic in a variety of cases. The proper form of administration is the *infusion* (half a troyounce to cold water Oj), in the dose of f℥ij, twice or thrice daily. Of the *fluid extract* (of which a fluidounce represents an ounce of the bark), the dose is f℥j–ij. The *syrup* is made by percolating five troyounces of the coarsely powdered bark with water till a pint of filtered liquor is obtained, and afterwards adding twenty-eight troyounces of sugar; it is an agreeable preparation, dose, f℥ss.

NECTANDRA.

The BARK of Nectandra Rodiei (*Nat. Ord.* Lauraceæ), the Greenheart tree, a large tree of Guiana, and the neighbouring countries of South America, has, within a few years, been introduced into medicine, under the name of *bebeeru* bark. It occurs in large, flat, heavy pieces, one to two feet long, from two to six inches broad, and three or four lines thick, of a grayish-brown colour on its outer surface, and a dark cinnamon on the inner. It has an intensely bitter, somewhat astringent taste, and contains tannic acid, resin, gum, &c., and two alkaloids, which have been isolated, termed *bebeeria* ($C_{19}H_{21}NO_3$), and *nectandria* ($C_{20}H_{23}NO_4$). Bebeeru bark is employed as a febrifuge and tonic in South America, and the *sulphate of bebeeria* has been used in Europe and this country with some success, in the treatment of intermittent fevers. The full dose is ℈j–ʒj.

The RHIZOME of Geum rivale, or Water Avens, and the ROOT of Spiræa tomentosa, or Hardhack (*Nat. Ord.* Rosaceæ), and the BARK of Prinos verticillatus, or Black Alder (*Nat. Ord.* Aquifolaceæ), are indigenous astringent tonics of considerable power.

PEPSINA—PEPSIN.

In connection with the subject of stomachic tonics, this article is entitled to brief mention. It is prepared from the rennets either of the calf, sheep, or pig, taken from the animal as soon as killed. These are washed under a thin stream of water. The internal membranes are then carefully scraped off, and macerated in water for two hours, at a temperature of 59° F., and then strained through a coarse cloth. The pepsin in the solution is then precipitated by acetate of lead, allowed to settle, and the supernatant liquid poured off; a current of sulphuretted hydrogen is passed through the semi-liquid deposit, which precipitates the lead in the form of sulphide. The pure pepsin remains in solution, which is then filtered, and evaporated to dryness at a uniform temperature of 113° F. Boudault's Pepsin has the highest commercial reputation. Pepsin is now a good deal used in dyspepsia and diarrhœa, and may be given in doses of 15 to 30 grains before each meal, suspended in syrup of orange-peel or other syrup, to disguise its disagreeable taste. It is probably more efficient in cases of children than of adults. When nourishment is to be given by the rectum (as when food is rejected by the stomach), the addition of pepsin and a little hydrochloric acid to animal broths for rectal injection is highly useful.

PANCREATINUM—PANCREATIN.

This is obtained from the pancreas of recently killed animals, by treating the colourless viscous juice with alcohol and drying the precipitate in vacuo. It is employed to promote the digestion of fatty matters, and may be administered in the form of emulsion, or dissolved in diluted alcohol or glycerin, or as a powder; it is a good addition to cod-liver oil. Dose, 2 to 5 grains.

MINERAL TONICS.

FERRI PRÆPARATA—PREPARATIONS OF IRON.

The preparations of IRON (FERRUM), termed *Ferruginea*, *Chalybeates*, and *Martial* preparations, are the most important of the mineral tonics. Besides their local tonic-astringent effect, and their general corroborant action on the cerebro-spinal system, which they possess in common with the other mineral tonics, they exercise a restorative influence on the composition of the blood, by increasing the number of its colouring particles, and the amount of its solid constituents. Iron is in fact a natural constituent of the blood, and is to be considered as a nutrient rather than a medicine. The effects of the chalybeates are best observed in conditions of the system in which there is a relative want of the red corpuscles of the blood. Under their use in such cases, while the digestive functions are promoted, the pulse becomes fuller and stronger, the skin assumes a healthy tint, the lips and cheeks become more florid, the temperature of the body is increased, and the muscular strength is greatly invigorated. On the other hand, the administration of the ferruginous preparations in health, or too long continued, is thought to produce symptoms of plethora, vascular excitement, and a tendency to congestion and hemorrhage; though it may be doubted whether the blood will assimilate more than the normal proportion of iron.

The red corpuscles of the blood act as carriers of oxygen, which they take up from the inspired air in the lungs, and it is now believed that the iron in the blood-corpuscles converts oxygen into ozone, a more active form of this element. The diseases in which chalybeates are most serviceable are those which depend on a deficiency of the red corpuscles of the blood, as the various forms of *anœmia*, particularly where this is connected with irregularity of the uterine functions; also, scrofula, tuberculosis, degeneration of the viscera, and cachectic states of the system, characterized by a pale, flabby condition of the solids. Many forms of nervous disorder, as neuralgia, chorea, hysteria, and epilepsy, are very decidedly controlled by the preparations of iron, and they probably constitute the best remedies in these affections, when attended with anæmia. Several of the preparations of iron are also much employed both as stomachics and astringents.

The following are the officinal preparations of iron:

FERRUM REDACTUM (*Reduced Iron*). Metallic iron is obtained for medicinal purposes in the form of an impalpable powder, by reducing the hydrated oxide (officinally subcarbonate), by passing a stream of hydrogen gas over it. It is a light, tasteless, iron-gray powder, insoluble in water, but completely soluble in diluted sulphuric acid, and it should be kept in a well-stoppered bottle, owing to its great liability to oxidation. This preparation, sometimes called Quevenne's Iron, is a mild chalybeate, and is a favourite prescription with many practitioners, in the treatment of chlorosis and other varieties of anæmia. Dose, gr. v to gr. x, three times a day, in the form of pill made with sugar and gum; it is sometimes prepared with chocolate in the form of lozenges. It is well adapted to prolonged use.

FERRI OXIDUM HYDRATUM (*Hydrated Oxide of Iron*). This preparation (*ferric hydrate*) ($Fe_2 6HO$) is made by precipitating the ferric hydrate from its combination in any tersalt of iron by means of ammonia. Officinally, the tersulphate of iron is employed for this purpose. When dry, it is a reddish-brown powder, and is not considered an eligible preparation for medicinal use. It is furnished in the form of a freshly precipitated, soft, moist, reddish-brown magma, for use as an antidote to arsenious acid.

FERRI SUBCARBONAS (*Subcarbonate of Iron*). This salt is obtained by the double reaction of solutions of sulphate of iron and carbonate of sodium. It is at first a white precipitate;

but, by exposure to the air, it becomes greenish, and afterwards rust-colored, being converted nearly entirely into the *hydrated oxide* by the absorption of oxygen, and the evolution of carbonic acid. It has a slightly styptic taste, is insoluble in water, but readily dissolves in hydrochloric and sulphuric acids and carbonic acid water. It is one of the most valuable of the ferruginous compounds, free from local irritation, and readily dissolved in the fluids of the stomach; and is much employed in chlorosis, chorea, neuralgia, and even pertussis and tetanus. Dose, gr. v to gr. xxx, three times a day.

Trochisci Ferri Subcarbonatis (*Troches of Subcarbonate of Iron*), are made with subcarbonate of iron five troyounces, vanilla thirty grains, sugar fifteen troyounces, and a sufficient quantity of mucilage of tragacanth—the mass to be divided into 480 troches; each lozenge contains five grains of the subcarbonate.

Emplastrum Ferri (*Plaster of Iron*), is made with subcarbonate of iron three troyounces, lead-plaster twenty-four troyounces, and Burgundy pitch six troyounces.

PILULA FERRI CARBONATIS (*Pill of Carbonate of Iron*).—*Vallet's Ferruginous Pill.* To protect the carbonate of iron (ferrous carbonate) ($FeCO_3$) from oxidation, it is prepared (as in the process last described) by dissolving the reacting salts in weak syrup instead of water; honey and sugar being afterwards added, to preserve it unaltered and bring it to the pilular consistence. This preparation, from its unchangeableness, is preferred to the ordinary subcarbonate, and is one of the most popular of the chalybeates. It contains nearly half its weight of ferrous carbonate. From five to twenty grains of the pilular mass may be taken in divided doses through the day.

Mistura Ferri Composita (*Compound Mixture of Iron*), is a mixture of the carbonate of iron (prepared by the reaction of sulphate of iron twenty grains and carbonate of potassium twenty-five grains), with myrrh sixty grains, spirit of lavender half a fluidounce, and rose-water seven fluidounces and a half, and sugar sixty grains to resist oxidation. It is a favourite chalybeate in chlorosis and amenorrhœa. Dose, f℥j to f℥ij, three times a day.

Pilulæ Ferri Compositæ (*Compound Pills of Iron*), are prepared with carbonate of sodium and sulphate of iron each eighteen grains, myrrh thirty-six grains, and syrup, the mass to be divided into twenty-four pills. Dose, from two to six pills three times a day. Both these preparations should be made only as wanted for use.

FERRI SULPHAS (*Sulphate of Iron*), known, in its impure state, as *green vitriol* or *copperas*, is prepared for medicinal use by dissolving iron wire in diluted sulphuric acid, with heat. It is *ferrous sulphate* ($FeSO_4 7H_2O$), and occurs in transparent, pale bluish-green crystals, of the form of the oblique rhombic prism, of an acrid, styptic taste, soluble in water, but insoluble in alcohol. By exposure to the air, they effloresce, absorb oxygen, and become yellowish-white, from the formation of ferric sulphate. When heated to 212°, they give out six of their seven equivalents of water, and are converted into a grayish-white mass, known as the *dried* sulphate. The alkalies and alkaline earths and their carbonates, nitrate of silver, acetate of lead, are incompatible with this salt. Sulphate of iron is one of the most active of the ferruginous preparations, but its local effects are powerfully astringent, and in a concentrated form it acts as an irritant poison. It is preferred to other chalybeates, where there is much relaxation of the solids, with excessive discharges; but it is not so well adapted to long-continued use, on account of its local irritant action. Topically, it is employed in substance and solution, as a styptic and astringent. Dose, gr. j to gr. v, in pill; of the *dried sulphate* (*ferri sulphas exsiccata*), gr. ss to gr. iij.

LIQUOR FERRI TERSULPHATIS (*Solution of Tersulphate of Iron*). This preparation is made by dissolving 12 troyounces of the sulphate of iron (ferrous sulphate) in a mixture of 2 troyounces and 60 grains of sulphuric and a troyounce and 360 grains of nitric acid, with water enough to make a pint and a half of solution. The nitric acid furnishes oxygen, which converts the iron from a ferrous to a ferric condition. It is $Fe_2 3SO_4$ (*ferric sulphate*). This solution is a clear, reddish-brown liquid, nearly devoid of odour, and of a sour, very styptic, and somewhat acrid taste. Its chief use is in making the hydrated oxide of iron, and it should be kept on hand, for the preparation of the antidote for arsenious acid. It may be used as a styptic, but for this purpose it is inferior to the next preparation.

LIQUOR FERRI SUBSULPHATIS (*Solution of Subsulphate of Iron*). This solution, known as *Monsel's Solution*, is made in the same way as the last preparation, except that only half the amount of sulphuric acid is used; the ferric oxide is therefore only partially saturated, and a subsalt results ($2Fe_23SO_4$) It has a syrupy consistence, a ruby-red colour, is inodorous, and has a very astringent but not acrid taste. It is a less irritant salt than the tersulphate, and may be used internally, in hemorrhage from the stomach and bowels, in the dose of from five to fifteen grains. Externally, it is one of the most efficacious styptics we can employ, and has been injected into varicose veins with success for the cure of varicose ulcers, and, applied by means of the atomizer, has been found efficient in hemoptysis. Diluted with water, it is a good local application to inflamed mucous surfaces.

FERRI CHLORIDUM (*Chloride of Iron*). This salt, which is *ferric chloride* (Fe_2Cl_6), is made by heating iron wire with muriatic acid (by which ferrous chloride is formed), and afterwards converting the ferrous chloride into ferric chloride by heating it with muriatic and nitric acids. It occurs in fragments of a crystalline structure, an orange-yellow colour, inodorous, of a strong chalybeate, styptic taste, deliquescent, and wholly soluble in water, alcohol, and ether. Internally, it is used chiefly in the form of the *tincture*. Externally, it is applied as a styptic, and in solution, of various strengths, as an astringent. One part, gradually added to six parts of collodion, forms a yellowish-red, limpid liquid, of valuable styptic properties.

Liquor Ferri Chloridi (*Solution of Chloride of Iron*), is prepared by dissolving iron wire (*three troyounces*) in muriatic acid (*eleven troyounces*), heating to the boiling point, then heating the liquid, after filtration, with muriatic acid (*six troyounces and a half*) and nitric acid (*a troyounce and a half*) and afterwards adding distilled water enough to make a solution measuring a pint. A reddish-brown liquid, having an acid and strongly styptic taste, and sp. gr. 1.355. It may be used internally, for the purposes of the chloride, in doses of ♏ij–vi, diluted, and externally as a styptic.

Tinctura Ferri Chloridi (*Tincture of the Chloride of Iron*), is made by mixing one part of *Solution of Chloride of Iron* with three parts of alcohol. It is a tincture of the chloride, though there is probably some reaction between the acid and alcohol, as the preparation has an ethereal odour. It is of a reddish-brown colour, and has a sour, styptic taste. It is one of the most effective of the chalybeates, acting locally as an energetic astringent and styptic, and, in large doses, as an irritant. Its indications, both general and topical, are very analogous to those of the sulphate, with the addition of some specific action on the urino-genital apparatus, which renders it applicable to the treatment of affections of these organs; it is especially useful in erysipelas. Dose, ♏x to ♏xxx, gradually increased to f℥j or f℥ij, and taken in some mild diluent.

FERRI IODIDUM (*Iodide of Iron*). This salt is *ferrous iodide* (FeI_2), and is made by the addition of iron filings to a mixture of iodine in distilled water. By evaporation, with as little contact of air as possible, green tabular crystals are obtained, of a styptic taste, volatile, deliquescent, and very soluble in both water and alcohol. But, by exposure to the air, the ferrous iodide undergoes decomposition, a portion of the iron parting with its iodine, and becoming oxidized. Hence, the salt is hardly fit for medicinal use, unless protected from decomposition, as in the officinal

Syrupus Ferri Iodidi (*Syrup of Iodide of Iron*), which is prepared by mixing iodine (2 *troyounces*) and iron wire (300 *grains*) in distilled water (3 *fluidounces*), and shaking the mixture until the solution has acquired a green colour. Into this solution, a pint of syrup, heated to 212°, is to be filtered, and, when the liquid has cooled, sufficient syrup is to be added to make the whole measure 20 fluidounces. It must be kept in well-stoppered two-ounce vials. It is a transparent liquid, of a pale-green colour, and furnishes an excellent alterative tonic, combining the effects of iodine and of iron, and is particularly applicable to the treatment of scrofula, visceral engorgements, phthisis, &c. Dose, 20 to 40 drops, three times a day.

Pilulæ Ferri Iodidi (*Pills of Iodide of Iron*), are made with iodine, iron wire, reduced iron, sugar, gum arabic, liquorice-root, liquorice, and an ethereal solution of balsam of Tolu. They keep very well. Each pill contains about one grain of iodide of iron, and one-fourth of a grain of reduced iron.

FERRI ET POTASSII TARTRAS (*Tartrate of Iron and Potassium*) ($Fe_2KC_4H_4O_6,H_2O$), is prepared by the addition of hydrated oxide of iron to a mixture of bitartrate of potassium in distilled water. It occurs in transparent scales of a ruby-red colour, which are wholly soluble in water. The tartaric acid and potash, in combination in this preparation, render it less constipating than the other chalybeates; and, from its agreeable taste, it is adapted to the diseases of childhood. It is, moreover, not incompatible with alkalies. Dose, gr. x to ʒss.

FERRI PHOSPHAS (*Phosphate of Iron*), is obtained by the double reaction of solutions of sulphate of iron and phosphate of sodium, and is *ferrous phosphate* (Fe_32PO_4). It is a bright, slate-coloured powder, insoluble in water, but soluble in the mineral acids; by exposure to the air it absorbs oxygen, with the production of ferric oxide, and acquires a blue colour. Dose, gr. v to gr. x.

FERRI PYROPHOSPHAS (*Pyrophosphate of Iron*), is a mixture of *ferric pyrophosphate* ($Fe_43P_2O_7,9H_2O$), and of citrate of ammonium. It occurs in apple-green scales, of an acid, slightly saline taste, and is very soluble in water. A good chalybeate. Dose, grs. ij–v. Given also as a *syrup*.

FERRI CITRAS (*Citrate of Iron*), may be prepared by the addition of hydrated oxide of iron to a solution of citric acid. It is *ferric citrate* ($Fe_2C_6H_5O_7$), and occurs in thin, transparent pieces, of a garnet-red colour, with a mild, acid, chalybeate taste, slowly soluble in cold water, but readily soluble in boiling water. Dose, gr. v to gr. x. It is officinal also in the form of *solution of citrate of iron* (*liquor ferri citratis*), a deep reddish-brown liquid, given in doses of 10 to 20 drops; and it is by evaporating this solution that the solid citrate is obtained.

LIQUOR FERRI NITRATIS (*Solution of Nitrate of Iron*), is prepared by the gradual addition of diluted nitric acid to an excess of iron wire. It is *ferric nitrate* ($Fe_2 6NO_3$), and is a pale, amber-coloured liquid, with a strong, astringent, acid taste. It is tonic and astringent, agreeing very well with the stomach, and is employed in the treatment of chronic diarrhœa, hæmatemesis, hemorrhage from the bowels, and uterine hemorrhage, particularly when anæmic symptoms are present. Dose, gtt. x to gtt. xx, two or three times a day, in dilution.

FERRUM AMMONIATUM (*Ammoniated Iron*), is prepared by evaporating a solution of chloride of iron and chloride of ammonium. It is a mechanical mixture of these salts, and is of an orange-red colour, wholly soluble in water and diluted alcohol. It contains a small and variable quantity of iron; but is considered a valuable deobstruent in glandular swellings, and in large doses is aperient. It is not now officinal. Dose, gr. iv to gr. xij, or more.

FERRI HYPOPHOSPHIS (*Hypophosphite of Iron*) (*ferric hypophosphite*) ($Fe_2 2PH_2O_2$), is obtained by the reaction of a solution of hypophosphite of sodium or ammonium with solution of tersulphate of iron. It is a white, amorphous powder, insoluble in cold water, soluble in hydrochloric acid, incompatible with the soluble salts of mercury and silver, but has the advantage of not being decomposed by the cincho-tannic acid of cinchona. This is a good chalybeate in diseases of degeneration of the nervous tissue, and has been also given in phthisis; other hypophosphites are combined with it. Dose, gr. x–xxx, three times a day.

FERRI OXALAS (*Oxalate of Iron*), (*ferrous oxalate*) (FeC_2O_4), is made by the reaction of solutions of oxalic acid and sulphate of iron. It occurs as a lemon-yellow, crystalline powder, almost destitute of taste, slightly soluble in water, but easily acted upon by the dilute acids, and decomposed by the alkalies and their carbonates. This chalybeate is of recent introduction, and has the advantage of being well borne by the stomach, of being readily absorbed, while it is nearly destitute of astringency, and not disposed to change like the ferrous salts generally. Dose, gr. ij–iij, in pill, three times a day.

Ferri Ferrocyanidum (*Ferrocyanide of Iron*), (Fe_4Fcy_3), or Pure Prussian Blue, is obtained by the action of ferrocyanide of potassium on solution of tersulphate of iron. It is of a rich dark-blue colour, without smell or taste, and is insoluble in water, alcohol, and the dilute mineral acids. Its effects on the economy in health are not very striking; but it has been used both as an antiperiodic tonic and in the treatment of neuralgia, chorea, &c. Dose, gr. v, three or four times a day.

Ferri Lactas (*Lactate of Iron*), is made by mixing diluted lactic acid with iron filings. It is *ferrous lactate* and occurs in greenish-white crystalline crusts or grains, of a mild, sweetish, ferruginous taste, sparingly soluble in water, and insoluble in alcohol. Used in chlorosis, and has a marked effect in increasing the appetite. Dose, gr. x–xx, in *pill*, *lozenge*, or *syrup*.

Ferri et Quiniæ Citras (*Citrate of Iron and Quinia*). This salt is prepared by precipitating quinia from the sulphate by ammonia, and afterwards dissolving it in a hot solution of citrate of iron. As found in the shops, it is probably a mixture of *ferric citrate* with a variable proportion of citrate of iron and quinia. It occurs in thin, transparent scales, of a reddish or yellowish-brown colour, with a tint of green, not very soluble in water, and of a ferruginous, moderately bitter taste. It combines the virtues of its two bases, and is thought to have an especial agency in diminishing the formation of urea by the kidneys, whence its use in uræmia. Dose, gr. v–x.

Ferri et Ammonii Citras (*Citrate of Iron and Ammonium*), is made by adding water of ammonia (6 *fluidounces*) to solution of citrate of iron (*a pint*), and evaporating. It occurs in the form of garnet-red, translucent scales, of a slightly ferruginous taste, and is readily soluble in water; it has antacid properties. Dose, gr. v–x.

FERRI ET STRYCHNIÆ CITRAS (*Citrate of Iron and Strychnia*), is made by mixing a solution of strychnia and citric acid (*each 5 grains*), in a fluidrachm of distilled water, with a solution of citrate of iron and ammonium (500 *grains*), in a fluidounce of water, and evaporating. It occurs in garnet-red scales, of a bitter, ferruginous taste, readily soluble in water. An excellent tonic—dose, gr. ij–iij, two or three times a day.

FERRI ET AMMONII SULPHAS (*Sulphate of Iron and Ammonium*) ($Fe_4 3SO_4,(NH_4)_2SO_4 24H_2O$). This salt, called also *ammonio-ferric alum*, is made by adding sulphate of ammonium to a hot solution of tersulphate of iron. It occurs in octohedral crystals, of a pale-violet colour, and sour astringent taste, efflorescent, and very soluble in water. Used in diarrhœa and chronic dysentery. Dose, gr. v–xv, two or three times a day.

FERRI ET AMMONII TARTRAS (*Tartrate of Iron and Ammonium*), occurs in transparent, garnet-red scales, of a sweetish taste, soluble in water, insoluble in alcohol and ether. A mild chalybeate. Dose, gr. x–xxx.

Various other combinations of iron have been from time to time introduced into the practice of medicine; but they are needlessly multiplied. The *arseniate*, *acetate*, *bromide*, *tannate*, and *valerianate*, are recommended by different therapeutists.

CUPRI PRÆPARATA—PREPARATIONS OF COPPER.

Metallic copper is inert. The salts of copper act locally as caustics, irritants, and astringents. When exhibited in small doses, they exert a corroborant influence over the cerebro-spinal system, and are employed to fulfil the indications to which *tonics* are applicable, as in the cure of ague, neuralgia, epilepsy, &c. In larger doses, they act as *emetics;* and, in excessive doses, they produce gastro-intestinal inflammation, and disorder of the nervous system; death, in fatal cases, is usually preceded by convulsions, paralysis, and delirium. They are employed therapeutically, both as external and internal remedies; externally, as stimulants, astringents, styptics, and caustics; internally, as tonics, astringents, and emetics. In cases of poisoning from the cupreous compounds, the best antidote is *albumen*, as white of eggs, milk, wheaten flour. The *ferrocynanide of potassium* is also very efficacious, forming with the cupreous compound an insoluble ferrocyanide of copper. This salt (which throws down a mahogany-coloured precipitate), ammonia (which strikes an azure-blue colour), sulphuretted hydrogen or sulphide of ammonium (which throws down a deep brownish-black precipitate), and metallic iron, (on which metallic copper is deposited from a cupreous solution), are tests for the soluble salts of copper.

CUPRI SULPHAS (*Sulphate of Copper*). This salt, known as *blue stone* and *blue vitriol*, is obtained by roasting the native sulphuret, or by combining the oxide of copper and sulphuric acid, and occurs also as a by-product in silver-refining. It is *cupric sulphate* ($CuSO_4 5H_2O$). It occurs in fine, prismatic, blue crystals, which, by exposure to the air effloresce slightly, and become covered with a greenish-white powder. It has a styptic, metallic taste, is entirely soluble in water, but insoluble in alcohol. It is employed as a *tonic* and *nervine*. It is an excellent remedy in obstinate intermittent fever, neuralgia, and essential nervous diseases, in doses of gr. ¼ to gr. j, or more, in pill, repeated so as not to occasion vomiting. As an *astringent*, it may be given in the same doses, and will be found extremely valuable in the treatment of chronic diarrhœa, dysentery, and enteritis, and chronic catarrh with profuse secretion. As an *emetic*, the dose is gr. iij to gr. v. Externally, it is used as an escharotic to fungous granulations, and in solution to arrest hemorrhages, mucous discharges, &c.

CUPRUM AMMONIATUM (*Ammoniated Copper*), (*Ammonio-sulphate of copper*) is made by rubbing together sulphate of copper and carbonate of ammonium. It has a deep azure-blue colour, a styptic, metallic taste, and an ammoniacal odour. Its action is very similar to that of sulphate of copper; but it is used principally as an antispasmodic tonic in nervous disorders,—epilepsy, chorea, hysteria, spasmodic asthma, &c. Dose, gr. ½, gradually increased.

CUPRI SUBACETAS (*Subacetate of Copper*), or *Verdigris*, ($Cu_2O2C_2H_3O_2$), occurs in pale, bluish-green or green masses or powder. The dose is gr. ⅛ to gr. ¼; but it is a powerful poison in an overdose, and hence is rarely given as a tonic. The powder is used as an escharotic, and an *ointment* is used.

ZINCI PRÆPARATA—PREPARATIONS OF ZINC.

Zinc in its metallic state is inert. Its compounds are very analogous in their effects on the system to those of copper, but are less energetic. The tests for soluble zinc salts are sulphide of ammonium, which throws down a white sulphide (the only white sulphide met with), the alkalies, alkaline carbonates, and ferrocyanide of potassium, all of which give white precipitates. The zinc preparations are employed topically as caustics, astringents, and desiccants; and internally as tonics, astringents, and antispasmodics, and in large doses, as emetics. In cases of poisoning (which are, however, very uncommon), albumen, demulcents and opiates are to be administered.

ZINCI SULPHAS (*Sulphate of Zinc*), or *White Vitriol*, is prepared by dissolving zinc in diluted sulphuric acid. It occurs in small, colourless, transparent, prismatic crystals, resembling those of sulphate of magnesium ($ZnSO_4,7H_2O$). They have a metallic, astringent taste, are soluble in water, and insoluble in alcohol. Dose, as a *tonic*, *antispasmodic*, and *astringent*, gr. j to gr. v; as an *emetic*, it is the promptest and safest that can be given in cases of narcotic poisoning, in the dose of gr. x to gr. xx. Externally, it is much used as a caustic, and in solution as an application to inflamed mucous membranes, in the strength of gr. j or ij to f℥ss of water.

ZINCI OXIDUM (*Oxide of Zinc*) is made by roasting zinc in the air. This is an impure form, known as *Commercial Oxide of Zinc* (*Zinci Oxidum Venale*), sometimes called *tutty*. A purer form is obtained by exposing precipitated carbonate of zinc to heat, which expels the carbonic acid and water. It is a yellowish-white powder (ZnO), insoluble in water, but soluble in diluted sulphuric and chlorohydric acids. It has been given in diarrhœa, and as an antispasmodic tonic, in doses of gr. ij to iij, gradually increased to gr. viij or x, and is highly esteemed in the treatment of epilepsy; but it is chiefly used externally as a dusting powder, or in the form of *ointment* (80 grains to ointment of benzoin 400 grains).

ZINCI ACETAS (*Acetate of Zinc*) is made by heating commercial oxide of zinc in a solution of acetic acid and distilled water, and occurs in white micaceous crystals ($Zn2C_2H_3O_2,2H_2O$), very soluble in water, and efflorescent in a dry air. It may be given internally as a tonic antispasmodic, in the dose of gr. j or ij, gradually increased; but it is chiefly used as a topical astringent in ophthalmia, gonorrhœa, leucorrhœa, &c., in the proportion of gr. ij to gr. vj, or more, to an ounce of water.

ZINCI CARBONAS PRÆCIPITATA (*Precipitated Carbonate of Zinc*), is obtained by the double reaction of solutions of sulphate of zinc and carbonate of sodium. It is a soft, white powder, a mixture of carbonate and hydrate ($ZnCO_3,2ZnH_2O_2$), similar in its action to the oxide, but is chiefly used as a dusting powder, and to make a mild astringent and desiccant *cerate* (a troyounce to ointment five troyounces).

CALAMINA PRÆPARATA (*Prepared Calamine*), obtained by heat from *calamine*, the native impure carbonate of zinc, is a pinkish powder, used as a desiccant, and in the form of a *cerate*, called Turner's cerate. *Calamine* is so frequently adulterated that it is now dismissed from the Pharmacopœia, though still much used.

LIQUOR ZINCI CHLORIDI (*Solution of Chloride of Zinc*), is prepared by dissolving zinc (6 *troyounces*), in muriatic acid, then adding nitric acid (150 *grains*), and evaporating to dryness; this is dissolved in distilled water (5 *fluid ounces*), with the addition of precipitated carbonate of zinc (150 *grains*), and, after filtration, enough distilled water is added to make the liquid measure a pint. The evaporation of this solution yields

ZINCI CHLORIDUM (*Chloride of Zinc*) ($ZnCl_2$), a whitish-gray, semitransparent, deliquescent mass, having the softness of wax, and soluble in water, alcohol, and ether. It has been employed internally in doses of gr. j or ij, as an antispasmodic tonic in chorea, epilepsy, and neuralgia. Its local action is that of a powerful caustic, and it is one of the best escharotics that can be exhibited, to produce healthy granulations in malignant or indolent ulcers, especially in lupus. It may be used as a lotion in the strength of gr. ij to f℥j of water, or dissolved in a little alcohol, or in the form of paste, made with one part of the salt to two or four of flour. A solution of the chloride of zinc is employed as an antiseptic, and is also injected into the bloodvessels of anatomical subjects to preserve them for dissection. Burnett's Disinfecting Fluid is a solution of about 200 grains in a fluidounce of water.

ZINCI IODIDUM (*Iodide of Zinc*) (ZnI_2), is made by digesting an excess of zinc with iodine diffused in water. It occurs in the form of a white deliquescent mass, or of fine needles, of a metallic styptic taste, very soluble in water. It has been used internally, as a tonic, antispasmodic, and astringent, in doses of gr. i–ij, best exhibited in the form of syrup. Externally, it is a most valuable local stimulant and escharotic, equal if not superior in effect to the chloride, and, although not officinal, is much used.

ZINCI VALERIANAS (*Valerianate of Zinc*) ($Zn2C_5H_9O_2$), is prepared by the double reaction of valerianate of sodium and sulphate of zinc. It occurs in white, pearly scales, having a faint odour of valerianic acid, and a metallic styptic taste. It dissolves in 160 parts of water and 60 of alcohol. Used in epilepsy and nervous affections, in the dose of one or two grains, repeated several times a day.

ARGENTI PRÆPARATA—PREPARATIONS OF SILVER.

In the metallic state, silver is wholly inert. The only preparation which is extensively employed is—

ARGENTI NITRAS (*Nitrate of Silver*). This salt ($AgNO_3$) is obtained by dissolving silver in diluted nitric acid. It is anhydrous, and occurs in transparent colourless, shining, heavy rhombic plates, which have a strongly metallic and bitter taste, are wholly soluble in distilled water, and become blackened by the action of light and organic matters. Its solution yields with chlorohydric acid or chloride of sodium a white precipitate, entirely soluble in ammonia.

Physiological Effects.—The topical action of nitrate of silver is that of a caustic or corrosive; and this effect is produced by its combining with the albumen and fibrin of the tissues. When applied to mucous membranes, it forms a compound with the animal matter of the mucus, which protects the tissues from the action of the caustic. Hence, large doses may be taken with considerable impunity by the stomach. But, in excessive quantity, it may occasion gastro-enteric irritation, with disturbance of the nervous system; and in these cases, the *antidote* is *common salt* (chloride of sodium), or any inert chloride, which produces, when in contact with the nitrate, nitrate of sodium and chloride of silver. In medicinal doses, nitrate of silver has a specific corroborant and antispasmodic action on the nervous system; and, after prolonged use, produces a peculiar indelible *blueness* or *slate-colour* of the skin.

Medicinal Uses.—*Internally*, nitrate of silver has been chiefly employed as an antispasmodic tonic in the treatment of epilepsy, and it is among the most reliable remedies that can be administered in this intractable affection; but its effect in discolouring the skin is an objection to its protracted use. It is also used in locomotor ataxia, chorea, and gastrodynia, and as an astringent in dysentery. But it is as an *external agent* that it is chiefly resorted to. It is the most efficacious application that can be made to inflamed mucous membranes, and either in the solid form or in solution, it is employed in every variety of inflammation of this tissue. It is also extensively used to produce healthy granulations in wounds and ulcers, to arrest the progress of erysipelatous inflammation and variolous pustules, in porrigo and other skin diseases, in strictures, and to destroy the virus of chancres and of poisoned wounds.

Administration.—The dose of nitrate of silver internally is gr. $\frac{1}{6}$, gradually increased to gr. iij or iv, three times a day, in pill made with some mild vegetable powder. For external use, solutions are made of various strengths, from gr. ij to ʒss, in an ounce of distilled water. An ointment is also employed.

ARGENTI NITRAS FUSA (*Fused Nitrate of Silver, Lunar Caustic*). For external use, in the solid form, nitrate of silver is melted and poured into small moulds.

ARGENTI OXIDUM (*Oxide of Silver*) (Ag_2O), is obtained by adding solution of potassa to a solution of nitrate of silver. It is a tasteless, olive-brown powder, very slightly soluble in water. Its uses are analogous to those of the nitrate, and it is employed in epilepsy, gastrodynia, chronic diarrhœa, uterine disease, &c. It is considered to be free from liability to discolour the skin. Dose, gr. ss to gr. ij, twice or thrice daily, in powder or pill.

BISMUTHI SUBNITRAS—SUBNITRATE OF BISMUTH.

This salt is prepared by first forming the ternitrate of bismuth by dissolving bismuth in diluted nitric acid; as metallic bismuth generally contains arsenic, the nitrate thus formed is converted into the carbonate, by the addition of solution of carbonate of sodium, whereby most of the arsenic is removed as soluble arseniate of sodium; the carbonate of bismuth is next dissolved in nitric acid, and the nitrate of bismuth is again formed; a little water is added to the mixed solution of nitrate and arseniate of bismuth, by which the subarseniate is deposited and separated; the addition of a large amount of water causes a deposition of subnitrate of bismuth; the supernitrate remaining in solution is lastly decomposed by ammonia, which takes most of the nitric acid, and precipitates the bismuth combined with the remainder, in the form of subnitrate. Subnitrate of bismuth, known as *pearl white* and *magistery of bismuth* ($BiONO_3,H_2O$) is a white, inodorous, tasteless powder, nearly insoluble in water. In large amounts (two drachms have produced death), it acts as a poison with symptoms like those of arsenical poisoning. Its medicinal properties are tonic, antispasmodic, and astringent, and it has been employed in intermittent fever; but it is now chiefly used to allay sickness and vomiting in chronic nervous affections of the stomach, to relieve the pain of gastralgia, and also as an astringent in subacute and chronic diarrhœa. Dose, gr. v to ℈j, or even ʒss, in powder or pill. Externally, it is a good remedy in skin diseases in the form of ointment. The *subcarbonate of bismuth* —*bismuthi subcarbonas* ($Bi_2O_2CO_3,H_2O$)—is recommended as a substitute for the subnitrate. It is thought to be more readily tolerated by the stomach, and is more soluble in the gastric juice, but it is less astringent. The *test* for a soluble salt of bismuth is a piece of paper wetted with a solution of sulphocyanide of potassium, and dried, which will produce a yellow spot at the point of contact.

CADMII SULPHAS—SULPHATE OF CADMIUM.

This salt is obtained by the addition of sulphuric acid to carbonate of cadmium; the latter salt being first procured by the reaction of carbonate of sodium upon nitrate of cadmium, previously made by dissolving cadmium in nitric acid and water. It occurs in transparent, colourless, prismatic crystals ($CdSO_4$), of an astringent, austere taste, and very soluble in water. In its effects on the system, it closely resembles sulphate of zinc, but it has been chiefly used in this country, as a collyrium (gr. j–ij to water f℥j), and has been found very efficacious in specks and opacities of the cornea.

CERII OXALAS—OXALATE OF CERIUM.

This salt ($Ce''C_2O_4,3H_2O$), is usually made by adding a solution of oxalate of ammonium to any soluble salt of cerium, and is also obtained from the mineral *cerite*. It occurs as a snow-white, granular powder, inodorous and tasteless, insoluble in water, alcohol, and ether, but dissolved by sulphuric acid. It is believed to resemble the salts of silver, bismuth, and zinc in its effects, and has lately been deservedly extolled in obstinate forms of vomiting, especially the vomiting of pregnancy. In chorea, and other neuroses, it is also highly recommended.

Dose, a grain three times a day, or oftener, in pill or suspended in water. The *nitrate of cerium* has also been employed, and is more soluble. Dose, somewhat less.

ACIDA MINERALIA—MINERAL ACIDS.

The diluted mineral acids are usually classed with tonics; but, although they exert a very considerable corroborant influence on the system, their action is in many respects peculiar and distinctive. In the concentrated form, they are corrosive. When properly diluted with water and swallowed in medicinal doses, they allay thirst, increase the appetite, and stimulate digestion. After absorption into the blood, they often produce a restorative effect in morbid conditions of the circulating fluid, and in their passage out by the secretions, act as astringents. They are employed—as tonics, usually in combination with the vegetable bitters, in dyspepsia, especially when it is dependent on a deficiency of the gastric fluid; as antalkalines, to correct the morbid alkalinity of the blood in typhoid and other essential fevers, and in purpura, scurvy, and analogous blood diseases; as astringents and styptics in hemorrhage from the stomach and bowels, and in colliquative discharges; to allay febrile heat and cutaneous irritation; in phosphatic lithiasis; and locally, as escharotics; and, in very dilute solution, they are injected into the bladder as lithontriptics. In cases of poisoning from the mineral acids, the alkaline earths and fixed oils are the proper antidotes.

Acidum Sulphuricum (*Sulphuric Acid*), (H_2SO_4), formerly called *Oil of Vitriol*, is obtained by burning sulphur, mixed with nitre, over a stratum of water contained in a chamber lined with sheet-lead. It is a dense, colourless, inodorous, corrosive liquid, of a strongly acid taste and an oily consistence, which unites with water in all proportions, with the evolution of heat. When of the sp. gr. 1.845, it contains one equivalent of water. It should have, as directed by the Pharmacopœia, the sp. gr. 1.843, when it contains 79 per cent of anhydrous acid. The diluted acid is readily detected by a soluble salt of barium, which precipitates a white insoluble barium sulphate. In the concentrated form, it is not employed internally, but is sometimes used externally as a caustic. When swallowed, it acts as a violent corrosive poison, usually staining the lips, mouth, and fauces with white or black sloughs; occasionally, the action of the poison is spent upon the upper part of the larynx, and death takes place from asphyxia, without the entrance of the poison into the stomach. The proper *antidote* is magnesia or chalk, or solution of soap, and mucilaginous drinks should be afterwards freely administered.

ACIDUM SULPHURICUM DILUTUM (*Diluted Sulphuric Acid*), contains two troyounces of sulphuric acid in a pint of acid diluted with distilled water. It is given as a tonic, refrigerant, and astringent, in the dose of from ten to thirty drops, three times a day, in water, and should be sucked through a tube to prevent injury to the teeth. This acid is a particularly valuable remedy in typhus and typhoid fevers, colliquative perspirations, cholera, and choleraic diarrhœa; and it is the best corrective for phosphatic lithiasis. Some observations have been made which seem to assign it prophylactic powers against epidemic cholera. It is used externally as a gargle, and wash to ulcers.

ACIDUM SULPHURICUM AROMATICUM (*Aromatic Sulphuric Acid*), or *Elixir of Vitriol*, is made by digesting six troyounces of sulphuric acid in a pint of alcohol, then percolating a troyounce of ginger and a troyounce and a half of cinnamon with alcohol till a pint of tincture is obtained, and mixing the tincture with the diluted acid. It is a reddish-brown liquid, with an aromatic odour and a pleasant acid taste; and is an agreeable substitute for the diluted sulphuric acid, administered in the same doses.

ACIDUM SULPHUROSUM (*Sulphurous Acid*), is made by heating sulphuric acid with charcoal and distilled water. The sulphuric acid is deprived of an equivalent of oxygen by the charcoal, and becomes sulphurous acid (H_2SO_3). It is a colourless liquid, having the smell of burning sulphur, and a sulphurous, sour, and somewhat astringent taste. It has been only of late years employed in medicine, and is believed to have a special influence in destroying parasitic life. Internally, it is very efficacious in sarcina ventriculi, or yeast vomiting; dose, fʒj, largely diluted with water. Externally, it is used in skin diseases (particularly those of a parasitic nature, either animalcular or cryptogamous)—diluted with two or three measures of water or glycerin. The *sulphite of sodium—sodii sulphis* ($Na_2SO_3,7H_2O$)—is used as a substitute for sulphurous acid, which is developed from the salt by any of the organic acids. It occurs in white efflorescent, prismatic crystals, of a sulphurous taste, soluble in four parts of cold and one part of boiling water. Dose, ʒj, three times a day; a solution (ʒi–f℥i of water) is a good local application in erysipelas. The *hyposulphite of sodium* ($Na_2S_2O_3,5H_2O$), is used for the same purposes. It occurs in white, tabular crystals, of a pearly lustre and sulphurous taste, which are very deliquescent, and very soluble in water and alcohol, and insoluble in ether. Dose, gr. x–xx, three times a day, and for *external use*, ʒj, dissolved in water f℥j. Both the sulphite and hyposulphite of sodium have been found efficacious in intermittent and remittent fevers. The sulphite is perhaps the more efficacious salt. *Potassii sulphis* (*sulphite of potassium*) ($K_2SO_3,2H_2O$), occurs in white, opaque fragments or powder, of a saline and sulphurous taste, very soluble in water; its uses and doses are the same as those of sulphite of sodium. The *sulphite of magnesium* ($MgSO_3,6H_2O$), is also employed in zymotic diseases, and is less unpalatable than the sodium salt, and besides contains a larger proportional quantity of acid. The sulphites of sodium, potassium, and magnesium are employed in the treatment of purulent infection. *Sulphites* of *calcium* and *ammonium* have been also recommended.

Acidum Nitricum (*Nitric Acid*) (HNO_3), is obtained by the action of sulphuric acid upon nitrate of potassium. When pure, it is colourless; but, as found in the shops, it is usually of a straw colour, owing to the presence of hyponitric acid. It should have a sp. gr. 1.420 (when it contains 60 per cent. of anhydrous acid), and is a corrosive, sour liquid, employed, in the concentrated form, as an escharotic to destroy warts and stimulate indolent sinuses, and, diluted, as an astringent wash or gargle. Cases of poisoning from this acid are to be treated with magnesia or soap, and mucilaginous drinks. In poisoning from nitric acid, the fauces and mouth are covered with yellow eschars. Internally, it is used in the form of

ACIDUM NITRICUM DILUTUM (*Diluted Nitric Acid*), which contains three troyounces of acid in a pint of diluted acid. This is given as a substitute for sulphuric acid, but is more apt to disagree with the stomach; it is also employed as an alterative in syphilis, and has been found useful in whooping-cough. Combined with laudanum and camphor-water, it is much used in the treatment of dysentery, under the name of *Hope's Camphor Mixture* (camphor water f℥viij, nitric acid fʒi, laudanum 25 drops; dose f℥ss, repeated). Dose, for internal use, 20 to 40 drops, three times a day, reduced with water.

ACIDUM MURIATICUM (*Muriatic Acid*), is an aqueous solution of hydrochloric acid gas (HCl), of sp. gr. 1.160, and is obtained by the action of sulphuric acid on solution of chloride of sodium or common salt. It is, when pure, a transparent, colourless liquid, but has often a yellow colour, owing to the presence of chlorine, iron, or other contaminations; it gives off dense white fumes when in contact with ammonia, and evolves chlorine gas when heated with peroxide of manganese. It has a corrosive taste, and a suffocating odour, and is an active poison, though less irritating than sulphuric and nitric acids. Magnesia or soap is the proper antidote. It is used, externally, as a caustic, and as an application in diphtheria, ulcerative and gangrenous stomatitis, &c.; internally, in the form of

ACIDUM MURIATICUM DILUTUM (*Diluted Muriatic Acid*), which contains four troyounces of acid in a pint of diluted acid. This is employed in typhoid and typhus fevers, malignant scarlatina, &c.; also to counteract phosphatic deposits in the urine, to prevent the generation of worms, in syphilis, in dysentery, and in some forms of dyspepsia. Dose, twenty to sixty drops, which may be given in infusion of rose.

ACIDUM NITRO-MURIATICUM (*Nitro-Muriatic Acid*). This acid is made by mixing three troyounces of nitric acid with five troyounces of muriatic acid, and consists of two compounds of chlorine and nitric oxide ($N_2O_2Cl_4$ and NOCl), mixed with free chlorine. It has a deep golden-yellow colour, and emits the smell of chlorine, which is the chief active constituent. *Internally*, it is employed as a stomachic tonic, and is thought also to be particularly efficacious in oxaluria, and in diseases of the liver and syphilis. It should not be given with mercurials. *Externally*, it is used as a bath, either local or general, in oxaluria, syphilis, and chronic hepatitis, for which purpose one or two ounces of acid may be added to a gallon of water. Dose, from two to five drops, properly diluted, and carefully increased.

ACIDUM NITRO-MURIATICUM DILUTUM (*Diluted Nitro-Muriatic Acid*), contains four troyounces of acid in a pint of diluted acid; dose, ten to twenty drops.

ACIDUM OXALICUM (*Oxalic Acid*) ($H_2C_2O_4,2H_2O$). This acid, which is found in many vegetables, as the sorrels, and is often deposited in the bladder as oxalate of calcium or *mulberry calculus*, is usually obtained by decomposing sugar or starch with nitric acid. It occurs in small, colourless, prismatic crystals, having a strongly acid taste, is soluble in water, and decomposable by heat without residue. It is used medicinally with success in typhoid fever, in scurvy, and purpura, and as an astringent to check the colliquative perspirations of phthisis, and the expectoration of chronic bronchitis. Dose, gr. ½ to gr. 1, three or four times a day. It is a virulent acronarcotic poison, in large amounts, acting with very great rapidity and certainty; and, as its crystals resemble those of Epsom salt, it is often sold by mistake for that purgative, from which it may be distinguished by its acid properties, and, in solution, by nitrate of silver (which yields a white precipitate, soluble in cold nitric acid), and by calcium salts (which precipitate white oxalate of calcium, soluble in nitric acid). The proper antidote is chalk or magnesia, mixed with water. *Salt of sorrel*, a crystalline compound of oxalic acid with acid potassium oxalate, produces analogous poisonous effects.

ORDER V.—ASTRINGENTS.

These are medicines which produce contraction and corrugation of the tissues. Their constitutional effects are somewhat analogous to those of tonics; as, like them, they increase the tone and vigour of the body, and exercise a control over various disorders of the nervous system. But they are chiefly employed to cure relaxation of the fibres and tissues, to subdue inflammation of superficial parts, and to arrest hemorrhage and excessive discharges from mucous membranes or other secreting surfaces. In checking morbid discharges from the bowels, astringents, while they diminish the secretions from the intestinal canal, do not, like opium, restrain the peristaltic movements; hence the necessity of combining them with opiates. They are divided into *Vegetable* and *Mineral* astringents. Most of the former owe their astringency to the presence of a principle termed TANNIC ACID, and differ from tonics in the absence of bitterness. The mineral preparations, usually classed among astringents, are those of alum and lead, and are distinguished from the mineral astringent-tonics, by their more decided astringency and a sedative action on the vascular system.

VEGETABLE ASTRINGENTS.

ACIDUM TANNICUM—TANNIC ACID.

This acid, which is the active principle of the vegetable astringents, is usually extracted from powdered nutgalls by the action of washed ether. The nutgall, made into a soft paste with ether, is enveloped in a canvas cloth, and is pressed between tin plates; the resulting cake is again mixed with washed ether and expressed; and the expressed liquids are mixed, evaporated, and dried; the water seems to be the solvent which extracts the tannic acid. It is a light, feathery, non-crystalline powder, of a yellowish-white colour, and a strongly astringent taste, is very soluble in water, and soluble, though less so, in alcohol and ether. It produces a white flocculent precipitate with solution of gelatine, a bluish-black precipitate with ferric salts, and white precipitates with solutions of the vegetable alkalies; and these substances are to be, therefore, considered *incompatible* with all the vegetable astringents. There is a variety of tannic acid (*mimo-tannic acid*), obtained from kino, catechu and some other substances, which strikes a *greenish-black* precipitate with the salts of iron, and is not convertible into gallic acid. Tannic acid is $C_{27}H_{22}O_{17}$; it is a glucoside, yielding, like many other substances, glucose, when boiled with diluted sulphuric or hydrochloric acid, the other product being gallic acid.

Effects and Uses.—Tannic acid is a powerful astringent, and is applicable to all the cases in which astringents are useful. It is now believed, however, that, owing to its coagulating influence on albumen, tannic acid is not absorbed in the stomach, and cannot produce constitutional effects until converted into gallic acid, but this is probably again changed in the blood into tannic acid by combination with glucose. It is used internally, in the treatment of diarrhœa, dysentery, cholera, hemorrhage, colliquative sweats, &c.; also as an enema in diarrhœa, dysentery, prolapsus ani, and fissure of the rectum; and, as a topical application, in hemorrhages, inflammations, and morbid discharges from mucous membranes, ulcers, &c. It is, perhaps, the best form in which the vegetable astringents can be employed, owing to the certainty and minuteness of the dose in which it can be given. Dose, gr. j to gr. iij, or iv, in pill, occasionally repeated. For external use, the *glycerite of tannic acid* (*glyceritum acidi tannici*), is employed; it is made by rubbing together and dissolving at a gentle heat 2 troy-ounces of tannic acid in half a pint of glycerin. *Ointment of tannic acid* (*unguentum acidi tannici*), is made by rubbing up 30 grains of tannic acid with a troyounce of lard.

ACIDUM GALLICUM—GALLIC ACID.

This principle is found in many of the vegetable astringents, but less uniformly than tannic acid, and is probably the result of changes which the latter has undergone. It is prepared by exposing a mixture of nutgalls in water to the air, when the tannic acid gradually absorbs oxygen and is converted into gallic acid; it is purified by being boiled in water and filtered through animal charcoal. It occurs in small, silky, nearly colourless crystals, having a slightly acid and astringent taste, and is soluble in boiling water, and slightly so in cold water. It is $H_3C_7H_3O_5,H_2O$.

Effects and Uses.—Gallic acid is a valuable astringent, which has of late been extensively employed in hemorrhagic disorders, as uterine hemorrhage, hemoptysis, hæmaturia, bloody diarrhœa, &c. Both tannic and gallic acids have been found useful in albuminuria. Gallic acid has but feeble local astringent powers, and is probably converted into tannic acid in the blood; given by the stomach, it is more efficacious than the latter acid. It may be given in doses of gr. ij to gr. v, in pill, every two or three hours. *Glycerite of gallic acid* is made by the same formula as that of *tannic acid.*

GALLA—NUTGALL.

Nutgall is a morbid EXCRESCENCE found upon Quercus infectoria, or the Gall-Oak (*Nat. Ord.* Corylaceæ), a small tree or shrub of Asia Minor. The Gall-nuts are produced by the puncture of the buds by a fly (*Cynips quercûsfolii* or *Diplolepis gallæ tinctoriæ*) to form a nidus for its eggs. This occasions an irritation and flow of juices to the part, resulting in the formation of a tumour round the larva, which, on attaining maturity, perforates the gall and escapes. Galls are produced chiefly in Syria and Asia Minor, and are imported from the Levant. They are brought also from Calcutta, being collected to some extent in India. Galls are spherical, about the size of a hickory-nut, but of varying dimensions, with small tubercles on their surface. The best are *bluish* or *black* externally, and grayish within, without odour, and of a very astringent, bitter taste. They yield their properties to both water and alcohol, but best to the former, and contain both tannic and gallic acids. *White* galls are collected after they have been perforated by the insect, and are inferior in astringency.

Effects and Uses.—Galls are powerfully astringent, but are not much used internally. In the form of infusion or decoction, they are employed as enemata in diarrhœa and dysentery, and also as gargles. Dose of the *powder*, gr. x to gr. xx. The *tincture* (four troyounces to diluted alcohol Oij) may be given in the dose of f℥j to f℥iij, but it is chiefly used as a chemical test. The *ointment* (one part to seven parts of lard) is a favourite application in hemorrhoids.

CATECHU.

Catechu, formerly called Terra Japonica, is an EXTRACT of the wood of Acacia Catechu, a small prickly tree of India (*Nat. Ord.* Fabaceæ). Twelve or fifteen varieties of the drug are described by pharmacologists; but it is usually met with in the shops, in masses of various shapes and sizes, of a rusty-brown colour externally, and varying internally from a reddish or yellowish-brown to a dark-brown colour. The best is of a dark colour, and is easily broken into small angular fragments, with a smooth glossy surface, bearing some resemblance to kino. It is without smell, and has an astringent, bitter taste. It contains about 50 per cent. of tannic acid (of the variety which strikes a *greenish-black* precipitate with the salts of iron), and about 30 per cent. of a peculiar extractive, called *catechuic acid*, to both of which it owes its peculiar properties.

Effects and Uses.—This is one of the most powerful and valuable of the vegetable astringents, possessing also mild tonic properties. It is much employed in diarrhœa, dysentery, hemorrhages, and in all cases of immoderate discharge, unattended with inflammatory action. It is a good deal used in relaxed conditions of the mouth and throat, to relieve the hoarseness of public speakers, also in aphthous ulcerations of the mouth, and spongy affections of the gums. Topically, it is employed as a styptic, and in solution as an injection in gonorrhœa and gleet, &c. Dose of the powder, gr. x to ʒss, in bolus or emulsion.

Infusum Catechu Compositum (*Compound Infusion of Catechu*), is made by adding boiling water (Oj) to powdered catechu (half a troyounce), and cinnamon (ʒj)—dose, f℥j to f℥ij, three or four times a day. Of the *tincture* (three troyounces to diluted alcohol Oij, with cinnamon two troyounces), the dose is fʒj to fʒiij.

KINO.

The term *Kino* is applied to the products of several trees. Five varieties are known. 1. East India kino, which is the most common, and is the INSPISSATED JUICE of Pterocarpus marsupium (*Nat. Ord.* Fabaceæ), a lofty tree of Malabar. 2. African kino, the original variety introduced into Europe, but not now met with; obtained from Pterocarpus erinaceus (*Nat. Ord.* Fabaceæ). 3. Jamaica kino, the *extract* of the wood and bark of Coccoloba uvifera, or Seaside Grape (*Nat. Ord.* Polygonaceæ), a small tree of South America and the West Indies. 4. South America or Caraccas kino, which is probably derived from Coccoloba uvifera. 5. Botany Bay kino, the *concrete juice* of Eucalyptus resinifera (*Nat. Ord.* Myrtaceæ), a large tree of Australia.

East India kino is met with in small, angular, shining fragments, of a dark-brown or reddish-brown colour, brittle, without smell, but with a very astringent taste. It contains tannic acid (of the second variety), kinoic acid (which is the red colouring matter), pectin, ulmic acid, and inorganic salts.

South American kino comes in large masses, externally very dark, and internally of a deep reddish-brown colour.

Jamaica kino is like the last, but contained in large gourds.

Effects and Uses.—Kino is a powerful astringent, and is much used in diarrhœa, chronic dysentery, leucorrhœa, gonorrhœa, hemorrhages, &c. Externally, it is employed as a styptic, and as a stimulant to indolent ulcers. Dose, of the *powder* gr. x to ʒss; of the *tincture* (ʒvj (mixed with an equal bulk of dry sand) to diluted alcohol, consisting of two measures of alcohol and one measure of water, f℥viij), f℈j or f℈ij may be given, and it is frequently added to chalk mixture in diarrhœa. It spoils by keeping.

KRAMERIA—RHATANY.

Rhatany is the ROOT of Krameria triandra (*Nat. Ord.* Polygaleæ), a shrub of Peru. It occurs in woody cylindrical pieces, of the thickness of a goose-quill to twice that size—many radicles being often united to a common head. They have a dark, reddish-brown bark, and a tough central ligneous portion, of a lighter red colour. They are without smell, but have a very astringent, slightly bitter, and sweetish taste, which is much stronger in the cortical than the ligneous portion; and, hence the smallest pieces should be preferred, as they contain the most bark. Rhatany yields a large proportion of tannic acid (of the second variety), and a peculiar acid, termed *krameric*, both of which probably contribute to its astringency. It imparts its properties to both cold and boiling water, but more fully to alcohol.

Effects and Uses.—Rhatany is powerfully astringent, with some tonic properties. It is much used in the treatment of diarrhœa, dysentery, hemorrhages, &c., and as an enema in fissure of the anus, hemorrhoids, leucorrhœa, &c. The powdered extract is an ingredient in many tooth-powders, and the tincture is also used as an astringent mouth-wash. Dose of the *powder* gr. xx to gr. xxx. But it is more employed in *infusion* (a troyounce to boiling water Oj), dose, f℥j or f℥ij; watery *extract*, dose gr. x to gr. xv; *fluid extract*, dose f℈ss–i; *tincture* (six troyounces to diluted alcohol Oij), dose f℈j to f℈ij; and *syrup* (twelve troyounces percolated with water till four pints of filtered liquor are obtained, which is to be evaporated to seventeen fluidounces, and in this thirty troyounces of sugar are to be dissolved by gentle heat), dose f℈j to f℥ss; or the syrup may be made by adding twelve fluidounces of the fluid extract to twenty-four fluidounces of syrup.

HÆMATOXYLON—LOGWOOD.

Logwood, or Campeachy wood, is the HEART-WOOD of Hæmatoxylon Campechianum (*Nat. Ord.* Fabaceæ), a medium-sized tree of Campeachy and other maritime parts of tropical America, and now naturalized in the West Indies. The portion used in medicine, and also as a dye, is the heart-wood, from which the bark and white sap-wood are removed, previously to exportation. It is imported in billets of different sizes, of a dark colour externally, and a deep-red internally; in the shops it is kept in chips or raspings. It has a sweetish, astringent, and rather peculiar taste, and a feeble, not unpleasant smell. It contains kino-tannic acid, a colouring principle called *hœmatin* or *hœmatoxylin*, volatile oil, resin, &c.

Effects and Uses.—It is a mild astringent, useful in chronic diarrhœa and dysentery, and particularly well adapted to the weakened condition of the bowels, which follows cholera infantum, and is also much employed in the diarrhœa of phthisis. It is given either in *decoction* (a troyounce to water Oij, boiled down to Oj), in the dose of f℥j to f℥ij to adults, and fʒj to fʒij to children; or watery *extract* in the dose of gr. x to ʒss, in solution.

QUERCUS ALBA—WHITE OAK. QUERCUS TINCTORIA—BLACK OAK.

The barks of several species of American oaks possess astringent properties, and are probably to be found in the shops, but the only officinal varieties are Quercus Alba, White Oak, and Quercus Tinctoria, Black Oak (*Nat Ord.* Amentaceæ). The INNER BARK is the portion used, but the leaves and acorns are also astringent. *White Oak-Bark* is distinguished by its whitish colour. When prepared for use, it is deprived of its epidermis, and is of a light brown colour and fibrous texture, with an astringent and bitterish taste. Water and alcohol extract its virtues, which depend mainly on the presence of tannic and gallic acids, with a bitter principle, termed *quercin.* *Black Oak-Bark* is more furrowed, has a darker colour, a more bitter taste, and stains the saliva yellow, when chewed; it is much employed as a dye, under the name of *quercitron.* It contains a larger proportion of tannic and gallic acids than the white oak-bark.

Effects and Uses.—A decoction of white oak-bark is a good remedy in diarrhœa and hemorrhoids, and is employed as an enema in hemorrhoids, and prolapsus and fissure of the anus, as a gargle in relaxation of the uvula, and as an injection in leucorrhœa. It is used as a bath in the bowel complaints of children; and a poultice of the ground bark is applied in gangrene. Black oak-bark is too irritating for internal exhibition: but for external use it is a stronger astringent than the white oak-bark. Of the *decoction* of *white oak* (*decoctum quercûs albæ*), (a troyounce to water Oj), f℥ij may be taken frequently.

GERANIUM.

One of the most powerful of the *indigenous* astringents is Geranium maculatum, Crowfoot, or Cranesbill (*Nat. Ord.* Geraniaceæ), a perennial herbaceous plant, growing in moist woody situations, with an erect stem, one or two feet high, three to five-lobed, incised, pale-green, mottled leaves, and large purple flowers, which appear in April and May. The part used is the RHIZOME, which should be collected in the autumn. This, when dried, occurs in wrinkled, rough pieces, from a quarter to a half an inch in thickness, furnished with slender fibres, of a dark-brown colour externally, and a pale-flesh colour within. It has an astringent, but not bitter taste, little or no smell, and contains tannic and gallic acids, with some mucilage.

Effects and Uses.—This is an excellent simple astringent, agreeing very well with the stomach, and might be advantageously substituted for more expensive foreign drugs. It may be used internally to fulfil the indications of kino, rhatany, &c., in bowel complaints and hemorrhages, and topically as an enema, gargle, injection, &c. It is also a valuable styptic. Dose in *powder*, gr. x to xx; of the *decoction* (a troyounce to water Oj), f℥j to f℥ij may be given; this is not officinal. A decoction

Fig. 15.

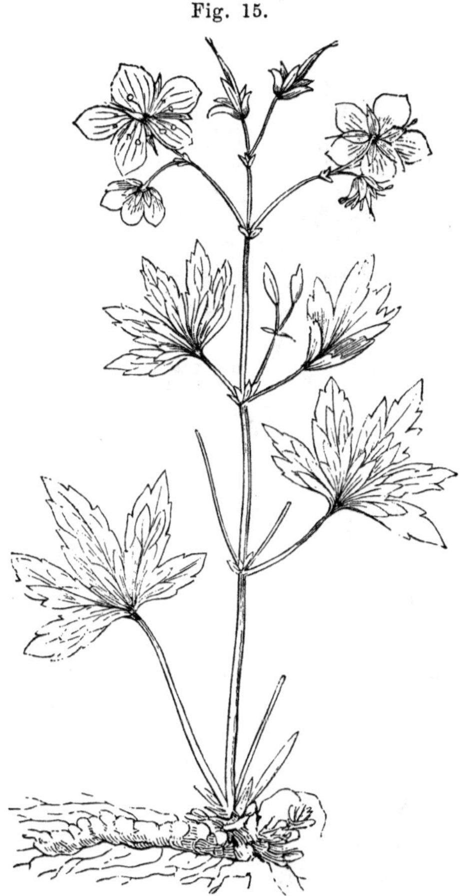

in milk is given to children. The *fluid extract* may be given in doses of ℥ss–℥i.

UVA URSI.

Arctostaphylos Uva Ursi, or Bearberry (*Nat. Ord.* Ericaceæ), is a small, trailing, evergreen shrub, with coriaceous, obovate leaves (somewhat like box leaves and red whortleberry leaves), about half an inch in length, pale rose-coloured flowers, appearing from June to September, and small red berries, which ripen during the winter. It is found in the northern

Fig. 16.

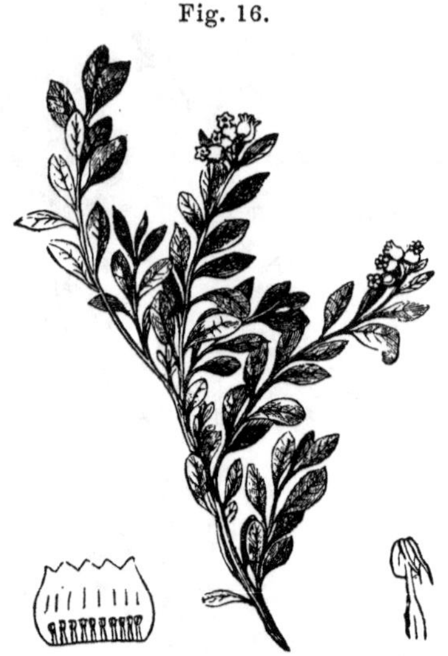

parts of Asia, Europe, and America. The LEAVES are the only part used. When dried, they have a faint hay-like odour, and a bitterish, astringent taste. They yield their virtues to water and alcohol, and contain tannic and gallic acids, a principle termed *ursin* (which is said to act as a diuretic in the dose of a grain), a crystallizable glucoside, termed *arbutin*, extractive, resin, gum, &c.

Effects and Uses.—Uva Ursi is astringent, tonic, and diuretic, and exercises a particular control over discharges from mucous surfaces. Hence, its employment in catarrh of the bladder, chronic bronchitis, with profuse discharge, &c. It is also applicable to the ordinary uses of the vegetable astringents. Dose of the *powder* ℈j to ℈ij, three times a day; but it is usually given in *decoction* (a troyounce to water Oj), of which f℥j to f℥ij may be taken three times a day. The *fluid extract* may be given in the dose of fʒss–fʒj.

CHIMAPHILA—PIPSISSEWA.

Chimaphila umbellata, Pipsissewa, Wintergreen, or Ground-Holly (*Nat. Ord.* Pyrolaceæ), is a small, indigenous, evergreen

Fig. 17.

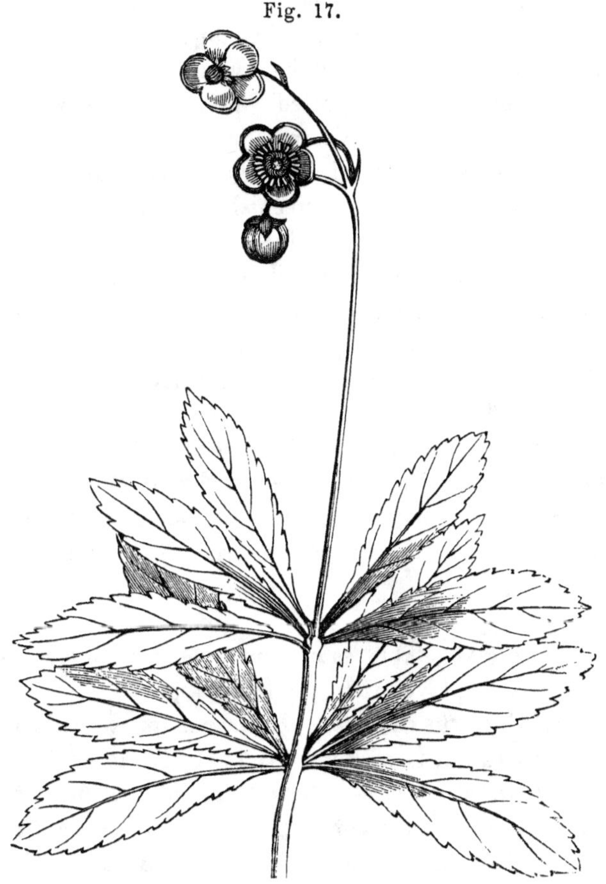

plant, common to the northern parts of Europe, Asia, and America, and found abundantly in woody situations in all parts of the United States. It has an erect stem, three to ten inches high, lanceolate, somewhat wedge-shaped, serrated, dark-green leaves, arranged in irregular whorls, and beautiful five-petaled flowers, of a white colour tinged with red, and a very agreeable perfume, which appear in June. The LEAVES are the officinal portion. In the fresh state, they have a fragrant smell when bruised, which they lose after drying. Their taste is bitterish and astringent, but somewhat aromatic. They contain tannic acid, bitter extractive, resin, and probably some acrid volatile constituent—as the fresh leaves, when bruised and applied to the skin, will cause redness and even vesication.

Chimaphila maculata, or Spotted Pipsissewa, possesses analogous properties to those of C. umbellata, from which it differs principally in the character of its leaves. They are of a deep olive-green colour, veined with greenish-white; and the flowers are a pure white, and appear in July.

Effect and Uses.—Pipsissewa is astringent and tonic, and also diuretic. It is employed in the disorders of the urinary organs to which uva ursi is applicable, and also for its diuretic properties in dropsy, attended with debility of the digestive organs. Indeed, it is classed by some therapeutists among the diuretics. It is usually given in *decoction* (a troyounce to water Oi), of which Oj may be taken in the twenty-four hours; and a *fermented decoction*, made with molasses, ginger, and yeast, is often used. The *fluid extract* may be given in doses of f℥ss–i.

The following vegetable astringents deserve notice, though less frequently employed than the foregoing:

GRANATI FRUCTÛS CORTEX (*Pomegranate Rind*). This is the RIND OF THE FRUIT of Punica Granatum, the Pomegranate tree (*Nat. Ord.* Myrtaceæ), a small tree of Northern Africa, Syria, and Persia, now naturalized in the warmer portions of Europe, the West Indies, our Southern States, &c. The rind of the fruit is a powerful astringent, but is little used internally, from its liability to occasion nausea. Dose, in *powder*, gr. xx to ℨss; but it is best given in decoction (a troyounce to water Oj), (not officinal), dose, f℥j.

ROSA GALLICA (*Red Rose*). ROSA CENTIFOLIA (*Pale Rose*). The PETALS of these two species of rose are officinal, but those of almost every other species of cultivated rose may be employed for the same purposes as rosa centifolia, which is not astringent. The red rose is a mild astringent, and is chiefly used in conjunction with sulphuric acid, in the *infusum rosæ compositum—compound infusion of rose* (half a troyounce to boiling water Oijss, diluted sulphuric acid f℥iij, sugar a troyounce and a half); dose, f℥ij to f℥iv. The *confection* is used as a basis for pills. *Mel Rosæ* (*Honey of Rose*), made with diluted alcohol and clarified honey, is used as an addition to gargles; the *syrup* is added to mixtures. The pale rose is slightly laxative. *Aqua Rosæ* (*Rose Water*), distilled from the pale rose is much employed in collyria, &c. *Unguentum Aquæ Rosæ* (*Ointment of Rose Water*) is made by melting together expressed oil of almond, 3 troyounces and a half, spermaceti, a troyounce, white wax, 120 grains, and then gradually adding Rose water, 2 fluidounces; this is a very soothing application, much used under the name of *cold cream*.

DIOSPYROS (*Persimmon*). The UNRIPE FRUIT of Diospyros Virginiana (*Nat. Ord.* Ebenaceæ), an indigenous tree, is employed in diarrhœa, dysentery, and uterine hemorrhage, in infusion, syrup, and vinous and acetous tinctures. The bark is bitter and astringent, but is not officinal.

TORMENTILLA (*Tormentil*). The RHIZOME of Potentilla Tormentilla (*Nat. Ord.* Rosaceæ), a European plant, is used in Europe as an astringent, in the dose of ʒss to ʒj, but is seldom or never employed in this country.

RUBUS (*Blackberry*). The BARK OF THE ROOT of Rubus villosus, and Rubus Canadensis (*Nat. Ord.* Rosaceæ), the former an erect, prickly shrub, and the latter a creeping brier, are very efficient mild astringents, which have been used with excellent effect in bowel-complaints, especially those of children. The astringency resides principally in the cortical portion, and hence the smallest roots should be preferred; of the *decoction* (not officinal), (a troyounce to water Oj), f℥ij may be taken frequently.

The *fluid extract* may be given in doses of fʒi–ij; the syrup is made by adding half a pint of the fluid extract to a pint and a half of syrup. Dose, a tablespoonful.

HEUCHERA (*Alum-root*). The RHIZOMES of Heuchera Americana and other species of Heuchera (*Nat. Ord.* Saxifragaceæ), indigenous plants known under the common name of Alum-root, with radical leaves somewhat like those of the maple, and numerous radical flower-stems, one to two feet in height, with rose-coloured flowers arranged in pyramidal panicles—possess very decided astringent properties, and may be used both externally and internally.

A large number of vegetable substances, both indigenous and foreign, have been used as astringents, in addition to those enumerated—the astringent principle being the most common medicinal quality with which plants are endowed.

The foregoing list comprises all the more important.

CREASOTUM—CREASOTE.

Creasote is a peculiar substance obtained from wood-tar, or from crude pyroligneous acid. When pure, it is a colourless, oleaginous liquid, with a caustic, burning taste, and a penetrating, disagreeable characteristic odour, like that of smoked meat. Its sp. gr. (U. S. P.) is 1.046; its formula is $C_8H_{10}O_2$. It forms two solutions with water, one of 1 part to 80 parts of water, the other of 1 part of water in 10 parts of creasote; and it is soluble, in all proportions, in alcohol, ether, naphtha, and acetic acid. It is distinguished from carbolic acid, by not coagulating collodion when mixed with it, and by not imparting a blue colour to a slip of pine wood dipped first into an alkaline solution of creasote, and, then, after drying, into muriatic acid. A remarkable property of creasote is its power of preserving meat, whence its name (from κρεὰς, flesh, and σώζω, I save).

Effects and Uses.—Creasote, in large doses, is an acro-narcotic poison. In small doses, it is styptic and astringent, and, though not very nearly allied to the vegetable astringent articles, which contain tannic acid, it is, perhaps, more generally administered for its astringent than for any other properties. It is an excellent remedy in hæmatemesis, and is also employed in hæmoptysis and other hemorrhages. It is very efficacious in allaying vomiting and gastric irritability, and has been exhibited for its astringent virtues with good effect in diarrhœa, diabetes, and chronic bronchitis, and as a nervine in epilepsy, hysteria, neuralgia, &c. Externally, it is applied, in various degrees of dilution, to indolent, sloughing, and foul ulcers; in several cutaneous affections; as a gargle in putrid sorethroat; and for the relief of deafness. In the concentrated form, it is a good styptic in capillary hemorrhages, and is applied with effect to the hollows of carious teeth, for the removal of the pain of toothache. There is no antidote in cases of poisoning from creasote, but stimulants are to be freely administered.

Dose, internally, one to two drops, frequently repeated, in pill, or diluted with mucilage.

For external use, from two to six drops, or more, may be added to a fluidounce of distilled water.

AQUA CREASOTI (*Creasote Water*) (ʒi to distilled water Oi), contains 3.72 minims in each fluidounce. Dose, fʒj–iv.

Creasote ointment contains half a fluidrachm of creasote in an ounce of lard.

ACIDUM CARBOLICUM—CARBOLIC ACID.

This substance, termed also phenic acid, phenylic acid, and phenylic alcohol, is a product of the distillation of coal-tar oil.

IMPURE CARBOLIC ACID (*Acidum Carbolicum Impurum*), is made by treating the impure coal-tar of commerce with a weak alkaline solution, when it is resolved, on the addition of water, into a light oil and a heavier alkaline liquid; the latter is separated and neutralized with muriatic acid, and the impure carbolic acid, which is disengaged, is afterwards distilled from dried chloride of calcium, to remove water, when, upon exposing the distillate to a low temperature, carbolic acid congeals in the form of a colourless crystalline mass.

In its pure state, it is solid at ordinary temperatures, crystallizing in minute plates or long rhomboidal needles, white or colourless, of a peculiar empyreumatic odour like that of creasote (but not identical with it), and an acrid burning taste; if even slightly impure, it has a reddish colour, or will acquire it, upon exposure. Its sp. gr. is 1.065, and it deliquesces upon exposure, and readily assumes the liquid state, in the presence of a little water, without dissolving in it. When quite pure, it melts at 106° F., forming an oily-looking colourless liquid, which boils at 359° F. It is soluble in 20 parts of water, and very soluble in alcohol, ether, acetic acid, glycerin, and the fixed and volatile oils. Its solution coagulates collodion, which distinguishes it from creasote. Although it combines with salifiable bases, it does not act as an acid upon colours, and would be properly designated as *phenylic alcohol*, or the hydrated oxide of phenyl (C_6H_5,HO).

Effects and Uses.—Carbolic acid is a local irritant, and, when applied to the skin or mucous membranes, produces severe pain, with a white eschar. Taken internally in large quantities, it acts as a powerful irritant poison, with an action on the brain, shown by contracted pupils, stertorous breathing, insensibility, coma, and frequently death, from asphyxia; its external application has destroyed life. As an antidote, in cases of poisoning, a saturated solution of saccharate of calcium has been lately recommended. In small doses, its local effects upon the gastro-enteric mucous membrane resemble those of creasote, and after absorption (as shown by experiments upon the lower animals), it exercises a decided influence upon the nerve-centres. Its most interesting property, however, is its destructive influence upon the lower forms of vegetable and animal life, through which it arrests fermentation, and produces a powerful disinfectant and antiseptic effect. It is used internally to check vomiting, as an astringent in diarrhœa, in sarcina ventriculi, as an anthelmintic, and in zymotic diseases as scarlatina, diphtheria, &c. As an external application, its uses are still more important. It is employed in the concentrated form as a caustic in hospital gangrene, and to produce local anæsthesia, and in various forms of dilution, as an application in diphtheria, in cutaneous eruptions (especially those of organic origin), as a dressing to foul ulcers, abscesses, and sinuses, to compound fractures, to carbuncles, to burns and scalds, to suppurating surfaces, with a view to the prevention of pyæmia, and, from its influence in coagulating albumen, as an hæmostatic. It is also a most valuable disinfectant. The dose, internally, is one or two grains, or, if liquefied by heat, one or two drops, in sweetened water or glycerin. For disinfectant purposes, the IMPURE LIQUID ACID (which contains from 70 to 90 per cent. of carbolic and cresylic acids jointly, with impurities derived from coal-tar), answers very well. Carbolates of sodium and potassium have been also employed. *Suppositories of Carbolic Acid* (*Suppositoria Acidi Carbolici*), contain each one grain of carbolic acid. *Glycerite of Carbolic Acid* (*Glyceritum Acidi Carbolici*), is made by rubbing together 2 troyounces of carbolic acid with half a pint of glycerin, until the acid is dissolved; of this 4 minims may be given internally. *Carbolic Acid Water* (*Aqua Acidi Carbolici*), contains 10 fluidrachms of the glycerite dissolved in distilled water enough to make the mixture measure a pint, dose, f℥ss–i. *Ointment of Carbolic Acid* (*Unguentum Acidi Carbolici*), contains 60 grains of carbolic acid in 420 grains of ointment.

Recently, SULPHO-CARBOLIC ACID and various salts of this acid have been employed. Sulpho-carbolic acid ($HC_6H_5SO_4$) is thought to be a more efficient antiseptic and disinfectant than carbolic acid alone. The SULPHO-CARBOLATE OF ZINC ($Zn(C_6H_5SO_4)_2H_2O$) is believed to combine the virtues of zinc-salts and carbolic acid, and has been used with success internally in diarrhœa, in the same doses as the sulphate of zinc, and externally, in aqueous solution of from 3 to 6 grs. to the ounce, as an injection in gonorrhœa, and as a dressing for wounds and ulcers. Sulpho-carbolates of sodium, potassium, magnesium, calcium, and quinia have also been employed; they are recommended as antiseptics in cholera and zymotic diseases generally. The sulpho-carbolate of lead might be used where the acetate of lead is indicated and the corrective action of carbolic acid is called for, while its solubility in glycerin and alcohol adapt it to external application.

MINERAL ASTRINGENTS.

PLUMBI PRÆPARATA—PREPARATIONS OF LEAD.

Metallic lead is considered inert. The sulphuret and sulphate are probably also inactive; but, with these exceptions, all the compounds of lead possess more or less activity. When administered in therapeutical doses, they act as astringents in the alimentary canal, checking secretion, and causing constipation. After absorption, they produce a diminution in the volume and frequency of the pulse and in the activity of the secreting functions, and frequently arrest sanguineous discharges, both natural and artificial. In excessive doses, several of the saturnine compounds are irritant and corrosive poisons, giving rise to gastro-enteric inflammation. The proper *antidotes* are sulphuric acid, or some alkaline or earthy sulphate, in solution in a large quantity of diluent. The hydrated sesquisulphuret of iron is also said to act as an antidote. The *tests* for lead are sulphuretted hydrogen, and a solution of iodide of potassium; the former strikes a black, and the latter a yellow precipitate, with soluble lead salts.

When the system becomes impregnated with lead, either from the too long-continued use of its preparations medicinally, from drinking water drawn through lead-pipes, or from exposure to its influence in lead-factories, &c., a peculiar kind of *chronic poisoning* is produced, which shows itself in a variety of symptoms. The most usual form of lead-poisoning is *colic*, sometimes termed *colica pictonum*, or *painter's colic*, which is characterized by sharp abdominal pains, with hardness and depression of the abdominal parietes, obstinate constipation, nausea, vomiting, &c. Next in frequency is *lead-arthralgy*, in which there are severe pains in the limbs, attended by cramps, hardness, and tension of the painful parts. *Lead-paralysis* is another, though less common variety of the disease, and is characterized by a loss of voluntary motion, owing to the want of contractility of the muscular fibres of the affected parts. It most frequently affects the upper extremities, and the extensor rather than the flexor muscles. Occasionally, functional *disease of the brain* is also observed as one of the consequences of lead-poisoning. The absorption of lead into the system is recognized by a saturnine coloration of the gums, of the mucous membrane of the mouth, and of the teeth. The *antidotical* treatment of chronic lead-poisoning consists in the internal administration of solutions of sulphuric acid and of soluble alkaline and earthy sulphates, and in the use of baths of sulphuret of potassium, dissolved in warm water, by which the salts of lead, deposited on the skin, are converted into the insoluble sulphuret. The iodide of potassium is employed as an *eliminative* remedy. For lead-colic, a combination of cathartics and opiates has been employed; but the best remedy is alum, in doses of ℨj or ℨij, every three or four hours, dissolved in some demulcent liquid. In the treatment of lead-palsy, strychnia and electricity may be used, but it is a very intractable form of the disease. The use of sulphuric acid lemonade is resorted to, by workmen in lead factories, as preventive of lead-poisoning. Milk has been found also to answer the same purpose. By passing a strong solution of the sulphuret of potassium or of sodium, heated to the temperature of 212° F., through leaden pipes, the interior surface will become coated with an insoluble sulphuret of lead, and the water distributed through them will be free from contamination.

Therapeutically, the preparations of lead are employed as astringents, sedatives, and desiccants. For internal use, the acetate is almost exclusively employed. It is a most valuable remedy in hemorrhages, from its combined sedative and astringent influence, and is also very serviceable in fluxes from the mucous membranes, particularly of the bowels. Topically, lead-washes are employed to relieve superficial inflammation, to arrest morbid discharges, and as desiccants. They are objectionable, however, as eye-washes, from their often forming precipitates of lead upon the cornea, which are highly injurious.

PLUMBI ACETAS (*Acetate of Lead*). This salt ($Pb2C_2H_3O_2$), known also as *Saccharum Saturni* or *Sugar of Lead*, is made by immersing lead in distilled vinegar, or litharge in pyroligneous or crude acetic acid. It occurs in colourless, needle-shaped crystals, which effloresce on exposure to the air. They have an acetous odour, and a sweetish, astringent taste, and are soluble in both water and alcohol. The mineral acids and their soluble salts, the alkalies and alkaline earths, and vegetable astringents, are *incompatible* with acetate of lead.

Effects and Uses.—The effects of this salt are those of the saturnine preparations, which have been already described. Its medicinal influence is sedative and astringent. In hemorrhages, it is more employed *internally* than any other remedy, usually in combination with opium. And this combination is also much resorted to in the treatment of diarrhœa, dysentery, and cholera, and may be prescribed with advantage to arrest the secretion of bronchitis and the night sweats of phthisis, and in the cure of internal aneurism. In yellow fever, it is employed to check the hemorrhagic condition of the gastric mucous membrane. It is a dangerous remedy in chronic diseases, from the liability to lead-poisoning. As a *topical* remedy, acetate of lead, in aqueous solution, is extensively employed to relieve inflammation and diminish morbid discharges.

Dose, gr. j or ij to gr. viij, two or three times a day. When applied to mucous membranes, the strength of the solution may be gr. ss to gr. j or ij, to water f℥j—for phlegmonous inflammation, ʒij to water Oj. *Suppositories of Lead* (*Suppositoria Plumbi*) contain each 3 grains of acetate of lead; for *suppositories of lead and opium*, see p. 58.

Liquor Plumbi Subacetatis (*Solution of Subacetate of Lead*). This preparation, frequently termed *Goulard's Extract*, is an aqueous solution of the diacetate of lead ($Pb_3O_22C_2H_3O_2$), and is made by boiling acetate of lead and litharge in distilled water. It is a colourless liquid, of sp. gr. 1.267, which is decomposed on exposure to the air, with the formation of insoluble carbonate of lead, and occasions a dense white precipitate with solution of gum. In other respects it resembles a solution of acetate of lead.

Uses.—It is chiefly employed, diluted, to promote the

resolution of external inflammation and arrest discharges from suppurating, ulcerated, and mucous surfaces. The officinal dilution is *Liquor Plumbi Subacetatis Dilutus*, commonly known as *lead-water*, and consists of solution f℥iij, to distilled water Oj. *Ceratum Plumbi Subacetatis*, or *Goulard's Cerate*, is made by mixing four troyounces of melted white wax with seven troyounces of olive oil, afterwards adding two fluidounces and a half of Goulard's extract, and thirty grains of camphor dissolved in a troyounce of olive oil; it is an admirable dressing to excoriated and blistered surfaces, burns, scalds, &c.

Plumbi Iodidum (*Iodide of Lead*) (PbI_2), is made by the double reaction of solutions of nitrate of lead and iodide of potassium. It is a bright-yellow, heavy, inodorous powder, volatilizable by heat, sparingly soluble in cold water, but more soluble in boiling water. It is chiefly used to reduce the volume of indolent tumours, and may be given internally in the dose of gr. iij or iv, or more, in pill; but it is principally employed externally in the form of *ointment* (ʒj to ointment 420 grains).

Plumbi Nitras (*Nitrate of Lead*) ($Pb2NO_3$) made by dissolving litharge in diluted nitric acid, occurs in white, nearly opaque, octohedral crystals, permanent in the air, of a sweet, astringent taste, and soluble in water and alcohol. It may be given *internally*, as a sedative astringent, in doses of gr. ¼ to gr. j, twice or thrice daily, in pill or solution. But its principal use is as a topical agent in the treatment of wounds, ulcers, and cutaneous affections. *Ledoyen's Disinfecting Fluid* is a solution of nitrate of lead ʒj in water f℥j.

Plumbi Oxidum (*Oxide of Lead*) (PbO) or *Litharge*, is prepared by blowing air through melted lead, and is also obtained in the process for extracting silver from argentiferous galenas. It occurs in minute yellowish or orange-coloured scales, insoluble in water, and is never employed *internally*. It is sometimes sprinkled over ulcers, but its chief use is in the preparation of *Emplastrum Plumbi* or *Lead-Plaster* (called also *diachylon*), which is made by boiling litharge (thirty troyounces) with olive oil (fifty-six troyounces) and water, and is, chemically, a mixture of oleate and margarate of lead. It serves as a basis for most of the other plasters. *Emplastrum Saponis* (*Soap-Plaster*), made by rubbing up soap (four troyounces) with lead plaster (thirty-six troyounces), is an excellent discutient. *Soap-Cerate* is made by melting together two troyounces of soap-plaster and two troyounces and a half of yellow wax, and afterwards adding four troyounces of olive oil.

PLUMBI CARBONAS (*Carbonate of Lead*), or *White Lead* ($PbCO_3$) is manufactured in this country by exposing lead to the fumes of vinegar or acetic acid, carbonic acid being derived from the fermentation of tan, in which the pots containing lead are packed; acetate of the protoxide of lead, as formed, is converted into carbonate. It is a white powder, without smell or taste, and insoluble in water, and, as it occurs in commerce, is a compound of the carbonate and hydrate of lead ($PbCO_3$+Pb2HO). It is never administered *internally*, but it is employed as a dusting powder—though there is danger of its absorption. *Unguentum Plumbi Carbonatis* (60 grains to ointment 420 grains), is a good application to burns, &c. White paint is used for the same purpose; but, when applied to a large surface, it may produce lead-poisoning.

ALUMEN—ALUM.

Alum is a double salt, a sulphate of aluminium and ammonium ($Al_2 3SO_4, Am_2SO_4, 24H_2O$). It is found native in Italy, in the neighbourhood of Rome, but is usually manufactured from aluminous schist, and sometimes by the direct combination of its constituents. It crystallizes in regular octohedrons; but it is commonly found in the shops in large, colourless, transparent crystalline masses, without any regular form. It has an astringent and sweetish acid taste; by exposure to the air it slowly effloresces; it is soluble in cold water, and more so in boiling water; and when heated, it undergoes the watery fusion, swells up, gives out its water of crystallization, and is converted into a white, spongy mass, called *dried alum*. The alkalies and their carbonates, lime-solution, magnesia and its carbonate, tartrate of potassium, acetate of lead, and the vegetable astringents, are *incompatible* with alum.

Besides the ammonia alum, there are varieties in which the ammonia is replaced by some other base, as potassa or soda; the alum of commerce was formerly the sulphate of aluminium and potassium ($Al_23SO_4,K_2SO_4,24H_2O$), but this has been superseded by ammonia alum.

Physiological Effects.—The immediate topical effect of alum is that of a powerful astringent, in virtue of a chemical action on the tissues. When it is applied to a part, in large quantities, the astriction is soon followed by irritation; and thus, taken internally in excessive doses, it gives rise to vomiting, griping, purging, and even inflammation of the gastro-enteric mucous membrane. After its absorption, it acts as an astringent on the system generally, and produces astriction of the tissues and fibres, and a diminution of secretion.

Medicinal Uses.—Alum is employed *internally* in hemorrhages, chronic diarrhœa, colliquative sweating, diabetes, &c., and it is sometimes combined with cubeb in the treatment of gleet, gonorrhœa, and leucorrhœa. It has been recommended in dilatation of the heart and aneurism of the aorta, and has also been given as an emetic in croup. Its use in lead-colic has been alluded to. As a *topical* remedy, it is extremely valuable as an astringent antiphlogistic, in ophthalmia, diphtheria, tonsillitis, &c.; to produce contraction of the tissues, in relaxation of the uvula, prolapsus ani, &c.; as a styptic in hemorrhages; and to arrest excessive secretion from the mucous surfaces. In hemoptysis and bronchitis, a strong solution of alum may be applied by atomization.

Dose, gr. x. to ℈j or ℈ij, in powder, or solution, or made into pills, with some tonic extract, and combined with an aromatic, as nutmeg, to prevent nausea. It may be agreeably given in the form of *whey*, prepared by boiling ʒij with milk Oj, and straining, of which the dose is f℥ij. *Topically*, it is employed in the forms of powder, solution, and poultice, the latter of which is made by rubbing up whites of eggs with alum, and is applied to the eye in ophthalmia, between folds of linen. *Dried alum* (*alumen exsiccatum*), is employed internally in the dose of gr. v–x, and externally as a mild escharotic.

ALUMINII SULPHAS (*Sulphate of Aluminium*) ($Al_2 3SO_4$, $9H_2O$), is employed externally as an astringent and antiseptic application to ulcers, an injection in gonorrhœa, &c. The aqueous solution is used to preserve bodies for dissection. A paste, made of a mixture of sulphate of aluminium and sp. nitrous ether, applied to the cavity of a carious tooth, is a good remedy for toothache.

ORDER VI.—STIMULANTS.

Stimulants are medicines, which produce a rapid and temporary exaltation of the vital functions. Their influence is most conspicuous in conditions of morbid depression, when a marked tolerance of their action is established, and large amounts are borne. In health, when the powers of the system are at the normal standard, stimulants soon induce depression. *Topically*, they irritate and inflame the parts to which they are applied, and hence are classed with *irritants*.

They are employed principally in disorders known as asthenic, and in all conditions of the system attended with exhaustion. From their action in arousing the energies of the nervous system, they exercise a control over many nervous disorders, particularly those of a spasmodic nature. They are also frequently given with a view to their action on some one or other of the secretions. As stimulants to the gastro-intestinal canal, they are administered to promote digestion (when they are called *stomachics*), and to dispel flatulence (when they are known as *carminatives*). Topically, they are employed as *rubefacients*, *vesicants*, &c.

The more powerful and rapid stimulants are called *diffusible*. In overdoses, they act as violent narcotics and sedatives. The diffusible stimuli usually employed are vinous and spirituous liquors, and the preparations of ammonia. Vegetable stimulants which contain a volatile oil, are termed *aromatics*, and are usually given as stomachics and carminatives. Their volatile oils are also employed as local irritants.

DIFFUSIBLE STIMULANTS.

ALCOHOL.

Alcohol is a product which results from a process termed the vinous fermentation, in substances containing grape-sugar. At a temperature of 80° F., the presence of a fermenting body converts a solution of grape-sugar into alcohol and carbonic acid. Starchy substances, being convertible into grape-sugar, also yield alcohol. Alcohol is obtained from vinous or fermented liquors, by repeated distillation. It is, chemically, a hydrated oxide of ethyl, C_2H_5HO. For officinal purposes, it should be of the specific gravity 0.835, when it contains about fifteen per cent. of water. It is a colourless, inflammable liquid, wholly vaporizable by heat, and unites in all proportions with water and ether. Contamination of fusel oil or amylic alcohol may be detected by agitation with concentrated sulphuric acid, when, if the alcohol become coloured, the presence of the impurity is indicated in proportion to the depth of the colour; or solution of nitrate of silver, with exposure to a bright light, will convert fusel oil into a black powder. *A stronger alcohol, alcohol fortius*, sp. gr. 0.817, is made by shaking officinal alcohol with heated carbonate of potassium. This is nearly free from water and fusel oil, and is used for pharmaceutical purposes.

Physiological Effects.—Alcohol is the intoxicating ingredient of all vinous and spirituous liquors. It is a powerful diffusible stimulant, the effects of which are most conspicuous in disease, while, in health, it soon begins to produce narcosis—in small doses, exciting the vascular and nervous systems, increasing the heat of the body, exhilarating the mental faculties, and stimulating the secretions; in larger amounts, disordering the stomach, destroying the control of the will over the voluntary muscles, and inducing incoherence, delirium, sopor, or other form of derangement of the intellectual functions; and, in excessive quantity, acting as a narcotic poison, producing coma and death.

The treatment in cases of poisoning from alcohol is the same as that which is to be pursued in cases of poisoning from opium. Ammonia is a physiological antidote. The habitual use of alcoholic narcotics in excess gives rise to a well-known train of mental and physical disorders: dyspepsia, visceral obstructions, cirrhosis of the liver, gout, dropsy, mania-a-potu, paralysis, and even confirmed insanity. *Topically*, alcohol acts as an irritant.

Medicinal Uses.—Alcohol, in the form of vinous and spirituous liquors, is employed to rouse and support the system in debility, asphyxia, syncope, the latter stages of acute attacks, typhoid and typhus fevers, asthenic and malignant diseases, exhausting hemorrhages and suppurations, gangrene, to counteract the effects of the bites of venomous reptiles, in mania-a-potu, and in poisoning from digitalis, tobacco, and other narcotics: also as a stomachic in colic, flatulence, indigestion, nausea, &c. In typhoid and typhus fevers, alcohol probably acts as a physiological antidote to the blood-poison, and should be given in the very first stage of the fevers. Indeed, the early administration of the preparations containing alcohol furnishes our best means of counteracting the depressing action of disease in general. As a topical application, alcohol is used to produce cold by its evaporation; as a styptic; to harden the cuticle over delicate parts; and as a stimulant. Mixed with white of eggs, it forms a good coating to bed-sores.

ALCOHOL DILUTUM (*Diluted Alcohol*), or *Proof Spirit*, consists of equal parts of alcohol and distilled water, and has a sp. gr. 0.941. It is used exclusively for pharmaceutical purposes.

VINUM (*Wine*). The fermented juice of the grape consists of water and alcohol in varying proportions, with volatile oil, œnanthic acid and ether, tannic, malic, and other acids, bitartrate of potassium, &c. Wine loses most of its cream of tartar by age. It is employed medicinally in typhus and typhoid fevers, exhausting chronic diseases, extensive suppurations, gangrene, &c. In typh-fevers, it constitutes our chief therapeutic resource, and may be administered to the amount of one or two pints, in the twenty-four hours, either pure, or in the form of *wine-whey*. This is made by adding from a gill to half a pint of white wine to a pint of boiling milk, separating the curd from the whey, and flavouring with sugar and spices.

The officinal wines are VINUM XERICUM (*Sherry Wine*), and VINUM PORTENSE (*Port Wine*). Port contains tannic acid, and is preferred in dysentery, diarrhœa, &c., for its astringency. *Madeira*, which is the strongest of the white wines, is an excellent stimulant, but may be objectionable from its acidity. *Champagne* is a pleasant stimulant, where gastric irritability is present. Madeira and Port contain about 23 per cent of alcohol; Sherry, 19 per cent.; Champagne, 13 per cent. As articles of diet, the stronger wines, when used in excess, often produce gout, dropsy, and diseases of the kidneys and liver; and, except in advanced age, and in feeble constitutions, or where the tuberculous diathesis exists, cannot but be considered as objectionable.

The *malt liquors* are useful where more permanent stimuli are called for, as in diseases tending to emaciation, chronic abscesses, &c. The best are porter and ale.

SPIRITUS VINI GALLICI (*Brandy*), is obtained by the distillation of wine. It contains about 50 per cent. of alcohol, with water, volatile oil, tannic acid, colouring matter, &c. It is the best stimulus, where a rapid and decided impression is called for, as in collapse, syncope, &c.; and, from the tannic acid which it contains, is useful in bowel-complaints. SPIRITUS FRUMENTI (*Whisky*), obtained from fermented grain by distillation, is of about the same alcoholic strength as brandy, and may be substituted for it; it does not contain tannic acid. RUM (*Spiritus Sacchari*), the ardent spirit obtained from sugar, is more sudorific than brandy. GIN (*Spiritus Juniperi*), is corn spirit flavoured with oil of juniper; and, owing to the oil of juniper, which it holds in solution, it is an active diuretic as well as stimulant and stomachic. *Arrack*, the spirit of Eastern countries, is prepared from a fermented infusion of rice. SPIRITUS MYRCIÆ (*Spirit of Myrcia*), *Bay-rum*, the spirit obtained by distilling rum with the leaves of myrcia acris, is a refreshing local application.

AMMONIÆ PRÆPARATA—PREPARATIONS OF AMMONIA.

Ammonia is a gaseous compound of hydrogen and nitrogen (NH_3), usually obtained by the action of lime on sal ammoniac (or chloride of ammonium). It is a powerful stimulant and local irritant, but is rarely used in medicine. The following preparations of Ammonia are employed as diffusible stimuli:

AQUA AMMONIÆ FORTIOR (*Stronger Water of Ammonia*). This is an aqueous solution of ammonia, of the specific gravity 0.900. It is a colourless liquid, wholly volatilizable by heat, of a caustic, acrid taste, and a very pungent odour of ammonia; and is too strong for medicinal use, internally, in its unmixed state, containing 26 per cent. of gaseous ammonia. It is a powerful corrosive poison, for which the diluted acids, as vinegar, lemon juice, &c., are the proper antidotes. It is used externally as a vesicant, and has the advantage over cantharides of a more speedy operation and non-affection of the urinary organs.

AQUA AMMONIÆ (*Water of Ammonia*), has a specific gravity of 0.960, containing nearly 10 per cent. of ammonia, and is employed as a stimulant, sudorific, antacid, and rubefacient. As a stimulant, ammonia is admirably adapted for speedily rousing the action of the vascular and respiratory systems, especially when it is an object at the same time to promote the action of the skin. For this purpose it is employed in low forms of disease, particularly in the typhoid exanthemata, in syncope, in asphyxia from narcotic poisons, and to counteract the effects of the bites of venomous reptiles. In dyspepsia, it is useful with a view to the relief both of acidity and flatulence. For internal use, other preparations of ammonia are generally preferred, and this is used chiefly as a rubefacient. Dose, internally, ten to thirty drops, largely diluted. As a *rubefacient*, the officinal *liniment* may be used (a fluidounce of water of ammonia to two troyounces of olive oil).

SPIRITUS AMMONIÆ (*Spirit of Ammonia*), is a solution of

ammonia in alcohol. It is given as a stimulant, antispasmodic, and carminative, in the dose of ten to thirty drops, diluted with water. But a pleasanter preparation, with similar properties, is

SPIRITUS AMMONIÆ AROMATICUS (*Aromatic Spirit of Ammonia*). This is made by dissolving a troyounce of carbonate of ammonium in three fluidounces of water of ammonia, previously mixed with four fluidounces of water, then dissolving two fluidrachms and a half of oil of lemon, forty minims of oil of nutmeg, and fifteen minims of oil of lavender, in a pint and a half of alcohol, afterwards mixing the two solutions, and adding water enough to make the whole measure two pints. It is a very agreeable antacid stomachic and stimulant, and may be given in the dose of thirty drops to f℥j, or more, diluted with water.

AMMONII CARBONAS (*Carbonate of Ammonium*). This salt, sometimes termed *volatile alkali*, is a *sesquicarbonate*, ($N_4H_{16}C_3O_8$), and is prepared by subliming a mixture of chloride of ammonium and chalk. It occurs in whitish, transparent masses, wholly dissipated by heat, of a pungent, ammoniacal odour, an acrid, alkaline taste, and is soluble without residue in water. On exposure to the air it becomes opaque, falls into powder, and deteriorates by the loss of ammonia.

Effects and Uses.—Its indications are the same as those of solution of ammonia, to which it is preferred for internal exhibition as a diffusible stimulant. It is especially valuable in pneumonia, and by some therapeutists is relied on to the exclusion of other medication in this disease. It has also been recommended in diabetes, and in scrofula, attended with a languid circulation. Dose, gr. v to xx, in pill, or preferably in solution with gum and sugar. Mixed with some aromatic oil (as that of bergamot or lavender), it is used as a *smelling salt*, in syncope, hysteria, &c.

ARNICA.

Arnica montana, Leopard's-bane (*Nat. Ord.* Asteraceæ), is a perennial, herbaceous plant, found in northern Germany and other northern countries of Europe, and also in the north-western portions of America. The FLOWERS are described by the U. S. Pharmacopœia as the officinal portion, but the article of commerce consists really of the HEADS, from which frequently the involucre has been removed; they are brought here from Germany. They are large, of a fine orange-yellow colour, of a strong, disagreeable odour, when fresh (which is diminished by desiccation), and an acrid, bitterish taste. The root also is used in Europe. Both contain a *volatile oil,* and an alkaloid principle termed *arnicina* has been found in them. Arnica is a stimulant, with emetic and cathartic properties in large doses. Its effects, internally, are not very well understood in this country, where it is little used, except *externally,* in the form of fomentation, or lotion, for the relief of bruises, sprains, and local paralysis. The *extract* (*alcoholic*), is given in doses of gr. v–x. This is chiefly used, however, in making a *plaster* (*emplastrum arnicæ,* one part of extract to two parts of previously melted resin plaster). The *tincture* (six troy-ounces to alcohol Ojss, water Oss, with, after percolation, the addition of diluted alcohol enough to measure Oij) is used as a local stimulant, often mixed with soap liniment.

PHOSPHORUS is obtained from the phosphate of calcium of *bone-ash,* by removing the lime with sulphuric acid, and afterwards deoxidizing the residuum by heating with charcoal. It is a translucent, highly inflammable, nearly colourless solid, resembling wax, without taste, but having a peculiar garlicky smell: sp. gr. 1.8. It is insoluble in water, and dissolves sparingly even in the oils, ether, and alcohol, but is readily soluble in chloroform. It emits, when exposed to the air, white fumes, which are luminous in the dark. In medicinal doses, phosphorus is a valuable stimulant to the nutrition of the tissues, and has been employed with advantage in cases of nervous exhaustion and degeneration of nerve-tissue, and especially in neuralgia. In overdoses, however, it is a most violent poison, being probably absorbed unchanged into the blood, and not converted into phosphoric acid, as was at one time supposed; it acts as a blood-poison, and among its effects is the production of acute fatty degeneration of the tissues. In cases of poisoning from phosphorus, after the administration of an emetic, *magnesia* should be given, suspended in large quantities of mucilaginous drinks. The oil of turpentine is also recommended as an antidote; it acts best when old; oxygenated water has been also used; oils and fats are to be avoided. Therapeutically, the dose is $\frac{1}{12}$ of a grain, dissolved in absolute alcohol, 3 or 4 times a day, to which some aromatic water may be added; melted resin, (24 parts to 1 part of phosphorus), is a good solvent.

THE PHOSPHURET OF ZINC has lately been employed in cases where the administration of phosphorus is indicated. It is prepared by passing the vapour of phosphorus over zinc heated to ebullition, in a current of dry hydrogen, and occurs as a gray, crystallized body, unaltered by moist air, and easily decomposed in the stomach, with the evolution of phosphuretted hydrogen. Dose, about gr. $\frac{1}{66}$.

AROMATICS.

Aromatics owe their virtues to the presence of oils obtained from them by distillation, and termed VOLATILE OILS (*olea volatilia*), sometimes also *distilled* and *essential* oils. These oils possess, in a high degree, the odour and taste of the plants from which they are procured. Locally, they are powerful irritants, and, taken into the stomach in overdoses, act as acrid poisons. They pass partially into vapour at ordinary temperatures, and are completely volatilized by heat; hence, decoctions and extracts are improper preparations of the aromatics. The distilled oils are inflammable, very slightly soluble in water, but soluble in alcohol and ether. Their ultimate constituents are usually, carbon, hydrogen, and oxygen; and, on exposure to the air, they gradually absorb oxygen, become thicker, less odorous, and of a deeper colour, and are finally converted into resins.

CAPSICUM.

Capsicum or Cayenne pepper is the FRUIT of Capsicum annuum, C. fastigiatum, and other species of Capsicum (*Nat. Ord.* Solanaceæ), American tropical plants, naturalized in most warm climates, and cultivated in our gardens. C. annuum is an annual, about two feet high, with an herbaceous, crooked, branching stem; ovate, pointed leaves; greenish-white flowers; and pendulous, pod-like berries of a crimson or yellow colour, two or three inches long. These pods, when dried and ground, form Capsicum, the best of which is the *African.* Powdered Capsicum has a bright-red colour, which fades upon exposure to light; an aromatic, peculiar smell, and a bitterish, acrid, burning taste. An alkaloid principle termed *capsicia*, slightly soluble in water, but very much so in alcohol, ether, and oil of turpentine, exists in capsicum, associated with resin and volatile oil.

Effects and Uses.—Capsicum is principally employed as a *condiment* and *stomachic*, and is very useful in torpid conditions of the digestive organs, or as an adjunct to other remedies, to rouse the susceptibility of the stomach. Its constitutional effect is not in proportion to its local effect, and it is therefore of no great efficiency as a diffusible stimulant. It has, however, been recommended in cynanche maligna and scarlatina anginosa. It is a good stomachic in the dyspepsia of drunkards. As a gargle, it is much employed in the sore throat of scarlatina, and also as a cataplasm to cause counter-irritation. Dose of the *powder*, gr. v to gr. x, in pill; of the *tincture* (a troyounce to diluted alcohol Oij), f℥j or f℥ij; of the *infusion*, which is used also for a gargle (half a troyounce to boiling water Oj) f℥ss. The *oleoresin* is a powerful rubefacient, and may be given internally in the dose of a drop.

PIPER—BLACK PEPPER.

Black pepper is the UNRIPE BERRIES of Piper Nigrum (*Nat. Ord.* Piperaceæ), a vine of the East Indies. The berries are gathered before they are quite ripe, and dried in the sun. They are wrinkled and black, in consequence of the drying of the pulp over the grayish-white seed, and in this state are known as *black* pepper. If permitted to ripen, and soaked in water till the outer coat is removed, they constitute *white* pepper. Pepper has an aromatic, peculiar odour, and a hot, spicy, pungent taste. Its properties are taken up by alcohol and ether, and partially by water. It contains a volatile oil, an acrid resin, and a peculiar alkaloid crystalline principle, called *piperin* or *piperia* ($C_{17}H_{19}NO_3$), which has been used as an anti-intermittent remedy.

Effects and Uses.—Pepper is a warm carminative stimulant, chiefly employed as a condiment; but it is also a useful stomachic, and a good adjunct to bark in the treatment of intermittent fevers. Dose, gr. v to gr. xx. Of the *oleoresin* the dose is 1–3 drops.

CINNAMOMUM—CINNAMON.

There are two varieties of cinnamon: Ceylon cinnamon, which is the prepared BARK of Cinnamomum Zeylanicum (*Nat. Ord.* Lauraceæ), a tree of Ceylon and Java; and China Cinnamon, or Cassia, the prepared BARK of Cinnamomum aromaticum (*Nat. Ord.* Lauraceæ), a tree of China. The most esteemed is the *Ceylon* cinnamon. To obtain this, the bark is peeled from branches which are three years old; the epidermis is afterwards scraped off; the smaller quills are introduced into the larger ones, and they are then dried in the sun and made into bundles. It is found in the shops in long, cylindrical pieces, which are very thin and smooth, and of a yellow-brown colour, and a splintery fracture. It has a fragrant odour, and a warm, sweetish, aromatic, slightly astringent taste. Its constituents are volatile oil, a little tannic acid, mucilage, an acid, lignin, &c. The greater part, however, of the cinnamon brought to this country is the *cassia* cinnamon. It has the general appearance, smell, and taste of true cinnamon. But its substance is thicker, its texture coarser, its fracture shorter, its colour darker, browner, and duller, and its flavour less sweet, and more pungent and astringent. Its properties are identical with those of the Ceylon variety.

Effects and Uses.—Cinnamon is an aromatic stimulant, with a slight astringency. It is used chiefly as a carminative, and as an addition to other medicines. Dose, gr. x to ʒss; of the *tincture* (three troyounces to two measures of alcohol with one measure of water Oij), the dose is fʒj to fʒiij. *Oleum cinnamomi* (*oil of cinnamon*), is of a light-yellow colour, which deepens by exposure to the air, with the development of an acid, termed *cinnamic;* dose, one or two drops. *Aqua cinnamomi* (*cinnamon water*), is prepared by rubbing up the oil with carbonate of magnesium, adding distilled water, and filtering.* It is used as a vehicle for other medicines. *Spiritus cinnamomi* (*spirit of cinnamon*), contains one part of the oil dissolved in fifteen parts of stronger alcohol; dose, ten to twenty drops. Cinnamon enters into a large number of preparations.

MYRISTICA—NUTMEG.

MACIS—MACE.

These products are portions of the FRUIT of Myristica fragrans (*Nat. Ord.* Myristicaceæ), a tree of the Moluccas, cultivated also in Java and Sumatra, and other parts of the East Indies, and introduced into the isles of France and Bourbon, and several of the West India islands. It bears a pyriform fruit, about the size of a small peach, which has a fleshy pericarp, opened by two longitudinal valves. Within this is the

* The *waters* of the aromatic oils are all made by rubbing up half a fluid-drachm of the oil with 60 grains of carbonate of magnesium, then with two pints of distilled water, and afterwards filtering.

ARILLUS, a scarlet reticulated membrane, which, when dry, becomes yellow-brown and brittle, and is termed *mace.* The KERNELS of the fruit are the *nutmegs.*

They are oval, of the size of an olive, of a greyish-brown colour, marked with furrows; and to preserve them from the attacks of an insect, they are steeped in a mixture of lime and water. Mace has a pleasant, aromatic smell, and a warm, bitterish, pungent taste. Nutmegs have a delightfully fragrant odour, and a warm, aromatic, grateful taste.

Nutmeg contains a volatile oil, and by expression yields a fatty substance, known as "butter of nutmegs." From mace, also, a volatile oil is obtained by distillation.

Effects and Uses.—Nutmeg is one of the most agreeable of the aromatic stimulants, and is much employed for its carminative virtues, also as a flavouring ingredient, and to obviate the griping effects of cathartics. It is said to have narcotic properties, and hence may be useful in bowel complaints. Mace is chiefly employed as a condiment. Dose of either, ℈j to ʒss. *Oleum myristicæ* (*oil of nutmeg*), is of a pale straw-colour; dose, 2 or 3 drops. *Spiritus myristicæ* is made by dissolving a fluidounce of the oil in three pints of stronger alcohol; dose, f℥j or f℥ij.

CARYOPHYLLUS—CLOVES.

Cloves are the UNEXPANDED FLOWERS of Caryophyllus aromaticus (*Nat. Ord.* Myrtaceæ), an evergreen tree of the Moluccas. They are from five to ten lines long, and from one line to one line and a half thick, the corolla forming a ball or sphere at the top, and the calyx a tapering, somewhat quadrangular base, resembling a nail, whence the common name, from the French *clou.* When good, they are of a dark-brown colour, with a yellowish-red tint; they have a strong, fragrant odour, a hot, acrid taste, and, when pressed with the nail, should give out oil. They contain a highly pungent volatile oil, tannic acid, resin, &c., and two crystalline principles, termed *caryophyllin* and *eugenin;* the oil consists of two oils, a heavy oil and a light oil, the heavy oil being termed *caryophyllic acid.*

Effects and Uses.—Cloves are among the most stimulating of the aromatics, but are chiefly used as a flavouring ingredient and as a condiment. Dose, gr. v to gr. x. The *infusion* (ʒij, to boiling water Oj) is a warm, grateful stomachic, and will often relieve nausea. The *oil*, *oleum caryophylli*, is pale, or yellowish, becoming darker by age; dose, 2 to 6 drops.

PIMENTA—PIMENTO.

Pimento, called also *Allspice*, is the UNRIPE BERRIES of Eugenia Pimenta (*Nat. Ord.* Myrtaceæ), a handsome evergreen tree of the West Indies and South America. It comes exclusively from Jamaica, and consists of round, brown, roughish berries, rather larger than black peppercorns, with an external hard, brittle shell, inclosing two dark-brown seeds. They have an aromatic, agreeable smell, and a strong, clove-like taste. They are principally used as a condiment. The oil, *oleum pimentæ*, has a brownish-red colour, and consists of a light and heavy oil, the latter identical with caryophyllic acid; dose, 3 to 6 drops.

OLEUM CAJUPUTI (*Oil of Cajeput*). The volatile oil of the leaves of Melaleuca Cajuputi (*Nat. Ord.* Myrtaceæ), a tree of the Moluccas, is a powerful diffusible aromatic stimulant, much employed in Eastern countries, and of late coming into use in the United States. It is a transparent oil, of a fine green colour, a lively penetrating odour, analogous to that of camphor and cardamom, and a warm, pungent taste. It is an admirable stomachic, for the relief of nausea, and is also used as an antispasmodic stimulant in low fevers, spasmodic cholera, &c.; dose, 1 to 5 drops.

OLEUM TEREBINTHINÆ—OIL OF TURPENTINE.

Oil of turpentine, commonly called *spirit of turpentine*, is obtained by distillation from the turpentine of Pinus palustris and other species of Pinus (*Nat. Ord.* Pinaceæ). When pure, it is a limpid, colourless, volatile, and inflammable liquid, of a strong, penetrating, peculiar odour, and a hot, pungent, bitterish taste. It is lighter than water, very slightly soluble in it, less soluble in alcohol than most other volatile oils, and readily soluble in ether.

Effects and Uses.—Oil of turpentine is stimulant, diuretic, blennorrhetic, and anthelmintic, and, externally, rubefacient. As a stimulant, it is a very valuable remedy in typhoid fever, particularly where the abdomen is tympanitic, the tongue dry, and the bowels are ulcerated. It is employed also with advantage in morbid discharges from mucous membranes, hemorrhages, rheumatism, nervous disorders, atonic dropsy, gleet, nephritic and calculous affections, and as an anthelmintic in tænia. Enemata of the oil of turpentine are particularly serviceable for the relief of tympanites. Externally, it is used for purposes of counter-irritation.

Dose, as a stimulant or diuretic, five to thirty drops, repeated; as an anthelmintic or as an enema, f℥ss to f℥ij.

ZINGIBER—GINGER.

Ginger is the RHIZOME of Zingiber officinale (*Nat. Ord.* Zingiberaceæ) a perennial, herbaceous plant, growing to the height of two or three feet, with long, lanceolate leaves, and yellow flowers. Its native country is unknown: but it has been cultivated in Asia from time immemorial, and was early introduced into the tropical regions of America. Ginger-root occurs in flattish, jointed, branched or lobed, palmate pieces, which rarely exceed four inches in length. In the young state, the roots are preserved in sugar, and form a very pleasant sweetmeat. When old, they are taken up, scalded in hot water, and dried, when they are known as *black ginger*. Sometimes they are scraped, previously to being dried, and are then called *white* or *Jamaica ginger*. The former comes from the East Indies; the latter from the West Indies. The powder of black ginger is yellowish-brown; that of white ginger, yellowish-white. Both varieties have a powerful, peculiar odour, and a warm, pungent, aromatic taste. They impart their virtues to water and alcohol, and contain a pale-yellow volatile oil, resin, starch, &c.

Effects and Uses.—Ginger is a pungent, aromatic stimulant, much employed as a stomachic in flatulency, and spasm of the stomach and bowels. It is also used as a condiment, and to correct the unpleasant taste and nauseating qualities of other medicines. A paste made of the powder and warm water is used as a counter-irritant. Dose, gr. x to gr. xx, in pill. The officinal preparations are: *infusion* (half a troyounce to boiling water Oj), dose f℥ij; *tincture* (eight troyounces to alcohol Oij), dose ♏x–xx; *fluid extract*—dose 20 to 30 drops; *syrup* (made by rubbing up a fluidounce of the fluid extract with 160 grains of carbonate of magnesium, 2 troyounces of sugar, and 42 fluidounces of water, and filtering, and then dissolving in the liquid 70 ounces of sugar at a gentle heat); *oleoresin*—dose, 1 to 2 drops; and *troches* (made by mixing the tincture (f℥j) with tragacanth (ʒij), sugar (ten troyounces), and a little syrup of ginger, and dividing into 240 troches).

CARDAMOMUM—CARDAMOM.

Cardamom is the FRUIT of Elettaria Cardamomum (*Nat. Ord.* Zingiberaceæ), a perennial plant, from six to nine feet high, found in the mountainous parts of Malabar. Three varieties of Malabar cardamoms are known in commerce: *shorts*, *short-longs*, and *long-longs*, all furnished by the same plant. They are ovate-oblong, from three to ten lines long, coriaceous, ribbed, and of a grayish or brownish-yellow colour; and contain a number of blackish or reddish-brown seeds, which have a pleasant, aromatic odour, and a warm, aromatic, agreeable taste. They yield a colourless volatile oil, a fixed oil, starch, &c.

Effects and Uses.—Cardamom is a very agreeable aromatic, devoid of acridity, and is much employed as a stomachic and carminative, and as an adjuvant and corrective of other medicines; dose gr. v–x. The *tincture* (four troyounces to diluted alcohol Oij) is the preparation chiefly used; dose, fʒj or fʒij. The *compound tincture* contains cardamom (360 grains), and also caraway (120 grains), cinnamon (300 grains), cochineal (60 grains), percolated with diluted alcohol till two pints and six fluidounces of tincture are obtained, which is afterwards mixed with two troyounces of clarified honey.

Pulvis Aromaticus (*Aromatic Powder*), consists of cinnamon and ginger, each two parts, cardamom and nutmeg, each one part. Dose, gr. x to xxx. *Confectio aromatica* (*aromatic confection*), consists of aromatic powder rubbed up with an equal part of clarified honey; it is a pleasant vehicle for other medicines.

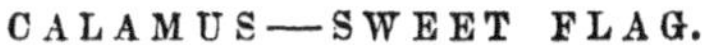

CALAMUS—SWEET FLAG.

Fig. 18.

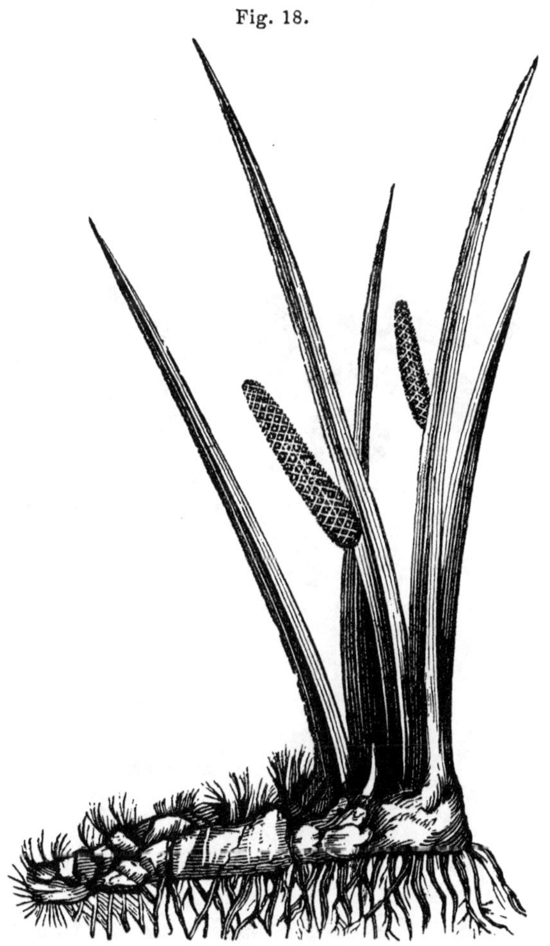

The rhizome of Acorus Calamus (*Nat. Ord.* Orontiaceæ), an indigenous marshy plant, with long, sword-shaped, radical leaves, is a valuable aromatic stimulant, with some tonic properties. It is found in the shops in somewhat flattened pieces, deprived of their epidermis, wrinkled, and of a yellowish-colour, and has a strong, fragrant odour, and a warm, bitterish, aromatic taste. It contains volatile oil, resin, extractive, &c. Dose, ℈j to ʒj, or it may be given in *infusion* (a troyounce to boiling water Oj)—not officinal.

GAULTHERIA.

Gaultheria procumbens, Partridge-berry, Deer-berry or Teaberry (*Nat. Ord.* Ericaceæ), is a small indigenous evergreen plant, with one, and sometimes two reddish stems, a few inches in height, bright-green, obovate, coriaceous, serrulated leaves,

Fig. 19.

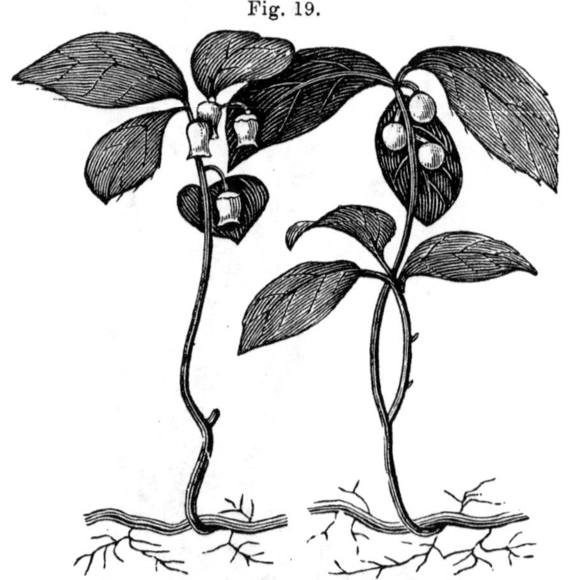

and white, ovate, five-toothed flowers, followed by scarlet berries. The LEAVES are the officinal portion, and contain a very stimulant volatile oil (*oleum gaultheriæ*), which, when first distilled, is colourless, but gradually becomes reddish, and is distinguished as being the heaviest of the volatile oils. An infusion of the leaves, and an essence or alcoholic solution of the oil, are in very general popular use as carminatives and stomachics.

AURANTII AMARI CORTEX—BITTER ORANGE PEEL.
AURANTII DULCIS CORTEX—SWEET ORANGE PEEL.

The RIND of the FRUIT of Citrus vulgaris, or Bitter Orange, and Citrus aurantium, or Sweet Orange (*Nat. Ord.* Aurantiaceæ), is much employed as a flavouring addition to other medicines. The *flowers* (*aurantii flores*) yield the delightful volatile oil termed oil of neroli, and are used in the form of *orange flower water* (*aqua aurantii florum*), as an agreeable vehicle, possessing slight antispasmodic virtues; *syrup of orange flowers* is made by dissolving 36 troyounces of sugar in 20 fluidounces of orange flower water; *confection of orange peel* (made by beating 12 troyounces of the grated sweet orange peel with 36 troyounces of sugar), and *syrup of orange peel*, are used as excipients and vehicles for medicines of unpleasant flavor; *tincture of* (bitter) *orange peel* contains 4 troyounces in 2 pints of diluted alcohol—dose, f℥i–ij.

The following aromatics, of the natural order LAMIACEÆ, are pleasant carminatives and stomachics:

LAVANDULA (*Lavender*). The FLOWERS of Lavandula vera, a small European shrub, cultivated in our gardens, about two feet high, with linear or lanceolate leaves, and purplish-gray flowers, which are gathered in June, and dried in the shade. They have an agreeable, fragrant odour, and a pungent bitter taste. The *oil*, which is of a pale-yellow colour, may be used in the dose of from one to five drops. But the preferred preparations are the *Spirit* (*Spiritus Lavandulæ*), made by dissolving a fluidounce of the oil in 3 pints of stronger alcohol, and the *Compound Spirit* (*Spiritus Lavandulæ Compositus*), which contains also oil of rosemary, cinnamon, cloves, nutmeg, and red saunders; dose, f℥j.

MENTHA PIPERITA (*Peppermint*), and MENTHA VIRIDIS

(*Spearmint*), are European plants, naturalized in the United States. The LEAVES and TOPS are employed; they have an aromatic odour, and a pungent, somewhat bitter taste, followed by a sensation of coolness. They contain volatile OILS, with some bitter extractive, &c. One to five drops of the *oils* may be given; but they are usually administered in the form of *spirit* (made by dissolving a fluidounce of the oil in 15 fluidounces of stronger alcohol, and afterwards macerating 120 grains of the mints in the solution), in the dose of ten to twenty or forty drops. A WATER is made by rubbing up either of the oils with carbonate of magnesium and water; the oil of peppermint is the stronger of the two. *Troches of Peppermint* are made by rubbing up a fluidrachm of oil of peppermint with 12 troyounces of sugar, and with mucilage of tragacanth, forming a mass to be divided into 480 troches.

ROSMARINUS (*Rosemary*). Rosmarinus officinalis, or Rosemary, a European evergreen shrub, cultivated in our gardens, contains a very stimulant *volatile oil*, which is chiefly used as an ingredient of rubefacient liniments. The LEAVES are used.

HEDEOMA (*Pennyroyal*). Hedeoma pulegioides, or Pennyroyal, is an indigenous annual plant, about a foot high, with oblong-lanceolate, serrated leaves, and small, pale-blue flowers, arranged in axillary whorls. The LEAVES and TOPS are used, which contain a light-yellow essential *oil*, similar in properties to the mint oils, but somewhat more powerful.

MONARDA (*Horsemint*). The LEAVES and TOPS of Monarda punctata, or horsemint, an indigenous plant. The essential *oil* is used chiefly as a rubefacient.

ORIGANUM. The HERB of Origanum vulgare, or common Marjoram. The essential *oil* is an ingredient in stimulating liniments.

MARRUBIUM (*Horehound*). Marrubium vulgare possesses combined stimulant, tonic, and expectorant properties, and, in large doses, proves laxative. It is chiefly used in cough syrups and candies. The LEAVES and TOPS are employed.

SALVIA (*Sage*). The LEAVES of Salvia officinalis, a European plant, cultivated in our gardens, are used as a condiment, and as a gargle in sore throat and relaxed uvula; they are slightly tonic and astringent, as well as aromatic.

THYMUS (*Thyme*). The HERB of Thymus vulgaris yields an essential oil, *oleum thymi*, which is often substituted for oil of origanum, and is used as an external application.

The following aromatic SEEDS are derived from plants of the natural order APIACEÆ:

FŒNICULUM (*Fennel*). The FRUIT of Fœniculum dulce, a European plant, cultivated in our gardens. It may be used in infusion; the dose of the *oil* is 5 to 15 drops. *Fennel water* is officinal.

CARUM (*Caraway*). The FRUIT of Carum Carui, a European plant, cultivated in this country. Dose of the *oil*, 1 to 10 drops.

ANISUM (*Anise*). The FRUIT of Pimpinella Anisum, originally a native of Egypt, but now cultivated throughout the south of Europe. Dose of the *oil*, 5 to 15 drops. *Anise water* is officinal. *Spirit of Anise* contains the *oil*, f℥i, in *stronger alcohol*, f℥xv. The *oil* of the fruit of Illicium anisatum, or Star Anise, an evergreen tree of Japan and China, possesses analogous properties to those of oil of anise, and is much used as a substitute for it.

CORIANDRUM (*Coriander*), the FRUIT of Coriandrum sativum, an annual plant of the south of Europe.

VANILLA.

This is the prepared, unripe FRUIT of Vanilla aromatica (*Nat. Ord.* Orchidaceæ), a climbing plant of Cuba and Mexico. The pods, when gathered, are yellow, but, by exposure to the sun, they assume a dark copper colour. They are cylindrical, somewhat flattened, wrinkled, six or eight inches long, three or four lines thick, and contain a soft, black pulp, in which numerous small black seeds are embedded. Vanilla has a strong, characteristic, highly pleasant odour, and a warm, aromatic, sweetish taste; the interior pulpy portion is most aromatic. The composition of vanilla is not determined, but its aroma is probably due to a volatile oil, developed in the curing of the pod.

It is a mild diffusible stimulant, chiefly used, however, as a perfume and flavouring ingredient.

ORDER VII.—SEDATIVES.

Sedatives are medicines which diminish the frequency of the action of the circulation. Their therapeutic influence is, probably, of a stimulant character; while abating irritability and relieving irregularity of the action of the heart, their primary effect is to restore its force and tone, when morbidly depressed. They are employed therapeutically to reduce excitement of the vascular system.

With sedatives may be included also the medicinal agents termed *refrigerants*, comprising nearly all the neutral alkaline salts, as well as those in which the acid predominates, and the vegetable acids. These substances have little power of diminishing the ordinary or healthy temperature; but they lower febrile heat, allay thirst, restore the secretions, and in this way are very useful adjuvants in the treatment of febrile complaints.

DIGITALIS.

Digitalis purpurea, or Purple Foxglove (*Nat. Ord.* Scrophulariaceæ), is a biennial European plant, cultivated in our gardens, with an erect stem three or four feet high, large ovate-lanceolate, crenate, downy, and veiny leaves, of a dull-green colour, and handsome bell-shaped crimson or purple flowers, arranged in a long terminal spike. The seeds and LEAVES are both active, but the latter only are employed, *from plants of the second year's growth;* and those from the European wild plants are preferred, as the cultivated variety is thought to be inferior in virtue. The petioles are removed, and the leaves are then dried in baskets, in a dark place, in a drying-stove. When dried, they have a dull-green colour, with a faint odour, and a bitter, nauseous taste, and afford a fine deep-green powder.

Both leaves and powder should be preserved in well-stoppered bottles, covered externally with dark-coloured paper, and kept in a dark cupboard. And, as their medicinal activity is impaired by keeping, they should be renewed annually. They contain a neutral principle termed *digitalin*, which possesses similar properties to those of the leaves.

DIGITALIN (*digitalinum*) is officinal, and is obtained by first preparing a strong alcoholic solution, adding acetic acid and a little animal charcoal, and filtering; to the liquor, filtered and partially neutralized by ammonia, a strong watery solution of tannic acid is added, so long as a precipitate is produced; the washed filter (which is tannate of digitalin), is mixed with oxide of lead and dried; it is then treated again with animal charcoal and digested at a gentle heat with stronger alcohol; the alcoholic solution is evaporated to dryness, powdered, and washed with ether, which removes impurities and leaves the digitalin. It is a white, or yellowish-white powder, odourless, but of a very bitter taste; readily soluble in alcohol, chloroform, and acids, but nearly insoluble in water and ether; dose from $\frac{1}{60}$ to $\frac{1}{30}$ of a grain.

Physiological Effects.—The ordinary results of the administration of digitalis, in *small and repeated doses*, are an increase in the secretion of urine and a reduction of the frequency of the pulse, sometimes accompanied by nausea; but these effects are not constant. The influence of digitalis over the pulse is more marked in weak and debilitated persons, than in those who are robust and plethoric. Its effects, too, in this particular, are more easily obtained in the recumbent than in the erect posture, owing to the less force required in the former position, to carry on the circulation. In the repeated use of small doses of this medicine, a *cumulative effect* is sometimes observed: its powers are not manifested for a certain time, and effects are suddenly produced, which are attributable to the whole amount administered, giving rise to dangerous and even fatal syncope. In morbid conditions of the circulation, where it is irritable, abnormally quick, or irregular, digitalis is considered to exercise a primary medicinal effect, in *steadying* the pulse and restoring its force and regularity, while it diminishes morbid frequency. As regards its diuretic action, it is probably rather indirect than direct, and is most conspicuous where dropsical effusions are removed under its influence. It increases the amount of solids eliminated in the urine, except that of urea and uric acid, which are diminished under its use; hence it is a good remedy in gout. When too long continued, or taken in *excessive doses*, digitalis acts as an acro-narcotic poison, producing effects similar to those of tobacco, lobelia, &c., as, vomiting, purging, severe abdominal pains, vertigo, disordered vision, dilated pupils, syncope, and finally delirium and stupor, death being usually preceded by convulsions. In such cases, after evacuating the stomach, the diffusible stimuli, as brandy and carbonate of ammonium, should be administered. The quantity of digitalis, however, that may be given, especially in disease, without destroying life, is considerable. Chemical analysis affords no certain tests of the presence of digitalis or its active principle, and, in cases of suspected poisoning, the *physiological* test is to be resorted to; in the celebrated *Pommerais* case, the criminal was condemned, from the evidence derived from the administration of an extract, obtained from the stomach and bowels of the deceased party, to small animals, in whom were produced vomiting and marked diminution of the number of heart-beats, with intermittent and irregular action.

Medicinal Uses.—From its action on the circulation, digitalis has been used in fevers, inflammations, and hemorrhages, where bloodletting is inadmissible, as in hectic fever, tubercular hemoptysis, &c. In the treatment of diseases of the heart and great vessels, it is a remedy of the greatest value, but is to be prescribed with discrimination. In dilatation of the heart, in fatty degeneration, and in failure or irritability of heart-action generally, digitalis, by increasing the force of the cardiac contractions and by abating irregular movement, is always useful; in uncomplicated hypertrophy, it is objectionable. In valvular, especially mitral disease, as well as aortic constriction, if the heart's action be feeble, it is indicated. It is greatly esteemed in the treatment of dropsy; and in the varieties of this disorder, resulting from heart-disease, it is more employed than any other remedy, from its combined cardiac and diuretic influence. In delirium tremens, digitalis has lately been given in large doses, with excellent effect. It is thought that a physiological antagonism exists between digitalin and the alkaloids aconitia and delphinia.

Administration.—Digitalis is best given in *powder*, of which the dose is gr. j, two or three times a day, to be gradually increased. An *infusion* is officinal (ʒj to boiling water Oss, with tincture of cinnamon f℥j), dose, f℥ij–iv; but water is a bad solvent. The *tincture* (four troyounces to diluted alcohol Oij), is a better preparation—dose 10 to 50 drops, two or three times a day, to be gradually increased; of the *extract* (*alcoholic*), the dose is one-fourth of a grain, to begin with; of the *fluid extract*, the dose is ♏j. If digitalis produces wakefulness, a little opium should be combined with it.

VERATRUM VIRIDE—AMERICAN HELLEBORE.

Veratrum viride, known as Swamp Hellebore, Meadow Poke, Indian Poke, &c. (*Nat. Ord.* Melanthaceæ), is an indigenous swampy plant, growing to the height of from three to six feet, with greenish-yellow flowers. The RHIZOME is the officinal portion; it is an inch or two in length, thick and fleshy, with numerous whitish radicles, and is usually found in the shops in small pieces or fragments, of a dingy white colour. It has a bitter, acrid taste, which leaves a permanent impression in the mouth and fauces. It yields its virtues to water and alcohol, and contains two alkaloids, one soluble in ether, the other insoluble in that menstruum, neither of them being identical (as was at one time supposed) with *veratria*. For the former alkaloid, the name *veratroidia* has been proposed; for the latter, *viridia*. Viridia has little or no local irritant action, produces neither vomiting nor purging, exerts no direct influence on the brain, but acts as a depressant of the spinal cord and of the circulation. Veratroidia is a local irritant, emetic, and sometimes a cathartic, and a depressant also of the circulation.

Viridia has been employed to produce the sedative action of veratrum viride, having the advantage of being free from the nauseating and emetic influence which the plant itself often produces. Dose, gr. $\frac{1}{6}$ every hour.

Effects and Uses.—American hellebore is an active local irritant. Taken internally, it somewhat promotes the flow of urine, and in doses of about five grains proves emetic. In continued doses it produces a *marked sedative action on the circulation*, irrespective of the nausea induced, which indeed may be prevented by careful administration. It has not generally proved laxative. No fatal effects are recorded from its use; stimulants invariably counteracting any excessive sedation. Within a few years past, this medicine has been largely used in our Southern States in inflammatory and febrile affections, particularly pneumonia and typhoid fever, with a view to its sedative action. It has been also used in cardiac affections, and in gout, rheumatism, and neuralgia. Dose, of the *powder*, gr. i–ij to begin with; of the *tincture* (sixteen troyounces to alcohol Oij), 8 or 10 drops; of the *fluid extract*, 4 or 5 drops.

VERATRUM ALBUM—WHITE HELLEBORE.

The RHIZOME of Veratrum Album (*Nat. Ord.* Melanthaceæ), a mountainous European plant, is found in the shops in small, rough, wrinkled, conical, cylindrical pieces, blackish externally, and whitish internally; its odour, in the dried state, is feeble; its taste at first sweetish, afterwards bitterish, acrid, and burning. It contains veratria, and other principles.

Effects and Uses.—White hellebore is a local irritant. In moderate doses, it stimulates the secretions, and depresses the pulse. In larger doses, it is a violent emetic and cathartic. It is an ancient remedy, now, however, from its severity of action, comparatively little used. Dose, gr. ij, to begin with. A *wine* is prescribed, and an *ointment*, in itch. As an *errhine*, it is sometimes mixed with five or six parts of powdered liquorice-root, or other inert powder.

VERATRIA ($C_{32}H_{52}N_2O_8$) is usually obtained from Cevadilla, the seed of Veratrum Sabadilla (*Nat. Ord.* Melanthaceæ), a plant of Mexico. It is made by evaporating a strong tincture of the seeds to the consistence of an extract, from which the alkaloid is dissolved by diluted sulphuric acid, and afterwards precipitated by magnesia. For purification it is dissolved in alcohol, from which it is evaporated, again converted into a sulphate, decolorized by animal charcoal, and finally precipitated by ammonia. When pure it is white, but it is usually a grayish or brownish-white powder, without odour, but very irritant to the nostrils, and of a bitter, acrid taste, producing a sense of tingling or numbness in the tongue; scarcely soluble in cold water, but readily soluble in alcohol. It has an alkaline reaction, and strikes an intensely red colour with concentrated sulphuric acid. The most delicate test for veratria is Trapp's—a permanent lilac-red colour, resembling a solution of permanganate of potassium, afforded by heating it in muriatic acid. Its effects are locally those of an irritant, and, when rubbed on the skin, it causes a sensation of heat and tingling. Taken internally, in small doses, it stimulates the secretions and depresses the pulse, and in excessive doses, it is a violent poison, producing tetanic symptoms: it is without narcotic action on the brain, producing death from paralysis of the spinal cord. Stimulants and ethereal inhalation would be the proper treatment in case of poisoning. *Veratria* has been used *internally*, in nervous disorders, dropsies, gout, rheumatism, &c., in doses of gr. $\frac{1}{12}$ to $\frac{1}{6}$ repeated; but it is most used *externally*, in the form of *ointment* (gr. xx to lard a troyounce), or dissolved in alcohol, as an application to rheumatic, paralytic, or neuralgic parts.

GELSEMIUM—YELLOW JASMINE.

Gelsemium Sempervirens, Yellow or Carolina jasmine (*Nat. Ord.* Scrophulariaceæ), is a beautiful climbing plant of our Southern States, with a twining, smooth, and shining stem, perennial petiolate, lanceolate leaves, and beautiful, very fragrant flowers, of a deep-yellow colour. The ROOT is used, and

14

occurs in the form of light, cylindrical or split pieces, about an inch in length, of a dingy yellowish-white colour, with occasionally remains of the darker epidermis, a faintly narcotic odour, and a bitterish, not unpleasant taste. It has been found to contain, with other principles, a peculiar alkaloid, termed *gelseminia,* which is the active principle and is a powerful poison, an amount of gelsemium estimated to contain one-sixth of a grain of gelsiminia having proved fatal to an adult woman.

Effects and Uses.—Gelsemium has been found to possess valuable sedative properties, without nauseating or purgative effects. In overdoses, it has produced death. It has been used in fevers, inflammations, essential spasmodic affections, as tetanus, and as an hypnotic in delirium tremens and other forms of morbid wakefulness. The *tincture* of gelsemium (four troyounces of the *root* to diluted alcohol Oj), is the form which has been heretofore employed, in the dose of 20 to 50 drops; but the *fluid extract* is now officinal, and should be preferred; dose 5 to 10 drops.

ANTIMONII PRÆPARATA—PREPARATIONS OF ANTIMONY.

ANTIMONII OXIDUM (*Oxide of Antimony*) (Sb_2O_3) is prepared from the sulphide by digesting first with muriatic acid, then adding a little nitric acid; next precipitating the terchloride formed with a large amount of water; afterwards decomposing the oxychloride thus obtained, by ammonia, by which the terchloride of the oxychloride is converted into teroxide. This is a heavy, grayish-white, insoluble powder. It has the general therapeutic properties of the antimonials, and, though not quite certain in its effects, as its solubility depends on the amount of hydrochloric acid, which may exist in the stomach, it is believed to produce the sedative operation of tartar emetic, with less nausea and derangement of the stomach. Dose, 2 or 3 grains repeated.

ANTIMONII ET POTASSII TARTRAS (*Tartrate of Antimony and Potassium*). This valuable salt, familiarly known as *tartar emetic* and *tartarized antimony*, is prepared by boiling water and cream of tartar with oxide of antimony. It occurs in colourless, transparent, rhombic, octohedron crystals, which become white and opaque from efflorescence on exposure to the air. When pure, its powder is perfectly white; but it is to be preferred in the crystalline state, as in this form it is less liable to adulteration. When dropped into a solution of sulphuretted hydrogen or sulphide of ammonium, the crystals should have an orange-coloured deposit formed on them, which is the tersulphide, and is distinguished from tersulphide of arsenic and all other precipitates, by forming with hot concentrated muriatic acid a solution, from which, when added to water, a white curdy precipitate of oxychloride of antimony is thrown down. The metal itself should, however, always be reduced, as by Marsh's test (see Arsenious Acid); antimoniuretted hydrogen is obtained, which burns with a bluish flame, and, if a piece of cold white porcelain be held low down in the flame, the metal is deposited in the form of a dull, black spot (surrounded by a grayish ring), soluble in sulphide of ammonium, which does not dissolve arsenic, and insoluble in a solution of hypochlorite of sodium or calcium, which readily dissolves arsenical spots. The powder of tartar emetic is sometimes adulterated with cream of tartar, which may be detected by adding a few drops of a solution of carbonate of sodium to a boiling solution of the antimonial salt, and, if the precipitate formed be not redissolved, no bitartrate of potassium is present.

Tartar emetic ($KSbC_4H_4O_7,H_2O$) is inodorous; has a nauseous, metallic taste; is soluble in 15 parts of cold and 3 parts of boiling water; insoluble in pure alcohol; and is decomposed by the pure alkalies, alkaline carbonates, and the vegetable astringents.

Physiological Effects.—Tartar emetic is a powerful *local* irritant. Applied to the skin, it occasions an eruption of pustules, resembling those of variola or ecthyma. When taken into the stomach, in full doses, it causes vomiting, purging, griping pains, &c.; and, in excessive quantity, it acts as an irritant poison, and has produced death, with great prostration, syncope, and even convulsions and delirium: very large doses have, however, been given medicinally with entire safety. The proper *antidote* is tannic acid; and opium, stimulants, and demulcents should be also administered. The *constitutional* effects of tartar emetic, when taken internally, in small doses, are an increase in the secretions and exhalations generally, especially from the skin; in somewhat larger doses, these effects are accompanied with nausea and vomiting, relaxation of the tissues (particularly the muscular fibres), a feeling of great feebleness and exhaustion, and a powerful sedative action on the circulation and respiration.

Medicinal Uses.—Tartar emetic is employed therapeutically as an emetic, nauseant, sedative, sudorific, and expectorant, and locally as a counter-irritant. As an *emetic*, it creates more nausea and depression than any other substance; and hence, while other emetics are to be preferred to it, when our object is merely to evacuate the contents of the stomach, with as little constitutional disturbance as possible, it is of the greatest value, when vomiting is resorted to as a means of making an impression on the system, and thereby checking the progress of disease. As a *nauseant*, tartar emetic is employed to relax the muscular system, in the reduction of dislocations, strangulated hernia, rigidity of the os uteri in labour, &c. As a *sedative antiphlogistic*, in large doses, it is a most powerful and valuable remedy in the treatment of acute inflammation, with fever, from its combined action in reducing the frequency of the circulation, moderating the heat of the skin, and promoting diaphoresis. When given in this way, at intervals, tartar emetic ceases to produce emesis, owing to *tolerance* of the medicine, especially in pneumonia, in which disease it has long been extensively resorted to; in the early stages of acute laryngitis and bronchitis, it is a remedy of great value. From gr. $\frac{1}{4}$ to gr. $\frac{1}{2}$ may be given every two hours, in gradually increasing doses, until some amelioration of the symptoms takes place, when the doses are to be again decreased. As a *diaphoretic*, it is very useful, in small doses (as from gr. $\frac{1}{16}$ to gr. $\frac{1}{4}$, repeated), in continued fevers, inflammation from wounds, injuries, &c.; and as an *expectorant*, in the same doses, it is employed in various pulmonary affections with advantage. As a *local irritant*, it is applied to the skin in the form of aqueous solution, ointment, or plaster, in chronic diseases of the chest, affections of joints, &c.

Administration.—The dose of tartar emetic, as an *emetic*, is gr. j or ij, and it is frequently combined with ipecacuanha. As a *sedative antiphlogistic*, gr. ¼ or ½, to gr. j or ij; as a *nauseant*, gr. ¼ to ½, and as a *diaphoretic and expectorant*, gr. $\frac{1}{16}$ to ¼, may be given in solution, and in each case repeated every two or three hours. For external use, the *ointment* (*unguentum antimonii*, 1 part to lard 4 parts) may be employed; or the *plaster*, made by mixing one part of tartar emetic with four parts of Burgundy pitch.

Vinum Antimonii (*Antimonial Wine*), is a solution of tartar emetic (gr. xxxij). in boiling distilled water (f℥j), and sherry wine (f℥xv). It is employed as an expectorant and sudorific, in the dose of from 10 to 30 drops, frequently repeated; and as an emetic for children, in the dose of 30 drops to f℥j, repeated every quarter of an hour.

ANTIMONIUM SULPHURATUM (*Sulphurated Antimony*), is prepared by boiling the native sulphide of antimony, previously purified by fusion, with a solution of potassa, and adding diluted sulphuric acid to the strained solution; the sulphate of potassium, which is formed, being afterwards washed away with hot water. It is a reddish-brown, odourless, almost tasteless, insoluble powder, and is chemically a mixture of teroxide (Sb_2O_3) and tersulphide (Sb_2S_3) of antimony. Its effects are analogous to those of tartar emetic; but it is chiefly employed as an *alterative* in cutaneous affections, secondary syphilis, &c., usually in conjunction with mercurials. Dose, as an *alterative*, gr. j to iij; as an emetic, gr. v to xx.

ANTIMONII OXYSULPHURETUM (*Oxysulphuret of Antimony*, or *Kermes Mineral*), is another mixture of tersulphide and teroxide of antimony, prepared by boiling tersulphide with an alkaline carbonate or caustic solution. It is an odourless, tasteless, purplish-brown, insoluble powder, sometimes employed as an antiphlogistic in pneumonia; but it is uncertain in its operation, and probably possesses no advantage over tartar emetic. Dose, gr. ½ to gr. ij, or iij.

By the addition of an acid to the liquor which remains after the precipitation of kermes, an orange-red, odourless, tasteless powder called *golden sulphur* of antimony, is obtained. It is a mixture of tersulphide and teroxide with some free sulphur, and acts like kermes, but is weaker. Dose, gr. j to gr. ij or iij.

Pilulæ Antimonii Compositæ (*Compound Pills of Antimony*), sometimes called *Plummer's pills*, contain equal parts of *sulphurated antimony* and of *calomel*, mixed with twice the amount of guaiac and molasses each. They are used as an alterative in syphilitic, rheumatic, and cutaneous affections. Six grains of the mass contain a grain of calomel and antimony each.

Pulvis Antimonialis.—An *antimonial powder* is prepared in imitation of the celebrated *James's powder*, by burning sulphide of antimony with hartshorn shavings or bone shavings. It is a white, gritty, tasteless, odourless powder, consisting of a mixture of antimonious acid and phosphate of calcium, with some teroxide of antimony and a little antimonite of calcium. It was formerly much employed in fevers; but it is unequal in its operation, owing its activity to the teroxide of antimony present. Hence, it has been dismissed from the U. S. Pharmacopœia. In the British Pharmacopœia, it is now directed to be made by mixing one part of oxide of antimony and two parts of precipitated phosphate of calcium. Dose, gr. iij to viij.

ANTIMONIATED HYDROGEN is a gaseous substance, which has lately been employed, with much success, by inhalation, in acute bronchitis and pneumonia. It is prepared by forming an alloy of a drachm of pure antimony and twice the quantity of pure zinc, which is to be mixed with a drachm of tartar emetic or chloride of antimony, and introduced into a bottle with a large tubulure; and from time to time, as the gas is wanted, from half a drachm to a drachm of muriatic acid is added. Muriatic acid gas is evolved at the same time, but this is prevented from reaching the respiratory orifices, by closing them with a sponge wet with an alkaline solution, which permits the antimoniated hydrogen to pass. The gas may be breathed for five minutes every hour.

POTASSII NITRAS—NITRATE OF POTASSIUM.

This salt, commonly called *nitre* and *saltpetre* (KNO_3), occurs in both the inorganized and organized kingdoms of nature. It is obtained, for medicinal use, principally by the purification of the native nitre of India; and it is also found in *saltpetre-caves* in various parts of the United States, associated with nitrate of calcium, from which it is separated by lixivation. It is artificially produced in several parts of Europe, in nitre-beds or saltpetre-plantations, by bringing together decayed organic animal and vegetable matters. And it is manufactured sometimes by the double decomposition of nitrate of sodium and chloride of potassium. Nitre is *refined* by re-solution and crystallization of the *crude* nitre. As purified for medicinal use, it is found in the shops in large transparent, colourless crystals, of the form of six-sided, striated prisms, with dihedral summits, which are unalterable in the air. They have no odour, a sharp, cooling taste, are wholly soluble in water, and insoluble in pure alcohol. They have no water of crystallization, but frequently have a portion of the mother liquid mechanically lodged in the spaces of the crystals, which may be driven off by heat, and the salt fused and cast into moulds, when it is termed *sal prunelle.*

Physiological Effects.—In *excessive doses*, nitre may act as a fatal poison, producing irritation of the alimentary canal and derangement of the nervous system; the symptoms are burning pain in the throat and stomach, bloody stools, a tendency to syncope, collapse, and death, sometimes preceded by dilated pupils, insensibility, and convulsions. There is no antidote for it, and cases of poisoning are to be treated by demulcents, opiates, stimulants, &c., after evacuation of the contents of the stomach. In *moderate doses*, it is a refrigerant, sedative, diuretic, and diaphoretic, and, in large or continued doses, laxative. Its refrigerant properties are best seen when the body is morbidly hot, as in fevers. When mixed with the blood, after absorption, it produces several chemical changes, the most important of which is an *antiplastic* effect, by impeding coagulation.

Medicinal Uses.—Nitre is a very valuable refrigerant and sedative remedy in fevers, inflammations, hemorrhages, &c. In fevers it is often prescribed with calomel and tartar emetic, under the name of *nitrous powders* (nitre gr. x, tartar emetic, gr. $\frac{1}{8}$, calomel gr. $\frac{1}{4}$ to $\frac{1}{2}$). In large doses, it was given formerly in acute rheumatism, and this practice has been lately revived with success in France. Dose, gr. x to ʒss. From ʒiv to ʒvj, are given in 24 hours, in acute rheumatism, and the quantity is increased to ʒviij, x, or xij. The fumes of paper, impregnated with nitre, are used with advantage in spasmodic asthma.

Sodii Nitras—Nitrate of Sodium. This salt, commonly called *cubic nitre*, is found in large deposits in South America, chiefly in Peru, but also in Brazil. The crude salt occurs in rather soft and pliable lumps, of white, yellow, or gray colour; it is often purified in Peru by solution, crystallization, and desiccation, but it is usually refined after importation. It occurs in colourless, rhombohedral crystals, slightly deliquescent, and wholly soluble in water ($NaNO_3$), without odour, and of a sharp, cooling, and bitter taste.

Effects and Uses.—Sodium nitre has been little used in medicine, its employment having been chiefly limited to dysentery, in which it is highly praised by German physicians, in amounts of from half a troyounce to a troyounce, in mucilaginous solution, during the day. Its effects are probably analogous to those of potassium nitre, though it no doubt requires larger doses.

REFRIGERANTS.

SODII BORAS—BORATE OF SODIUM.

Borax occurs as a native product in several localities, the most important of which for a long time was Thibet, in Asia;

it is also made artificially by the direct combination of native boracic acid (obtained from the lagoons of Tuscany), with soda. The supply of the United States is now, however, exclusively derived from Borax Lake, in California, about one hundred miles north of San Francisco. Borax ($2NaBO_2,2HBO_2,9H_2O$), occurs in the form of hexahedral prismatic crystals, terminated by triangular pyramids, of a sweetish alkaline taste, and an alkaline reaction. It is wholly soluble in water, and slowly effloresces, and has the property of rendering cream of tartar very soluble in water.

Effects and Uses.—Borax is a mild refrigerant and diuretic, and has had emmenagogue virtues attributed to it. Dose, gr. xxx. It has been given in infantile diarrhœa as an enema, and is used externally in cutaneous affections, especially as a detergent in aphthous affections of the mouth in children, mixed with equal parts of sugar. *Glycerite of borate of sodium* (*glyceritum sodii boratis*), is made by rubbing up two troyounces of borate of sodium in half a pint of glycerin; *honey of borate of sodium* (*mel sodii boratis*), is made by mixing sixty grains of borate with a troyounce of clarified honey—both these preparations are used chiefly as applications to the mouth and throat.

POTASSII CITRAS—CITRATE OF POTASSIUM.

This salt (formerly known as *salt of Riverius*), is made by saturating a solution of citric acid with bicarbonate of potassium, and evaporating to dryness. It is white, granular, inodorous, of a saline, slightly bitterish, but not unpleasant taste, deliquescent, and wholly soluble in water, ($K_3C_6H_5O_7$). It is an excellent refrigerant diaphoretic, much employed in febrile affections. Dose, gr. xx–xxv; ʒvj are usually dissolved in water Oss, and f℥ss of the solution is administered every hour or two. The salts of the alkalies with vegetable acids, as citrates, tartrates, and acetates, during their passage through the body, are converted into carbonates.

Liquor Potassii Citratis (*Solution of Citrate of Potassium*) is made by dissolving half a troyounce of citric acid and 330 grains of bicarbonate of potassium in half a pint of water—dose, f℥ss.

Mistura Potassii Citratis (*Mixture of Citrate of Potassium*, or *Neutral Mixture*), is made by saturating fresh lemon-juice with bicarbonate of potassium: or, when the lemon-juice cannot be had, a solution of citric acid, flavoured with oil of lemon, may be used as a substitute. This preparation contains some free carbonic acid, which renders it more grateful to an irritable stomach than the ordinary solution of the citrate. Under the name of *effervescing draught*, the citrate of potassium is often prepared extemporaneously (half a fluidounce of fresh lemon juice with an equal measure of water, added to a solution of 120 grains of carbonate of potassium in 4 fluidounces of water), and is given in the state of effervescence; it is an excellent remedy for irritable stomach with fever.

LIQUOR AMMONII ACETATIS—SOLUTION OF ACETATE OF AMMONIUM.

This solution, termed also *Spiritus Mindereri*, or *Spirit of Mindererus*, is made by saturating diluted acetic acid with carbonate of ammonium, and is a solution of the acetate of ammonium ($NH_4C_2H_3O_2$). When pure, it is a colourless liquid, with a saline taste; it should be always freshly made when dispensed. In small doses, it is refrigerant; in larger doses, diaphoretic, diuretic, and perhaps resolvent. It is employed in febrile and inflammatory affections, sometimes in conjunction with nitre or tartar emetic, sometimes with camphor and opium. Dose, f℥ss to f℥j, every two, three, or four hours, in sweetened water.

SPIRITUS ÆTHERIS NITROSI—SPIRIT OF NITROUS ETHER.

This preparation, commonly known as *Sweet Spirit of Nitre*, is a solution of nitrous ether in alcohol. It is now made by adding to stronger alcohol about a tenth of its bulk of sulphuric acid, rather more of nitric acid, with some copper-wire or turnings, and distilling at 180° F.; the distillate is mixed with alcohol, and the mixture is to be transferred to well stopped bottles and protected from the light. In this reaction nitric acid is reduced to nitric peroxide by the indirect agency of the copper: thus, $C_2H_5HO+HNO_3+H_2SO_4+Cu=C_2H_5NO_2$ (nitrous ether)$+2H_2O+CuSO_4$. It is a volatile, inflammable liquid, of a pale-yellow colour inclining slightly to green, having a fragrant, ethereal odour, free from pungency, and a sharp, burning taste. It mixes with water and alcohol in all proportions; sp. gr. 0.837, and it contains five per cent. of nitrous ether. It should not be long kept, as it becomes strongly acid by age.

Effects and Uses.—Sweet Spirit of Nitre is antispasmodic, refrigerant, diaphoretic, and diuretic. It is much used in febrile affections, and, from its diuretic properties, is often combined with other diuretics in the treatment of dropsies. From its pleasant taste and smell, it is very acceptable to children. Dose f℥ss to f℥j, frequently repeated. The inhalation of sweet spirit of nitre has produced dangerous and even fatal effects; pallor of the face, livid discoloration of the lips and fingers, weakness of the pulse, muscular prostration, præcardial oppression and headache, are the symptoms described; a case is recorded in which death was attributed to the inhalation of the ether from a broken bottle in a sleeping apartment.

ACIDA VEGETABILIA—VEGETABLE ACIDS.

The vegetable acids are refrigerant, and, when properly diluted, form useful drinks in fevers, &c. Those chiefly employed are *acidum aceticum* (*acetic acid*), *acidum citricum* (*citric acid*), and *acidum tartaricum* (*tartaric acid*). ACETIC ACID ($HC_2H_3O_2$) is employed internally only in the form of *diluted acetic acid* (one part of strong acid to seven parts of distilled water), or *vinegar* (*acetum*). *Acetum destillatum* (*distilled vinegar*) may be substituted for *diluted acetic acid*. Externally, strong acetic acid (sp. gr. 1.047, and containing 36 per cent. of monohydrated acid) is employed as an escharotic to remove warts, in the cure of lupus, &c. Acetic acid is less used internally as a refrigerant than citric acid, from its liability to produce colic and diarrhœa, except in typhus, scarlet, and other malignant fevers, owing to its supposed possession of antiseptic virtues. Spongings with vinegar and water are useful to relieve the heat of skin in fevers, and the vapour is grateful to the sick. The dose of vinegar is f℥j–iv. Concentrated acetic acid is a corrosive poison, for which the alkalies and their carbonates, soap, &c., are the antidotes. CITRIC ACID may be agreeably administered in the juice of lemons, limes, sour oranges, and tamarinds. When these cannot be obtained, a solution of citric acid (℈j to water Oj) may be substituted. Citric acid is manufactured from lemon or lime juice, by saturating it with carbonate of calcium, and afterwards decomposing the citrate of calcium, which is formed, by the addition of sulphuric acid. It occurs in colourless crystals ($H_3C_6H_5O_7, H_2O$), having the form of rhomboidal prisms with dihedral summits, freely soluble in water, and soluble in alcohol; ℥ixss, added to distilled water Oj, form a solution of the average strength of lemon-juice. In the dose of f℥j every hour or two, *lemon-juice, limonis succus* (the juice of the fruit of Citrus Limonum), has been employed with success in acute rheumatism and gout, and, though an uncertain remedy, is occasionally of undoubted efficacy. Properly diluted and mixed with sugar, it forms the delightful refrigerant known as lemonade. Lemon-juice is the best known remedy for scurvy. It has also proved of advantage in jaundice and torpor of the liver. *Syrup of citric acid* consists of 120 grains of powdered citric acid and four minims of oil of lemon rubbed up with a fluidounce of syrup, and afterwards dissolved in a pint and fifteen fluidounces more of syrup, at a gentle heat. *Lemon syrup*, which is pleasanter, is made by dissolving 48 troyounces of sugar in a pint of strained lemon-juice mixed with a pint of water, at a gentle heat. TARTARIC ACID is the acid of grapes, and is extracted from tartar, or crude cream of tartar. It is a white crystallized solid, in the form of irregular six-sided prisms ($H_2C_4H_4O_6$), and is found in the shops as a fine white powder.

It is soluble in water and alcohol, Being cheaper than citric acid, it may be used as a substitute for that acid. It is employed in making *soda* and *Seidlitz powders*. Tartaric acid yields a precipitate (cream of tartar) with a solution of carbonate or other neutral salt of potassium, while citric acid yields none.

ORDER VIII.—SPINANTS.

Under the term Spinants or Spastics, are comprised medicines which are employed to excite muscular contraction. Of this class, the most important articles are vegetable substances containing the alkaloids strychnia and brucia, which are employed therapeutically in torpid or paralytic conditions of the muscular system—and ergot, which is used to excite muscular contractions of the uterus.

NUX VOMICA.

Strychnos Nux vomica, or Poison-Nut (*Nat. Ord.* Apocynaceæ), is a middling-sized tree of the coast of Coromandel and other parts of India, which bears a round, smooth berry, the size of a pretty large apple, of a rich orange colour, and containing numerous seeds embedded in a juicy pulp. The SEEDS are the officinal portion; but the bark also is poisonous, and is known as *false angustura bark*, from its having been confounded with angustura bark. The seeds are round, peltate, less than an inch in diameter, nearly flat, or convex on one side and concave on the other, and surrounded by a narrow annular stria. They have two coats: a simple, fibrous, outer coat, covered with short, silky hairs, of a gray or yellowish colour, and a very thin inner coat, which envelopes the nucleus or kernel. This is hard, horny, of a whitish or yellowish colour, and of very difficult pulverization. The seeds have no odour, but an intensely bitter taste, which is stronger in the kernel than in the investing membrane. They impart their virtues to water, but more readily to diluted alcohol, and contain two active *alkaloid* principles, *strychnia* (which is officinal), and *brucia*, both of which exist in combination with an acid called strychnic, or igasuric; another alkaloid, termed *igasuria*, much more soluble in water than the two first named, has been lately extracted from nux vomica.

STRYCHNIA ($C_{21}H_{22}N_2O_2$) is obtained by the following process: Nux vomica is digested and boiled in water acidulated with muriatic acid, and the resulting muriate of strychnia and brucia is decomposed by milk of lime. The strychnia is separated from brucia and impurities by boiling alcohol, from which it is deposited when cool, the brucia being left in solution. It is then converted into a sulphate by the addition of diluted sulphuric acid, next decolorized by purified animal charcoal, and again precipitated by solution of ammonia. Thus obtained, it occurs as a white or grayish-white powder (but may be made to crystallize in the form of white, brilliant, rhombic prisms), of an intensely bitter taste, almost insoluble in water, slightly soluble in cold alcohol, but readily soluble in boiling alcohol. The usual *test* for strychnia is the bichromate of potassium, which, added to a solution of strychnia in concentrated sulphuric acid, produces a violet colour, which after a time changes to wine-red, and then to reddish-yellow. A still more delicate test is a solution of permanganate of potassium (gr. 1) in sulphuric acid (grs. 2000). In both these tests, the reagent is nascent oxygen. The presence of morphia in excess may disguise the colour test; here chloroform should be used to separate the strychnia from morphia. The physiological test should always be resorted to: if a small frog be placed in an ounce of water, containing $\frac{1}{100}$ of a grain of strychnia salt, in two or three hours it will undergo tetanic spasms, and soon die. The effects of strychnia are similar to those of nux vomica, but more violent; its local action is that of an irritant. It is employed for the same purposes as nux vomica, and should be given in very minute doses, as gr. $\frac{1}{32}$ to $\frac{1}{16}$ to begin with, to be gradually increased and repeated. The salts of strychnia may be also employed in the same doses, but they are more soluble, and therefore more active. For *endermic* use, gr. $\frac{1}{40}$ of strychnia may be used; it is best used in amaurosis hypodermically, $\frac{1}{60}$ of a grain to begin with.

STRYCHNIÆ SULPHAS (*Sulphate of Strychnia*), is made by dissolving a mixture of strychnia in distilled water, with diluted sulphuric acid, and evaporating. It occurs as a white salt, in colourless, prismatic crystals, efflorescent, odourless, very bitter, readily soluble in water, sparingly soluble in alcohol, and insoluble in ether. It responds to the tests for strychnia, and may be used for the same purposes, and in the same doses.

Physiological Effects.—In very small and repeated doses, nux vomica has a tonic and diuretic effect, and sometimes operates slightly on the bowels and skin. In somewhat larger doses, the stomach is often disturbed; and in still larger doses, the muscular system becomes disordered. A sense of weight and weakness in the limbs, and increased sensibility to external impressions of all kinds, manifest themselves, with depression of spirits and anxiety; the limbs tremble, and slight convulsive movements of the muscles appear. If the medicine be continued, convulsive paroxysms of the whole muscular system ensue, with erotic desires, painful sensations in the skin, and occasionally eruptions: the pulse is not much affected. In paralytic patients, the effects of the medicine are principally observed in the paralyzed parts. When taken in excessive doses, it produces tetanus, asphyxia, and death, the intellect being usually unaffected, up to the fatal termination. There is no chemical antidote, unless, perhaps, tannic acid, and the ioduretted iodide of potassium; after evacuating the stomach, opium, conium, ether, chloroform, extract of Indian hemp, camphor, chloral, calabar bean, bromide of potassium, or atropia, may be exhibited, as physiological antidotes.

Medicinal Uses.—This medicine is our chief resource in torpid or paralytic conditions of the motor or sensitive nerves, or of the muscular fibre. When, however, paralysis is the result of inflammation of the nervous centres, it is injurious, and accelerates organic changes. It is most beneficial in those forms of paralysis which are independent of structural lesion, as lead palsy or paralysis from drunkenness. In paralysis, arising from cerebral hemorrhage,—after the absorption of the effused blood, and the paralysis remains, as it were from habit,—the cautious employment of nux vomica is often attended with advantage. In amaurosis, free from cerebral complication, it is very useful; and it is occasionally serviceable in other nervous affections. It has also been found beneficial in chorea, constipation, dysentery, cholera, diarrhœa, impotence, incontinence of urine, and spermatorrhœa; and in small doses it has been used with excellent effect as a general tonic, where there is loss of nerve-power, and as a stomachic in dyspepsia.

Administration.—Dose of the *powder*, gr. ij or iij, in pills, several times a day, and increased till an effect is produced; of the *extract* (alcoholic), gr. ½ to gr. j, to be repeated and increased; of the *tincture* (eight troyounces to alcohol Oij), gtt. v to xx, and this is sometimes used as an embrocation to paralyzed parts. A tolerance of nux vomica and strychnia is rapidly established in the system.

IGNATIA.

The SEED of Strychnos Ignatia, or St. Ignatius' Bean, a tree of the Philippine Islands, contains a large proportion of strychnia, and possesses medicinal properties analogous to those of nux vomica. It is used in this country in the form of *extract* (alcoholic), which may be given to fulfil the same remedial indications as extract of nux vomica, in the dose of half a grain to a grain, three times a day.

TOXICODENDRON (*Poison-Oak*). The LEAVES of Rhus Toxicodendron, or Poison-Oak (*Nat. Ord.* Anacardiaceæ), an indigenous shrub from one to three feet high, and other species of Rhus, possess properties somewhat analogous to those of nux vomica, and have been employed with success in paralysis. They contain a peculiar *acid* principle (*toxicodendric acid*), to which their poisonous and medicinal activity is due. Dose, gr. j to gr. iij, or more, to be repeated and increased. In cases of poisoning, the irritation of the skin is relieved by glycerite of carbolic acid, or alkaline solutions.

ERGOTA—ERGOT.

Ergot is now known to be a fungus growing from the diseased ovary of Secale cereale, or Rye, (*Nat. Ord.* Graminaceæ). The U. S. Pharmacopœia styles it the SCLEROTICUM OF CLAVICEPS PURPUREA, replacing the grain of secale cereale. Its predisposing cause is unknown, and it is not peculiar to rye, many other grasses being subject to it, as abortion in grazing animals has been frequently produced by their eating grasses affected with ergot. The ergot usually projects out of the glum or husk of the plant, beyond the ordinary outline of the spike or ear. It should not be collected until some days after it has begun to form, as it is thought not to possess full activity until about the sixth day of its formation. As found in the shops, it consists of cylindrical or somewhat prismatical tapering grains, curved like the spur of a cock, of a purplish colour externally, and of a yellowish or grayish-white colour within. Its smell is peculiar and nauseous; its taste is at first faint, but becomes bitterish, acrid, and disagreeable. It yields its virtues to water and alcohol, and does not keep well, being liable to the attacks of a minute worm.

Numerous analyses have been made of ergot, but there is still uncertainty as regards its active principles. The *oil of ergot* is not now believed to be, when pure, the medicinal constituent. A volatile alkaloid, termed *secalia* (identical with *prophylamia*,* the odorous principle of pickled herring), exists in ergot; and, lately, two fixed alkaloids (*ergotina* and *ecbolina*), have been discovered, in combination with an acid termed *ergotic*. Ecbolina is believed to be the principle which causes uterine contraction, half a grain of it having been found to produce the effect of 30 grains of ergot.

Physiological Effects.—The effects of ergot, in medicinal doses, are most conspicuous on the female system, in which it excites powerful contractions of the uterus. *After labour has*

* *Prophylamia* (C_3H_7HHN) has been used in rheumatism and neuralgia, in doses of two drops in some aromatic water, every two hours.

15

commenced, in ten or twenty minutes from its administration, it increases the violence, frequency, and continuance of labour pains, which usually never cease until the child is born. Administered *before labour*, it frequently originates the process, though its effects in this respect are less constant. And even on the *unimpregnated uterus*, it produces painful contractions, and evinces an influence over morbid conditions of the organ, by checking uterine hemorrhage, and expelling polypi. It is believed to cause contraction of the bloodvessels generally, and especially of the spinal cord. In large doses, it produces vomiting, purging, and a marked sedative effect on the circulation, and in excessive quantity it acts as an acro-narcotic poison on both sexes. When it is used for a length of time as an article of food, it produces a peculiar morbid condition, termed ergotism, which assumes two forms, one attended with convulsions, the other with dry gangrene of the limbs.

Medicinal Uses.—The chief employment of ergot is to promote the action of the uterus in parturition, when its expulsatory efforts are feeble and inefficient. It is, however, admissible, only when there is a *proper conformation of the pelvis and soft parts*, when the os uteri, vagina, and os externum are dilated or readily dilatable, and when the presentation of the child is such as to offer no great mechanical impediment to delivery. It is also useful—when from any cause it is important to accelerate delivery; in women subject to flooding, given just before delivery; to promote the expulsion of the placenta, when it is retained from a want of contraction of the uterus; to expel clots, hydatids, polypi, &c.; to restrain uterine hemorrhage, whether puerperal or non-puerperal; to excite and promote abortion, &c.; and locally as a styptic. It has been employed, too, in hemorrhages generally, in gonorrhœa, dysmenorrhœa, paralysis of the bladder, purpura, and several other diseases; lately, with marked success, by hypodermic injection, in the cure of aneurism and varix, and of fibroid tumours of the uterus; and also in paralysis dependent upon congestion of the spinal cord. By many, ergot is believed to exercise a dangerous sedative influence on the *child* during labour (owing to the interference of the passage of blood from the placenta, during violent uterine contraction), and its use may occasionally produce fœtal death, which timely resort to the forceps would have prevented.

Administration.—Ergot may be given in labour, in the dose of ℈i, in *powder*, every twenty minutes, till its effects are produced, or three doses are taken; in other diseases, the dose is from three to five grains. The *fluid extract* (made with diluted alcohol, acetic acid, and glycerin), is the best preparation (a fluidounce representing a troyounce of ergot),—dose, 20 to 30 drops. The *wine* (vinum ergotæ), contains 4 fluidounces of fluid extract, in 28 fluidounces of sherry wine. Dose f℥j to f℥ij. For hypodermic use, a non-officinal preparation, termed *ergotin*, is used, which is made by exhausting ergot with water, evaporating to a syrupy consistence, precipitating the gummy principles with alcohol, filtering, and evaporating to the consistence of a soft extract. Dose, internally, 2 or 3 grains; hypodermically, a solution of 45 grains in glycerin and distilled water, each 105 minims, may be used, 20 or 30 drops at once.

GOSSYPII RADICIS CORTEX—BARK OF COTTON ROOT.

Gossypium herbaceum (*Nat. Ord.* Malvaceæ), is a native of Asia, extensively cultivated in tropical and semi-tropical countries, and with great success in the South Atlantic and Gulf districts of the United States. By cultivation, different varieties of this plant have been produced. The ROOT has long been recognized by Southern physicians as possessing decided influence in exciting uterine contractions. A *decoction* (made by boiling four troyounces of the inner bark of the root in a quart of water to a pint), has been used in doses of a wineglassful repeated. The only officinal preparation is the *fluid extract*, dose, f℥–ij. COTTON, the well-known filamentous substance separated from the seed of the varieties of gossypium, is a useful application to burns, and parts affected with erysipelas and rheumatism.

CLASS II.—ECCRITICS.

ORDER I.—EMETICS.

Emetics (from εμεω, I vomit), are medicines which are employed to promote vomiting; when they are used merely to excite nausea, they are termed *nauseants*. When an emetic is administered, usually within fifteen or twenty minutes afterwards, a feeling of distress, relaxation, and faintness is experienced, with coolness and moisture of the skin, and a small, feeble, irregular pulse. These symptoms increase, till the contents of the stomach are ejected. During the act of vomiting, the face becomes flushed, the pulse is full and frequent, and the temperature of the body is increased. After vomiting is over, the skin is moist, the pulse soft and feeble, the patient becomes languid and drowsy, and, under peculiar circumstances, alarming and even fatal syncope has been induced. Vomiting is a reflex spinal act. Dr. Marshall Hall gives the following summary of its mechanism: "During the act of vomiting, 1, the larynx is closed; 2, the cardia is opened; and 3, all the muscles of expiration are called into action; but, 4, actual expiration being prevented by the closure of the larynx, the force of the effort is expended upon the stomach, the cardia being open, and vomiting is effected."

Susceptibility to the action of emetics differs in different individuals and in different diseases. In fevers, and where gastric irritation is present, their influence is increased; and, on the other hand, when the brain is oppressed by disease or by narcotic medicines, the stomach is exceedingly insensible to their action.

Emetics are employed therapeutically: 1, to evacuate the stomach, for the purpose of removing poisons, undigested food, &c.; and with this view, the emetics should be selected which occasion least nausea and distress; 2, to expel foreign bodies lodged in the throat or œsophagus; 3, to excite nausea and thereby depress the vascular and muscular systems; 4, to relieve spasm, as in spasmodic croup; 5, to promote secretion and excretion, &c.; and 6, sometimes, to break up a train of morbid association, by giving a shock to the system, as in the forming stage of certain fevers, as typhus and scarlatina, and of delirium tremens. They are improper in congestion of the brain, pregnancy, hernia, &c. The act of emesis is promoted by the free use of tepid drinks; excessive vomiting may be checked by demulcents, opiates, counter-irritation to the stomach, &c.

VEGETABLE EMETICS.

IPECACUANHA.

Ipecacuanha is the ROOT of Cephaëlis Ipecacuanha (*Nat. Ord.* Cinchonaceæ), a small shrubby perennial plant of Brazil, where it grows to the height of about five or six inches. The roots, as met with in the shops, are in pieces about the size of a quill, several inches long, of an irregular, twisted, contorted shape, with numerous circular rings or rugæ, from which they have been termed *annulated.* When broken, they are seen to consist of two distinct parts—a thin ligneous axis or centre, which is nearly inert, and a thick cortical layer, which has an herbaceous, acrid, rather bitter taste, and a slightly nauseous odour. A distinction is made of *brown*, *red*, and *gray* ipecacuanha, from differences in the colour of the epidermis, but they are all derived from the same plant, and are the same in properties and composition; the *brown* is the most common variety in our market. The powder is of a light grayish-fawn colour, and has a peculiar nauseous odour, which in some persons excites violent sneezing, in others dyspnœa. Ipecacuanha imparts its virtues to both water and alcohol, but they are injured by decoction. Its emetic property depends on the presence of a peculiar alkaline principle, termed *emetia* ($C_{30}H_{44}N_2O_8$), a whitish, inodorous, slightly bitter substance, sparingly soluble in water and ether, and very soluble in concentrated alcohol and chloroform. It produces vomiting in the dose of gr. ¼, and in overdoses may occasion dangerous and even fatal symptoms. Occasionally, a sophisticated root, that of *Psychotria emetica,* derived from New Granada, is found in the markets; this is not *annulated*, but longitudinally *striated*, and contains less than half the quantity of emetia, found in the genuine root (10½ per cent.).

Effects and Uses.—In full doses, ipecacuanha is a mild and certain emetic, well adapted to the treatment of spasmodic croup and acute bronchitis in children, and to all cases where a simple evacuation of the stomach is desired. In smaller doses, it produces nausea, depression of the pulse, expectoration, and diaphoresis, and with these views it is employed in the treatment of pulmonary affections, dysentery, and inflammatory disorders generally. In still smaller doses, it is useful as a tonic and stomachic. Ipecacuanha was first introduced as a remedy in dysentery, and, after being for a time laid aside, has been again recently used with marked success.

Administration.—Dose, as an *emetic*, gr. xv to gr. xx, often combined with a grain of tartar emetic; as a *nauseant*, gr. ss to gr. ij, three or four times a day; as an *expectorant* or *diaphoretic*, gr. $\frac{1}{4}$ to gr. $\frac{1}{2}$, repeated; as a *tonic*, gr. $\frac{1}{10}$, repeated. The *fluid extract* is used as an addendum to expectorant and diaphoretic mixtures, a fluidounce representing an ounce of the root; as an emetic, dose f℥ss–i; the *wine* (*vinum ipecacuanhæ*), contains two fluidounces of *fluid extract* in 30 fluidounces of sherry wine; dose, as an emetic, f℥ss–i; one part of *fluid extract*, mixed with fifteen parts of simple *syrup*, makes *Syrupus Ipecacuanhæ*, an excellent preparation for children—f℥j, containing gr. xxx of ipecacuanha; for a child a year or two old, f℥ss–j, may be given as an *emetic*, and v–xx drops, as an expectorant. *Pulvis Ipecacuanhæ Compositus*, *Compound Powder of Ipecacuanha*, or *Dover's Powder* (see Opium, p. 58). *Troches of Ipecacuanha* contain also arrow-root, sugar, and tragacanth (ipecacuanha and tragacanth each two drachms, arrow-root two troyounces, sugar eight troyounces, made into a mass with syrup of orange peel, which is to be divided into 480 troches, each containing one-third of a grain of ipecacuanha).

SANGUINARIA—BLOODROOT.

The RHIZOME of Sanguinaria Canadensis, or Bloodroot (*Nat. Ord.* Papaveraceæ), a small, indigenous plant, with radical, cordate, lobate leaves, and a handsome, white, eight-petalled flower, which appears in early spring—is usually classed with emetics. When dried, it is in flattened pieces, much wrinkled and contorted, of a reddish-brown colour, with a faint narcotic odour, and a bitterish, very acrid taste. It yields its virtues to water and alcohol, and loses them rapidly by keeping. An active alkaline principle, *sanguinarina* ($C_{37}H_{64}N_4O_8$), has been

Fig. 20.

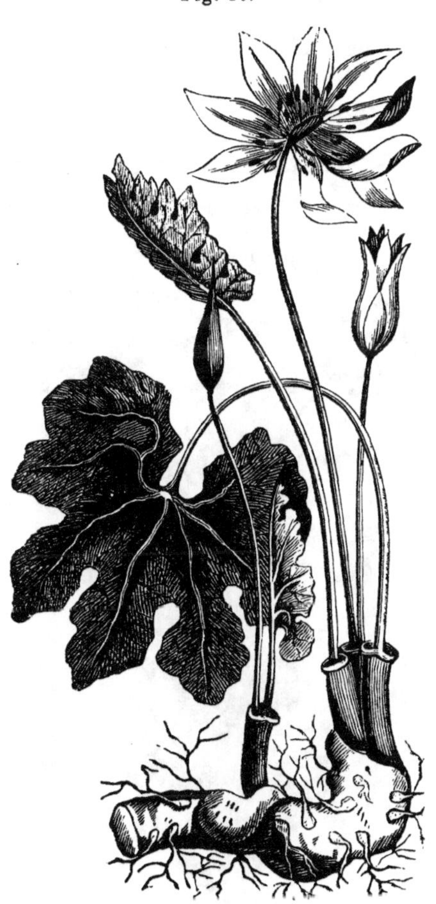

obtained from it, which possesses the properties of the root, and two other alkaloids have been discovered in it.

Effects and Uses.—Bloodroot is an acrid emetic, and, in large doses, an acro-narcotic poison. Locally, it acts as an irritant, and upon fungous surfaces as an escharotic. It is not much used as an emetic; but is occasionally employed with this view, in croup and diphtheria, or as a nauseant in pulmonary affections. Dose, as an *emetic*, gr. x to xx, in pill; or in *infusion* (half a troyounce to boiling water Oj—not officinal), of which f℥ss is the dose. *Tincture* (four troyounces to diluted alcohol Oij)—dose, as an emetic, f℥iij or iv; as an *expectorant*, 30 to 60 drops. The *Vinegar* (*Acetum*) is of the same strength as the tincture.

EUPHORBIA COROLLATA—LARGE FLOWERING SPURGE.

Fig. 21.

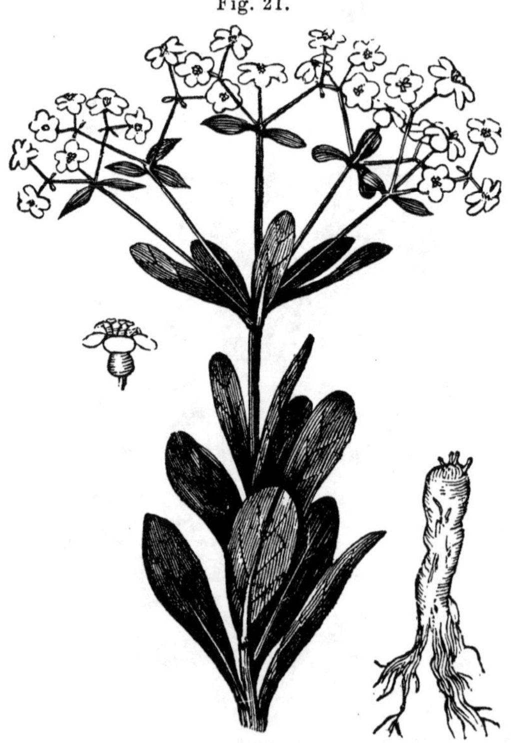

EUPHORBIA IPECACUANHA (*Ipecacuanha Spurge*). The ROOTS of these indigenous plants (*Nat. Ord.* Euphorbiaceæ), possess emetic properties; but they are apt to operate on the bowels, and, in overdoses, prove extremely violent. Dose, gr. x to xv.

GILLENIA.

Gillenia trifoliata, Indian Physic, or American Ipecacuanha (*Nat. Ord.* Rosaceæ), is an indigenous herbaceous plant, with a perennial root, consisting of a number of fibres, arising from a tuber; one or more stems, two or three feet high, of a reddish-brown colour; trifoliate leaves; and white flowers, with a tinge of red. West of the Allegheny Mountains, another species, G. stipulacea, is found, which is identical with the trifoliata in its properties, and is distinguished from it by having its lower leaves pinnatifid. The officinal portion of both is the ROOT. As found in the shops, it consists of pieces not thicker than a quill, wrinkled, of a reddish-brown colour, and composed of an easily separable and pulverizable cortical portion, and a comparatively inert internal ligneous cord, which should be rejected. The bark has a feeble odour, and a nauseous, bitter taste, and makes a light brownish powder.

Effects and Uses.—Gillenia is a safe and efficacious emetic, resembling ipecacuanha in its action, and, like it, in small doses proves a useful diaphoretic, expectorant, tonic, &c. Dose, as an *emetic*, gr. xxx; as an *expectorant* or *diaphoretic*, gr. ij to iv; and as a *tonic*, gr. ¼.

SINAPIS (*Mustard*). The POWDERED SEEDS of Sinapis nigra and Sinapis alba (*Nat. Ord.* Brassicaceæ), in doses of from a teaspoonful to a tablespoonful, are very useful emetics, particularly in atonic conditions of the stomach.

TOBACCO and LOBELIA act as emetics in large doses, but their employment is attended with danger, owing to the great prostration which they produce (see pp. 71, 73). SQUILL also possesses emetic powers, but it is too irritating for use in this respect.

MINERAL EMETICS.

TARTAR EMETIC. Dose, gr. j to gr. ij (see p. 210).
SULPHATE OF ZINC. Dose, gr. x to gr. xx (see p. 150).
SULPHATE OF COPPER. Dose, gr. iij to gr. v (see p. 149).
ALUM. Dose, a teaspoonful (see p. 183).

ORDER II.—CATHARTICS.

Cathartics (from καθαιρω, I purge), termed also *purgatives*, are medicines which produce evacuations from the bowels. Some operate by increasing the peristaltic motion of the intestines; others stimulate the mucous follicles and exhalants, and occasion watery evacuations, whence they are termed *hydragogues*. The more violent of the hydragogues, if given in overdoses, produce inflammation of the alimentary canal, characterized by violent vomiting and purging, abdominal pain and tenderness, cold extremities, and sinking pulse. From their activity, they are denominated *drastics*. Different cathartics affect different parts of the alimentary canal unequally, some acting more particularly on the upper portion, some on the lower, and others affecting all parts equally. Mercurial preparations purge chiefly by inducing a flow of bile from the liver.

Cathartics may be arranged into five groups: 1. *Laxatives*, which gently evacuate the contents of the bowels, without causing any obvious irritation, or affecting the general system. 2. *Saline cathartics*, which increase both the peristaltic action of the bowels and the effusion of fluids from the mucous surface, but are devoid of any excitant action on the general system, and are therefore adapted to the treatment of febrile and inflammatory cases. 3. *Mild acrid cathartics*, which are acrid, but not sufficiently violent in their local action to cause inflammation. 4. *Drastics*, comprising the more powerful and irritating cathartics, which, in large doses, act as acrid poisons. 5. *Mercurial cathartics.*

Cathartics are employed *therapeutically*,—1. To evacuate the bowels in constipation, and remove noxious matters, as retained feces, undigested food, morbid secretions, worms, poisons, &c. 2. To depurate the blood, as in typhus fever, uræmia, &c. 3. To relieve inflammation, congestion, and plethora, by the depletion of the bloodvessels, which results from increased secretion and exhalation from the gastro-intestinal canal. 4. To promote absorption. 5. To affect remote organs, particularly the brain, through the agency of revulsion and counter-irritation. 6. To stimulate the secretion of the liver and pancreas, by irritating the orifice of the ductus communis choledochus. 7. In the treatment of diarrhœa. 8. To relieve spasm of the bowels. 9. To restore the catamenia, by the irritating influence which they exert on the pelvic vessels. The more active cathartics are contraindicated in cases of inflammation or ulceration of the gastro-intestinal mucous membrane, peritonitis, the advanced stages of typhoid fever, pregnancy, &c.

The operation of cathartics is promoted by the addition of small doses of emetics and of the bitters. By combining those which act upon different portions of the alimentary canal, their operation is rendered less irritant, without any diminution of purgative efficiency. The griping and nauseating tendency of the drastic cathartics may be corrected by the addition of aromatics; carbonic acid water is a grateful vehicle for administering the saline preparations. Cathartics operate most speedily and favourably when given on an empty stomach, and susceptibility to their action is diminished during sleep, and increased by exercise. Mild diluent beverages promote their operation. In the event of hypercatharsis, opium should be administered by the mouth or rectum.

LAXATIVES.

Several articles of diet have a laxative operation on the bowels, and are useful in cases of habitual costiveness, as most of the ripe and dried fruits,—particularly tamarinds, peaches, apples, raisins, figs, and prunes,—West India molasses, honey, bran, cracked wheat, Indian and oatmeal, &c.

The following medicinal substances are usually arranged under the head of *laxatives*, and are employed in cases where we wish to open the bowels with the least possible irritation,—as in children and pregnant women, in inflammations or surgical operations about the abdomen and pelvis, in typhoid fever, hernia, piles, affections of the rectum or womb, &c.

TAMARINDUS—TAMARIND.

This is the PRESERVED FRUIT of Tamarindus Indica (*Nat. Ord.* Fabaceæ), a large tree of the East Indies, extensively cultivated also in the tropical portions of America. It comes to the United States chiefly from the West Indies. The preserved pods, as found in the shops, consist of a dark-coloured adhesive mass, formed of pulp, fragments of the pods, seeds, and syrup, of a sweetish acidulous taste. They contain a good deal of citric acid, with some tartaric and a little malic acid. An infusion of the pulp (half an ounce to a pint of boiling water), sweetened, makes a pleasant refrigerant and laxative drink; half an ounce to an ounce of the pulp is a good laxative. It enters into the *confection of senna.*

MANNA.

Manna is the CONCRETE SACCHARINE EXUDATION, in *flakes*, of Fraxinus ornus, and of Fraxinus rotundifolia (*Nat. Ord.* Oleaceæ), small trees of Sicily and southern Italy. It is obtained from incisions into the stems of the trees. The best kind is produced during the height of the season, when the juice flows vigorously, and from the upper stems, where it is less fatty. It is called *flake manna* or *manna cannulata*, and consists of pieces from one to six inches long, one to two inches wide, and from half an inch to an inch thick, of irregular form, but more or less stalactitic, hollowed out on one side (from the shape of the tree or substance on which they are concreted), of a white or yellowish-white colour, an odour like that of honey, and a sweet, afterwards rather acrid taste. A commoner manna, called *common manna*, or *manna in sorts*, is obtained from incisions later in the season, and from the lower stems. It occurs in small pieces, which seldom exceed an inch in length, and are softer, more viscid, and darker than the flake manna. A still inferior variety is termed *fat manna*, and consists of small, soft, viscid fragments, of a dirty, yellowish brown colour, mixed with a few pieces of the flake manna. Manna is soluble in both water and alcohol, and contains a white, crystalline, saccharine principle, termed *mannite* ($C_6H_{14}O_6$), not susceptible of alcoholic fermentation (found also in mushrooms, the olive tree, and other plants), some sugar, and a resin, to which it probably owes most of its purgative effect.

Effects and Uses.—In moderate doses, manna is nutritive; in larger, mildly laxative. It is principally given to children, to whom its sweet taste renders it acceptable; and it is sometimes combined with the more active cathartics. It may be taken in substance, or dissolved in warm milk or water. Dose for an adult, ℥j to ℥ij; for children, ʒj to ʒiij.

CASSIA FISTULA—PURGING CASSIA.

This is the FRUIT of Cassia Fistula (*Nat. Ord.* Fabaceæ), a large tree of Egypt and the East Indies, now naturalized in the West Indies and South America. It consists of long, woody, dark-brown pods, about an inch in diameter, and nearly two feet in length, which contain numerous seeds imbedded in a soft black pulp. The PULP is the part used, and has a faint, nauseous odour, and a sweet, rather pleasant, mucilaginous taste. It is, in small doses, a mild, agreeable laxative, but its chief use is as an ingredient in the *Confection of Senna.* Dose, ʒj to ℥j.

OLEUM OLIVÆ (*Olive Oil*). The well known FIXED OIL obtained from the FRUIT of Olea Europæa, or Olive Tree (*Nat. Ord.* Oleaceæ), is nutritive, demulcent, emollient, and laxative. It is frequently prescribed as a constituent of laxative enemata.

OLEUM AMYGDALÆ EXPRESSUM (*Expressed Oil of Almond*), is used for the same purposes as olive oil.

OLEUM RICINI—CASTOR OIL.

Castor oil is the FIXED OIL obtained from the SEED of Ricinus communis, or Palma Christi (*Nat. Ord.* Euphorbiaceæ), a small perennial tree of India, now naturalized in many warm climates, and cultivated extensively in the United States. In this country, it is an annual plant, about five or six feet in height, with round, thick-jointed, furrowed stems, of a purplish colour above; large peltato-palmate leaves, divided into seven or nine segments, on long round footstalks; and prickly, three-celled capsules, with a seed in each cell. The seeds are ovate, about the size of a small bean, and of a gray colour, marbled with reddish-brown spots and stripes. They possess considerable acridity, and, in large quantities, have produced death. They consist of a thin outer pellicle, an inner, hard, blackish shell—both of which are inert—and a white oleaginous *kernel*, which contains the acrid principle.

Castor oil is obtained by expression, by decoction, and by the agency of alcohol. The first method is the best, and is that which is pursued in this country, where large quantities are made both for home consumption and exportation; heat should not be employed in preparing it, as it renders it rancid. Thus procured, it is nearly colourless, or of a pale-yellow colour, of a thick viscid consistence, a faint, unpleasant odour, and a mild, nauseous taste, and becomes rancid and thick by exposure to the air. It is not soluble in water, but is extremely soluble in alcohol, readily so in ether, and forms soaps with alkalies. Its composition is not well understood; its constituents would seem to be mainly *ricinolein* (a saponifiable oil resembling olein), and a little stearin and palmitin.

Effects and Uses.—Castor oil is a mild and tolerably certain laxative, operating, when pure, without uneasiness in the bowels. It is admirably adapted to all cases where a free evacuation of the bowels is desired, without abdominal irritation, as in dysentery, pregnancy, typhoid fever, &c., and is an excellent purgative for children. The *leaves* are said to possess *galactagogue* properties, and are applied to the breasts, in the form of decoction, to induce the secretion of milk.

Administration.—For adults the dose is f℥ss to f℥j; for children fʒj to f℥ss. To cover its unpleasant flavour, it is sometimes taken floating on spirit, coffee, mint-water, compound spirit of ether, &c., or made into an emulsion, or mixed with the froth of porter or a little oil of bitter almonds.

FLAXSEED OIL and MELTED BUTTER are laxative in the same doses as castor oil.

SULPHUR.

Sulphur exists in both kingdoms of nature. It is procured by the purification of native sulphur, and by the decomposition of the native sulphurets. The sulphur of commerce is generally obtained in the former way, chiefly from Sicily, and is termed *crude sulphur;* it comes also from Romagna in Italy, and from California, and very recently, considerable deposits of sulphur have been found in the island of Saba, one of the Dutch West Indies. After importation, it is purified by sublimation, and is known as SUBLIMED SULPHUR—SULPHUR SUBLIMATUM. It is sometimes sublimed in the form of an impalpable powder, when it is called the *flowers of sulphur.* Sometimes it is cast in wooden moulds and forms the roll sulphur or brimstone of commerce. Sublimed sulphur contains more or less sulphuric acid, and for medicinal use, it is further purified by washing, when it constitutes the SULPHUR LOTUM or WASHED SULPHUR of the Pharmacopœia. As met with in the shops, it is a fine bright-yellow powder, with a feeble odour and taste, insoluble in water, but soluble in alcohol, ether, chloroform, alkaline solutions, and the oils: and, when perfectly pure, it is wholly volatilized by heat, and ought not to change the colour of litmus paper.

Effects and Uses.—In small and repeated doses, sulphur is a gentle stimulant to the skin and mucous membranes; and in larger doses, it acts as a mild purgative, without exciting the pulse or occasioning griping. It is probably absorbed by being converted in the small intestine, by the alkali of the bile, into a sulphide; after its continued use, the intestinal gases give off sulphuretted hydrogen. It is employed in the cases to which laxatives are applicable, and also as an alterative diaphoretic in chronic cutaneous diseases, rheumatism, and gout, and as an expectorant in pulmonary affections. It is considered a specially useful laxative in hemorrhoids. To increase its cathartic effect, it is often combined with cream of tartar or magnesia. *Externally*, it is a valuable remedy in various skin diseases, particularly *scabies*.

Administration.—Dose, ʒj to ʒiij or ʒiv, in syrup, treacle, or milk. *Externally*, it is applied in the form of vapour-bath or *ointment*. *Unguentum Sulphuris* consists of one part of sulphur and two parts of lard, rubbed together until thoroughly mixed.

Sulphur Præcipitatum (*Precipitated Sulphur*, or *Lac Sulphuris*), is prepared by boiling together sulphur, slaked lime, and water, and afterwards precipitating the sulphur by muriatic acid. It is a finer and softer powder than sublimed sulphur, is of a paler yellow colour, with a grayish tint, and is not gritty between the teeth. When exposed to the air, however, it is liable to become contaminated with sulphuric acid, and, as found in commerce, it is often adulterated with sulphate of calcium. Its effects, uses, and doses, are the same as those of sublimed sulphur.

Potassii Sulphuretum (*Sulphuret of Potassium*), or *Liver of sulphur* is prepared by rubbing together one part of dried sulphur with two parts of carbonate of potassium, afterwards melting the mixture, and pouring it when cold into a bottle. Its composition is variable and uncertain. When freshly and carefully prepared, it is of a liver colour, has an acrid, alkaline, disagreeable taste, and forms an orange-yellow solution with water. This salt and the other sulphides probably act like sulphur; they are perhaps in part decomposed by the acids of the stomach, but any liberated sulphur must be again combined with the alkali of the bile. Taken in large quantities, the potassium sulphuret is considered to be a corrosive poison, capable of producing fatal gastro-enteric inflammation. The sulphides are considered to be expectorant, diaphoretic, and alterative. They have been especially recommended in the scrofulous abscesses of children—the sulphide of calcium being preferred; dose, for an adult, 2 to 10 grains, several times a day. They are used externally in scaly skin diseases, in the form of *ointment* (ʒss to ℥i of lard), and of *baths*.

SALINE CATHARTICS.

MAGNESIA.

Magnesia, sometimes called *calcined* magnesia, from the mode in which it is prepared, is procured by exposing the carbonate of magnesium to a red heat, till the carbonic acid is wholly expelled. It is a light, fine, white, colourless, odourless powder (MgO), of a feeble earthy taste, very slightly soluble in water, and more soluble in cold than in hot water. *Henry's Magnesia*, a patent English medicine, has the advantage over the ordinary magnesia, of greater density and softness, and more ready miscibility with water. Magnesia, prepared by Husband, and Ellis, of Philadelphia, is very similar in properties to Henry's.

Effects and Uses.—Magnesia is antacid and laxative. A good deal of its cathartic effect is the result of its combination with the free acids of the stomach and intestines, in which soluble magnesian salts are formed. When taken in large quantities, and for too long a period, it sometimes accumulates in the bowels; and hence it is best to increase its solubility by giving it with lemonade. It is an excellent laxative where much acidity exists in the stomach; and is particularly useful in infantile cases. As an antacid, it is employed in heartburn, sick headache, and nephritic complaints. Dose, as a *laxative*, ʒj; as an *antacid*, ℈j, in water or milk. Of Henry's, half the quantity.

MAGNESII CARBONAS—CARBONATE OF MAGNESIUM.

Carbonate of magnesium, sometimes called *magnesia alba*, is prepared by decomposing sulphate of magnesium with an alkaline carbonate. As found in the shops, it is a combination of carbonate of magnesium and hydrate of magnesium, ($3MgCO_3$, $Mg2HO,4H_2O$). It occurs in the form of light, white, cubical cakes or powder; is inodorous, almost insipid, and nearly insoluble in water, but soluble in carbonic acid water.

Its *effects and uses* are nearly the same as those of calcined magnesia; but, from its effervescence with the acids of the stomach, it is apt to create flatulence, though sometimes, on this account, more acceptable to delicate stomachs. Dose, as a *laxative*, ʒj to ʒij; as an *antacid*, gr. x.

MAGNESII SULPHAS—SULPHATE OF MAGNESIUM.

This salt, commonly called *Epsom Salt*, from its having been first procured from the Epsom mineral water in England, occurs in native crystals, and is a constituent of sea-water and many saline springs. It is obtained in England from *dolomite*, or magnesian limestone; and also from *bittern*, or the residual liquor of sea-water, from which common salt has been separated. In this country, it is extensively manufactured at Baltimore and Philadelphia, by the action of sulphuric acid on *magnesite*, the silicious hydrate of magnesium. It is usually met with in small acicular crystals, which are colourless, transparent, and odourless, but have an extremely bitter taste. They effloresce on exposure to the air, are very soluble in water and insoluble in alcohol. The chemical composition of the salt is one equivalent of acid, one of magnesia, and seven of water of crystallization ($MgSO_4,7H_2O$).

Effects and Uses.—Epsom Salt is a mild, safe refrigerant purgative, which, from its cheapness, is by far the most commonly employed of all cathartics. It is sometimes combined with senna, sometimes with the bitter infusions, and is most agreeably administered in solution in carbonic acid water. Dose, ʒj.

LIQUOR MAGNESII CITRATIS—SOLUTION OF CITRATE OF MAGNESIUM.

The citrate of magnesium is employed medicinally, only in solution, with a slight excess of acid, and in the effervescing state. It is prepared according to the following formula: 400 grains of citric acid are dissolved in 4 fluidounces of water, and in this solution 200 grains of carbonate of magnesium are stirred until dissolved; this solution is filtered into a strong twelve-ounce bottle, containing 2 fluidounces of syrup of citric acid; to this are added 40 grains of bicarbonate of potassium, and water enough nearly to fill the bottle, which must be closed with a cork, secured with twine; the mixture must be occasionally shaken, to insure the solution of the bicarbonate. The effervescing solution has a pleasant acid taste, without anything disagreeable. It is a very grateful cathartic, and is much employed as a substitute for Epsom salt. Dose from a half to a whole bottle.

SODII SULPHAS—SULPHATE OF SODIUM.

Sulphate of sodium, commonly called *Glauber's Salt*, is a constituent of many mineral springs, and is prepared in various chemical processes. It occurs as a residuum in the manufacture of muriatic acid, made by adding sulphuric acid to chloride of sodium; and it is obtained from sea-water in the winter season. It is found in colourless, six-sided, very efflorescent crystals, which are inodorous, but have a cooling, saline, very bitter taste. It is soluble in water, more readily in hot than in cold water, and is insoluble in alcohol. Its chemical composition is one equivalent of soda, one of acid, and ten of water ($Na_2SO_4,10H_2O$).

Its *effects and uses* are very similar to those of Epsom salt, but it is more bitter and nauseous, and is now little used. It has an antiplastic action on the blood. Dose, ℥j; in an effloresced state, ℥ss.

MANGANESII SULPHAS—SULPHATE OF MANGANESE.

This salt is made by heating the native black oxide with concentrated sulphuric acid, and consists of one equivalent of sulphuric acid and one of protoxide of manganese ($MnSO_4,5H_2O$). It occurs in rhombic, prismatic crystals, of a pale-rose or pink colour, transparent, and of an astringent, bitterish taste. It is very soluble in water, insoluble in alcohol.

In its *effects* it is said to resemble *Glauber's Salt,* acting also as a cholagogue. Dose, as a purgative, ℥i–ij. As a tonic, it has been given in doses of gr. v–xx.

SODII PHOSPHAS—PHOSPHATE OF SODIUM.

This salt is prepared by digesting powdered burnt bone with diluted sulphuric acid, and decomposing the resulting superphosphate of calcium with carbonate of sodium. It occurs in large, rhombic, colourless, transparent, very efflorescent crystals ($Na_2HPO_4,12H_2O$), which are wholly soluble in water, and insoluble in alcohol, and have a pleasant saline taste, resembling that of common salt.

Effects and Uses.—Phosphate of sodium is a mild saline cathartic, well adapted, from its agreeable taste, to the cases of children and delicate persons, but too expensive for general use. It is a constituent of the blood in health, and has been recommended in cholera as a restorative of deficient saline matters, and also in diseases where there is a deficiency of phosphatic matter in the bones. Dose, as a *cathartic,* ℥vj to ℥xij, in broth or soup; as an *alterative,* ℈j or ℈ij, three or four times a day.

POTASSII SULPHAS—SULPHATE OF POTASSIUM.

This salt exists in both kingdoms of nature, and is obtained artificially from the residuum of the distillation of nitric acid from nitrate of potassium and sulphuric acid. It occurs in small, hard, colourless, inodorous crystals (K_2SO_4), of a saline, bitter taste, which have no water of crystallization, and are unalterable in the air. They are moderately soluble in water, and are insoluble in alcohol.

Effects and Uses.—In small doses, it is considered a mild and safe cathartic; but, in large doses, it has proved a violent and even fatal poison, producing symptoms of cholera. It is thought to act as a *lactifuge*, or represser of milk, and is administered with this view in France. Dose, as a cathartic, gr. xv to ʒj, or ʒij; but it is little employed in this country. From its hardness and dryness, it is useful to promote the trituration and division of powders, and for this purpose is employed in making Dover's powder.

POTASSII BITARTRAS—BITARTRATE OF POTASSIUM.

This salt, well known as *Cream of Tartar*, and termed also the acid tartrate of potassium, exists in many vegetable juices, particularly the juice of grapes, from which it is obtained. It is deposited in an impure form, during fermentation, on the sides of wine-casks, and in this state occurs in crystalline cakes, of a reddish colour, known as *argol* or *crude tartar.* This is purified by solution and crystallization, and forms a white crystalline mass or powder, termed cream of tartar ($KHC_4H_4O_6$). It is without smell, has an acidulous and gritty taste, is very slightly soluble in water, and insoluble in alcohol; when heated in a close vessel, it is converted into black flux, a compound of charcoal and carbonate of potassium.

Effects and Uses.—In small doses, it is diuretic and refrigerant; in larger doses, cathartic; and in excessive doses, it will produce gastro-intestinal inflammation. It is employed to form a refrigerant drink, and as a gentle aperient, in fevers; and as a diuretic and hydragogue cathartic in dropsies. Dose, as an *aperient*, ʒj or ʒij; as a *cathartic*, ℥ss to ℥j; as a *diuretic*, ℈j to ʒj, in repeated doses. It enters into the *compound powder of jalap.*

POTASSII TARTRAS—TARTRATE OF POTASSIUM.

This salt, formerly called *Soluble Tartar*, is obtained by saturating the excess of acid in cream of tartar with carbonate of potassium. It occurs in white deliquescent crystals or grains, ($K_2C_4H_4O_6$), of a saline, somewhat bitter taste, and is very soluble in water. It consists of two equivalents of potassa and one of acid. It is a gentle cathartic and diuretic, at present not much used. Dose, ℥ss to ℥j.

POTASSII ET SODII TARTRAS—TARTRATE OF POTASSIUM AND SODIUM.

This salt, commonly called *Rochelle Salt*, is made by saturating the excess of acid in cream of tartar with carbonate of sodium. It occurs in large, transparent, colourless, prismatic, slightly efflorescent crystals, of a mildly saline and bitter taste, readily soluble in cold water, and still more so in hot water ($KNaC_4H_4O_6,4H_2O$). It is a mild and pleasant aperient, well adapted to gouty cases, and cases of uric acid lithiasis, but it renders the urine alkaline, and should not therefore be given to persons suffering with phosphatic deposits in the urine. Dose, ℥ss to ℥j. It is usually exhibited in the form of *Pulveres Effervescentes Aperientes* (*Aperient Effervescing Powders*), or *Seidlitz Powders*, which consist of Rochelle salt (ʒij) and bicarbonate of sodium (℈ij), in a blue paper, and tartaric acid (gr. xxxv), in a white paper. They are taken, dissolved in half a pint of water, while the liquid is in a state of effervescence, and form a very agreeable, mild aperient. They should not be kept in a damp place.

MILD ACRID CATHARTICS.

RHEUM—RHUBARB.

Rhubarb is the ROOT of Rheum palmatum, and of other species of Rheum (*Nat. Ord.* Polygonaceæ). It is not known with certainty what species yields the officinal rhubarb, but it is attributed by most writers to R. palmatum, a perennial plant, with large, roundish, cordate, half-palmate leaves, growing spontaneously in Chinese Tartary and Mongolia, and cultivated in Europe and this country, together with several other varieties, for the leaf-stalks, which make excellent tarts. Rhubarb roots are prepared for the market by being cleansed, deprived of their cortical portion, cut into pieces, pierced through their centre, strung upon a cord, and dried in the sun. Three principal sorts were long known: Chinese, Russian or Turkey, and European. The first two were obtained, by different routes, from Central Asia. 1. *Chinese rhubarb* is the common variety, and is imported principally from Canton; it is said to be derived from Rh. officinale. It occurs in roundish pieces, sometimes flattened, of a dirty brownish-yellow colour externally (the cortical portion apparently scraped off), having a ragged fracture (which presents red, yellowish and white veins), and it is often perforated with holes, with portions of the cord on which it was dried occasionally remaining. It has a peculiar odour, an astringent, somewhat bitter taste, is gritty when chewed, and tinges the saliva of a yellow colour; its powder is yellowish, with a reddish-brown tinge. 2. *Russian rhubarb* had probably the same source as the Chinese, but it was selected with greater care, and was rigorously inspected by the Russian government. It was carried in caravans through Russia to St. Petersburg, whence it was exported. The pieces are irregular in shape, and are often angular, from the cortical portion having been cut off and not scraped. They are less heavy and compact than the Chinese, of a livelier colour both externally and internally, and are perforated with larger holes, which have been made for the purpose of inspection. The taste and smell are very like those of the Chinese, but are more aromatic; the powder is bright yellow. Russian rhubarb has, however, within a few years past disappeared as an article of commerce, the Russian government having abandoned the inspection long practised on the frontiers of Bucharia, whence the supply was derived. 3. *European rhubarb* is of uncertain quality, and is seldom found in the shops. The kind most frequently met with is English rhubarb, which is thought to be derived from Rh. Rhaponticum, and generally comes in pieces five or six inches long, and about an inch thick, and is called *stick rhubarb.* It is lighter, more spongy, and redder than the Asiatic varieties, with a feebler odour and less bitter taste, and when broken exhibits a more compact and regular marbling; lately, the production of English rhubarb has much increased, and its quality has improved.

Rhubarb imparts its virtues to both water and alcohol, but they are impaired by long boiling. Its most important chemical constituents are—*chrysophanic acid*, a yellow, odourless, tasteless, granular substance; two, or perhaps three *resins*, soluble in alcohol, and insoluble in water; and *bitter extractive.* It is supposed that the therapeutical properties of the drug depend chiefly on the conjoint operation of these principles. It contains also tannic and gallic acids, sugar, pectin, oxalate of calcium, &c.

Effects and Uses.—In small doses, rhubarb is an astringent tonic. In larger doses, it is a slow and mild cathartic, occasionally causing griping and accelerating the pulse, but never inflaming the mucous membrane of the alimentary canal like the drastics; it tinges the milk and urine yellow. It is much employed as a purgative in *diarrhœa*, in which it is particularly useful from its secondary astringent effect, and in *dyspepsia*, attended with costiveness, where it acts both as a stomachic and laxative. It is not adapted to febrile or inflammatory cases. In the bowel complaints of children, rhubarb deservedly enjoys great popularity, and it is also highly esteemed in infantile scrofula. Made into a cataplasm, and applied to the abdomen, it acts as a purgative on children.

Administration.—Dose, as a *stomachic laxative*, gr. v to gr. x; as a *purgative*, ℈j to ʒj. The following are the officinal preparations: *Infusion* (ʒjj to boiling water Oss), dose, f℥j to f℥ij, repeated; *Extract* (alcoholic), dose, gr. x to gr. xxx; *Fluid Extract*, dose, fʒss, containing half a drachm of the root; *Tincture* (℥iij to diluted alcohol Oij, with cardamom ʒss); *Tinc-*

ture of Rhubarb and Senna (containing rhubarb a troyounce, senna 120 grains, coriander and fennel each 60 grains, liquorice 30 grains, raisins 6 troyounces, to diluted alcohol Oiij, and popularly known as *Warner's Gout Cordial*); *Tincture of Rhubarb and Aloes* and *Tincture of Rhubarb and Gentian* are no longer officinal; the dose of all the tinctures is f℥ss to f℥j, and they are chiefly adapted to low forms of disease and persons accustomed to the use of stimulants; *Pills of Rhubarb* (rhubarb 72 grains, beaten with water into a pilular mass with soap 24 grains, and divided into 24 pills); *Compound Pills of Rhubarb* (rhubarb 48 grains, aloes 36 grains, myrrh 24 grains, oil of peppermint 3 minims, beaten with water into a pilular mass, and divided into 24 pills); *Compound Powder of Rhubarb* (containing 2 parts of rhubarb, 6 parts of magnesia, and 1 part of ginger); *Syrup* (fluid extract 3 fluidounces mixed with syrup 29 fluidounces); *Aromatic Syrup* (rhubarb two troyounces and a half, cloves and cinnamon each half a troyounce, nutmeg 120 grains, percolated with diluted alcohol till a pint of tincture is obtained, and this mixed with six pints of syrup—much used in infantile cases under the name of *Spiced Syrup of Rhubarb*), dose for an infant fℨi; and *wine* (rhubarb two troyounces, canella 60 grains, Sherry wine 14 fluidounces, and diluted alcohol enough to make a pint—dose fℨi–f℥ss). Roasting impairs the cathartic power of rhubarb, and is said to increase its astringency.

JUGLANS (*Butternut*). The INNER BARK of the ROOT of Juglans cinerea, or Butternut (*Nat. Ord.* Juglandaceæ), an indigenous forest tree, possesses cathartic properties, resembling those of rhubarb. It is of a fibrous texture, a white colour, gradually changing to dark brown, a feeble odour, but a bitter, somewhat acrid taste. Dose of the bark, or of the *extract*, which is preferred, gr. x to gr. xxx.

ALOE—ALOES.

Aloes is the INSPISSATED JUICE of the LEAVES of Aloe spicata, Aloe Socotrina, Aloe vulgaris, and other species of Aloe (*Nat. Ord.* Liliaceæ), succulent, herbaceous plants, growing in warm countries. The finest kinds are obtained by exudation: those prepared by expression and by boiling are inferior. Three principal varieties are known in commerce: Cape, Socotrine, and Barbadoes aloes, the first two of which are the most used in the United States. 1. *Cape aloes* (*aloe Capensis*), which is much the most common, is obtained from the Cape of Good Hope, where it is collected indiscriminately from A. spicata and other species. It has a shining, resinous appearance, is of a deep-brown colour, with a greenish tint, translucent at its edges, and has a glossy or resinous fracture. Its powder is greenish-yellow; its odour is strong and disagreeable, but not nauseous. 2. *Socotrine aloes* (*aloe Socotrina*), when genuine, is the choicest variety. It is produced in the island of Socotra, and on the eastern coast of Africa, from A. Socotrina, and occurs in pieces of a yellowish or reddish-brown colour, becoming darker on exposure to the air, with a smooth and conchoidal fracture, the interior being lighter-coloured than the exterior. Its powder is golden-yellow; its odour peculiar, but not unpleasant, and its taste bitter and disagreeable, but aromatic. *Socotrine aloes* should always be preferred, and is the variety directed by the Pharmacopœia in all preparations into which aloes enters. *Hepatic aloes* is probably an inferior variety of Socotrine, and is seldom met with in our shops. It is of a reddish-brown colour, but darker and less glossy than the Socotrine. 3. *Barbadoes aloes* (*aloe Barbadensis*), comes from the West Indies, the product chiefly of A. vulgaris; it is imported in gourds. Its colour is not uniform, varying from a dark-brown or black to a liver colour. It has a dull fracture; makes an olive-yellow powder; and is distinguishable by its particularly disagreeable, nauseous odour. The taste of all the varieties of aloes is intensely bitter, and very tenacious.

Aloes yields its virtues to water and alcohol. A proximate neutral, crystalline principle, termed *aloin*, has been extracted from it, which was at one time supposed to be the cathartic principle; but it is now believed that this is a soluble, brown, uncrystallizable substance which is found largely in aloes.

Effects and Uses.—Aloes, in small doses, is tonic, and, in large doses, purgative. As a cathartic, it is remarkable for the slowness of its operation, and its special action on the large intestine and the pelvic viscera generally. Hence, it is objectionable in cases of disease of the genito-urinary apparatus, pregnancy, &c.; and, on the other hand, is useful in amenorrhœa. It stimulates the hepatic secretion also. It is principally employed in cases of dyspepsia, accompanied by costiveness, dependent on a torpid condition of the large intestine or liver. It is also useful as a revulsive in cerebral affections, and has proved efficacious as an anthelmintic. It was once thought that it was objectionable in hemorrhoids, but, this affection being now considered to depend upon *relaxation* of the veins of the rectum, aloes has been administered in it, upon theoretical views, and with very good results. As a purgative, it holds an intermediate rank between rhubarb and senna.

Administration.—Dose, gr. v to gr. x–xx, in pill; it is usually given in combination with other cathartics. Aloes is so often mixed with impurities, that, for medicinal use, it is best employed under the form of *aloe purificata* (*purified aloes*), which is prepared by straining and evaporating an alcoholic solution of Socotrine aloes. The officinal preparations are: *Pills of Aloes*, consisting of equal parts of aloes and soap, one pill containing two grains of aloes; *Pills of Aloes and Mastic*, four parts of aloes to one part of mastic and red rose, each, (the *Lady Webster pill*, each containing two grains of aloes); *Pills of Aloes and Assafetida*, consisting of 32 grains each of aloes, assafetida, and soap, divided into 24 pills, useful in flatulent constipation; *Pills of Aloes and Myrrh*, or *Rufus's Pills*, aloes four parts, myrrh two parts, and aromatic powder one part, made into pills with syrup, employed in amenorrhea, each pill containing 2 grains of aloes; *Powder of Aloes and Canella*, known as *hiera picra*, four parts of aloes to one of canella; *Tincture* (a troyounce to alcohol Oss, distilled water Ojss, with liquorice three troyounces), dose, f℥ss to f℥jss; *Tincture of Aloes and Myrrh* (aloes and myrrh each three troyounces to two pints of alcohol); *Wine of Aloes* (aloes a troyounce, cardamom and ginger each 60 grains, to a pint of Sherry wine): *Suppositories of Aloes* contain each two grains of aloes—they may be used with a view to the removal of ascarides.

LEPTANDRA.

The ROOT of Leptandra Virginica, Culver's Root, or Culver's Physic (*Nat. Ord.* Scrophulariaceæ), an herbaceous, perennial plant, three or four feet high, with leaves in whorls, and a long spike of white flowers, is now ranked as a valuable cholagogue cathartic. It consists of a dark-brown rhizome, from two to four lines in thickness, several inches in length, with numerous long slender radicals. The odour is feeble and disagreeable, the taste bitterish, and somewhat nauseous and acrid. Water and alcohol extract its virtues, which depend on a peculiar principle termed *leptandrin.* Dose of the *powdered* root, gr. xx to ʒj; of an impure resin (made by precipitating a tincture of the root), gr. ij–iv; a *fluid extract* also has been used.

SENNA.

Senna consists of the LEAFLETS of several species of Cassia (*Nat. Ord.* Fabaceæ), small shrubs, which grow in the tropical regions of Asia and Africa. The species recognized as officinal are C. acutifolia, C. obovata, and C. elongata; and besides these. C. lanceolata, and C. Æthiopica, are also generally received as sources of the drug. The commercial varieties of senna, which are found in the United States, are the Alexandria, the Tripoli, the India, and the Mecca senna. 1. *Alexandria senna,* which comes from the port of this name in Egypt, is made up chiefly of the leaflets of C. acutifolia (which are yellowish-green, acute in shape, and less than an inch in length), intermingled with the pods, leafstalks, flowers, &c., of this plant. It contains also leaflets of C. obovata, known by their rounded, obtuse summits; and is, moreover, occasionally adulterated with the leaves of Cynanchum oleæfolium, distinguishable, by their greater length, thickness, and firmness, from the genuine leaves. 2. *Tripoli senna,* brought from Tripoli, consists of the leaflets of C. Æthiopica, which are shorter, less acute, thinner, and more fragile than those of C. acutifolia, and are generally much *broken up.* 3. *India senna* is produced in Arabia, but comes into commerce through the ports of

Hindostan. It consists of the leaflets, intermixed with the leafstalks and pods, of C. elongata, and is readily recognized by the long, narrow, *pike-like* shape, and dark hue of the leaflets. A finer variety of India senna, cultivated at *Tinnevelly*, in Hindostan, has been known for some years past, which is distinguishable from the common sort of India senna, by the bright-green colour of the leaflets. 4. *Mecca senna* is a variety lately introduced, and consists of leaflets, intermediate in length between those of C. acutifolia and C. elongata, and has in mass a yellowish, tawny hue. Its source is not known with certainty, but it is probably the product of C. lanceolata. Cassia obovata has been lately found growing wild in abundance in Jamaica.

Commercial senna is prepared for use by separating the leaflets from the stalks, adulterations, &c.; the pods possess cathartic properties, but are less active than the leaves. The odour of senna is faint and sickly; its taste, bitter, sweetish, and nauseous. It imparts its virtues to water and alcohol, its infusion being of a reddish-brown colour. The chemical composition of senna has long been an unsettled point. By the latest analysis, it has been found to contain a glucoside, *cathartic acid* ($C_{180}H_{192}N_4SO_{82}$), which is insoluble in water, stronger alcohol, and ether, but which enters readily into watery solution with alkaline and earthy bases, in which state it exists in senna; this is actively cathartic. Catharto-mannite, sennepicrin, and a reddish-brown compound, soluble in ether, resembling chrysophanic acid, have been also obtained; and there is probably another purgative principle, which has not been isolated.

Effects and Uses.—Senna is a prompt, efficient, and safe cathartic, well adapted to febrile and inflammatory cases; it operates on the entire track of the intestinal canal, and produces watery, feculent discharges. Its tendency to gripe may in a great measure be counteracted by combining aromatics or neutral salts with it; the addition of bitters promotes its cathartic activity.

Administration.—The dose in *powder* is ʒss to ʒij; but it is usually given in *infusion* (a troyounce to boiling water Oj with coriander, ℨj), one-third for a dose, repeated. *Confectio sennæ* (made with senna, coriander, sugar, figs, and pulps of prunes, tamarinds, and purging cassia), is an excellent mild cathartic, much used for pregnant women; dose, ℨij. Of the *fluid extract* the dose is fℨi to f℥ss; a *fluid extract* of spigelia and senna is used as an anthelmintic.

CASSIA MARILANDICA—AMERICAN SENNA.

Fig. 22.

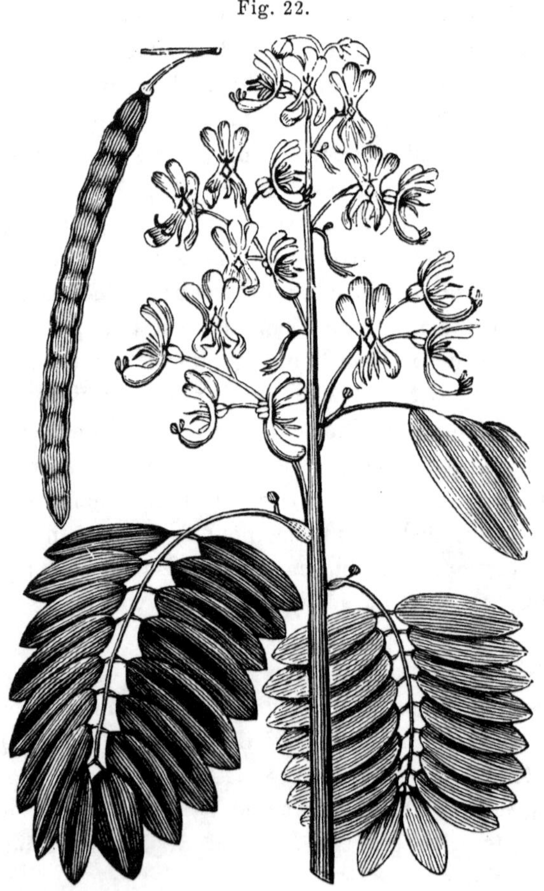

Cassia Marilandica, American Senna, or Wild Senna (*Nat. Ord.* Fabaceæ), possesses cathartic properties similar to those of imported senna, but is less active. It is an indigenous plant, common in the Southern and Western States, growing to the height of three or four feet, with alternate leaves, composed of from eight to ten pairs of oblong, lanceolate, pale-green leaflets, and bearing handsome golden-yellow flowers and a pendulous fruit two to four inches long. An *infusion* of the LEAFLETS is given in doses one third larger than those of senna.

SAMBUCUS—ELDER.

Several portions of Sambucus Canadensis, our indigenous *common elder* (*Nat. Ord.* Caprifoliaceæ), a well-known shrub, from six to ten feet high, found in all the Atlantic States, possess medicinal properties. The *flowers*, which are officinal, are employed internally as a diaphoretic; externally as a discutient. The INNER BARK, which is without smell, and has a taste at first sweetish, afterwards slightly bitter, acrid, and nauseous, and contains a resin, with valerianic acid, and other principles, is a hydragogue cathartic, and in large doses emetic. It is deemed a valuable remedy in dropsy, particularly in dropsy dependent on albuminuria, in which affection specific alterative virtues are attributed to it. It is given in *decoction* (an ounce boiled with two pints of water to a pint); dose, f℥iv. An infusion in cider is popularly employed.

DRASTIC CATHARTICS.

JALAPA—JALAP.

Jalap is the TUBER of Ipomæa Jalapa or Exogonium purga, (*Nat. Ord.* Convolvulaceæ), a climbing plant of Mexico, which derives its name from the city of Jalapa, near Vera Cruz. The tubers are imported usually entire, but sometimes in slices. When entire, they vary in size and shape from a walnut to a large pear, are hard and heavy—externally, brown and wrinkled, and internally, grayish, with brown, concentric rings; they are often furrowed with vertical incisions, made to promote drying.

They have a heavy, rather nauseous smell, and a sweetish, subacrid, disagreeable taste. They yield their virtues partly to water, partly to alcohol, and completely to diluted alcohol. In the shops, jalap is kept in the state of powder, which is of a yellowish-gray colour. Its active principle is a peculiar *resin*, which consists of two portions, both of which are cathartic, one soft and soluble in ether, the other, which has been termed *rhodeoretin*, insoluble in ether; it contains also gum and starch, which is apt to be attacked by worms, the worm-eaten pieces becoming thus the most active.

Effects and Uses.—Jalap is a powerful hydragogue cathartic, operating with great promptness, and often causing much pain. In overdoses, it may produce dangerous hypercatharsis. It is employed as a hydragogue in dropsy, when it is often combined with cream of tartar; as a revulsive in cerebral and other affections, and to increase the activity of calomel in bilious fever. Dose, gr. xv to xxx; in combination, gr. x. Of the *extract*, which is made with alcohol and water, and contains the resin and gum, the dose is one-half that of jalap. The *compound powder of jalap* (*pulvis jalapæ compositus*), contains one part of jalap and two parts of cream of tartar. The *resin* is extracted by solution in alcohol, and afterwards precipitated from the tincture by water (16 troyounces of jalap percolated with alcohol to a pint and a half, then reduced to six fluidounces by distillation, and precipitated with seven pints of water); dose, from four to eight grains. The *tincture* (six troyounces to alcohol, diluted with one-half a measure of water, Oij), is added to cathartic mixtures. Dose, f℥i–f℥ss.

PODOPHYLLUM—MAY-APPLE.

Podophyllum peltatum, May-apple or Mandrake (*Nat. Ord.* Ranunculaceæ), is a very common indigenous, herbaceous plant, with a long creeping, perennial root, and an upright stem about a foot high, separating at the top into two petioles, each supporting a large peltate leaf, divided into five or six lobes. At the fork of the petioles, it bears a single flower, which appears in May, the fruit ripening in September. The RHIZOME, which is the part used, is found in the shops in wrinkled, jointed, cylindrical pieces, about two lines in diameter, of a brown colour externally, and yellowish within. The powder is yellowish-gray, and has a sweetish smell; its taste is at first sweetish, afterwards

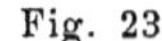

Fig. 23.

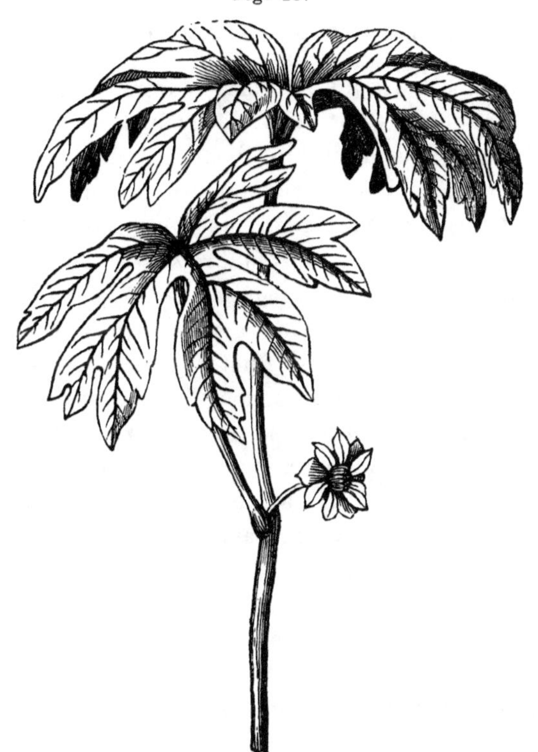

bitter, acrid, and nauseous. Diluted alcohol is the best solvent of podophyllum, which has been found to contain, with the alkaloid *berberina*, two *resinous* cathartic principles, both soluble in alcohol, but one only soluble in ether.

Effects and Uses.—This is an active hydragogue cathartic, with an especial determination to the upper portion of the alimentary canal, and a pretty decided cholagogue action, which is, however, probably produced by duodenal irritation. It is an ingredient in several cathartic nostrums. Dose, in *powder*

℈j; of the *extract* (prepared with alcohol and diluted alcohol), gr. v to gr. xv; of the *resin* (made in the same way as the *resin* of jalap, except that the water, used to precipitate the resin from its alcoholic solution, is previously mixed with two fluidrachms of muriatic acid), gr. ¼ to gr. j.

SCAMMONIUM—SCAMMONY.

Scammony is a RESINOUS EXUDATION from the ROOT of Convolvulus Scammonia (*Nat. Ord.* Convolvulaceæ), a twining plant of Syria. The finest kind is the product of exudation from the sliced root; but most of the drug which reaches us is probably obtained by expression. It comes from the Levant. Genuine scammony, termed *Virgin Scammony*, occurs in light, irregular, friable pieces, of various shades of colour from dark-ash to dark-olive, covered with a whitish-gray powder, and breaking with a bright-greenish fracture; they should not effervesce with an acid. The scammony of the shops, which is always more or less adulterated, is in hard, heavy, saucer-shaped cakes, from four to six inches in diameter (sometimes broken into pieces), of a dark ash or slate colour. The powder is light-gray; the smell disagreeable, like that of old cheese, the taste at first feeble, afterwards bitterish and acrid. Scammony is a gum-resin, its active ingredient being *resin*, which constitutes from 80 to 90 per cent. of the weight of good scammony. Its proper solvents are alcohol and ether.

A factitious scammony, made in France, and known as *Montpelier Scammony*, is occasionally imported into the United States. It is blacker than the genuine article, has a feeble, balsamic odour, and a very bitter, nauseous taste.

Effects and Uses.—Scammony is an energetic hydragogue cathartic, operating sometimes with great violence, and seldom given, except in combination with other cathartics. Dose, gr. v to gr. xv of the pure drug, gr. x to gr. xxx of the drug of the shops; of the *resin* (made by digesting six troyounces of scammony with successive portions of boiling alcohol until exhausted, mixing the tinctures, afterwards reducing the mixture to a syrupy consistence by distilling off the alcohol, and then precipitating with a pint of water), gr. iv to gr. viij. This is much used in the form of *compound extract of colocynth.*

HELLEBORUS (*Black Hellebore*). The ROOT of Helleborus Niger, Black Hellebore, or Christmas Rose (*Nat. Ord.* Ranunculaceæ), a mountainous European plant, at one time enjoyed much reputation as a hydragogue cathartic and emmenagogue; the small fibres, or roots, are about as thick as straw, and have a somewhat nauseous odour, and a bitter, unpleasant acrid taste; they contain two active principles, *helleborin* and *helleborein* (glucosides). Black hellebore is now little used, and only as an emmenagogue. Dose of the *powdered root*, gr. x to gr. xx; of the *extract* (*alcoholic*), gr. v to gr. x; of the *tincture* (four troyounces to diluted alcohol Oij) f℥ss to f℥j.

COLOCYNTHIS—COLOCYNTH.

Colocynth is the FRUIT (deprived of its rind) of Citrullus Colocynthis or bitter cucumber (*Nat. Ord.* Cucurbitaceæ), an annual plant of the south of Europe and parts of Asia and Africa, resembling the common watermelon. The fruit has a thin, but hard rind, but is *peeled* and dried for exportation, and comes to us from the Levant. It consists of light, whitish, spongy balls, about the size of a small orange, filled with numerous seeds. For medicinal use, the *pulp* only is employed, and the seeds, which are inactive, are rejected. The pulp has a feeble odour, and a nauseous, intensely bitter taste. It yields its virtues to both water and alcohol, and contains a peculiar glucoside principle termed *colocynthin*, resin, &c.

Effects and Uses.—Colocynth is a violent hydragogue cathartic, acting sometimes very harshly even in small doses, and in overdoses producing dangerous, and occasionally fatal enteric inflammation. Its chief use is to unload the bowels in obstinate constipation. The dose is gr. v to gr. x. It is seldom, however, administered alone. The *extract* (*alcoholic*), is made by depriving 48 troyounces of colocynth of seeds, grinding, macerating in 8 pints of diluted alcohol for four days, expressing, percolating the residue with diluted alcohol till the tincture and expressed liquid measure 16 pints; the alcohol is then recovered, and the residue evaporated to dryness and powdered. This is used chiefly in the preparation of the *compound extract*, which is made by mixing three troyounces and a half of alcoholic extract, twelve troyounces of purified aloes, three troyounces of resin of scammony, a troyounce and a half of cardamom, and three troyounces of soap; this is a favourite prescription, but it is apt to gripe, and it is well to combine some aromatic with it, as a little oil of cloves or capsicum—dose, gr. v–x.

GAMBOGIA—GAMBOGE.

Gamboge is a GUM-RESIN, procured from Garcinia morella, var. pedicellata (*Nat. Ord.* Guttiferæ), a tree of Siam and Cochin-China. The juice is said to be collected, as it exudes from the wounded bark of the tree, in cocoa-nut shells, and is afterwards rolled into cylinders, or transferred to earthen jars to dry; it is sometimes also received into the hollow joints of the bamboo. It is imported from Canton and Calcutta, and occurs in cylindrical rolls from one to three inches in diameter, of an orange colour, known as *pipe gamboge*, or in irregular masses (which are less pure), weighing two to three pounds or more, called *cake* or *lump gamboge.* Good gamboge is opaque, brittle, inodorous, nearly insipid, and breaks with a vitreous fracture; its powder is bright-yellow. It is a gum-resin, forming a yellow, opaque emulsion with water, and a golden-yellow solution with alcohol; it contains from 20 to 25 per cent. of gum, and from 75 to 80 per cent. of a resin termed *gambogic acid* ($C_{20}H_{23}O_4$).

Effects and Uses.—Gamboge is a powerful hydragogue, and in overdoses has proved fatal. Sometimes it vomits, and, in large amounts, has produced death merely from depression. It is employed in obstinate constipation—in dropsies, combined with cream of tartar or jalap—and has been given to destroy tænia. Dose, gr. ij to gr. vj. It is usually prescribed with other and milder cathartics, to promote and accelerate their action. *Compound cathartic pills* (pilulæ catharticæ compositæ), are made by mixing 32 grains of compound extract of colocynth, 24 grains of extract of jalap and calomel each, and 6 grains of gamboge, and with water forming a pilular mass to be divided into 24 pills. Three of the pills, containing $10\frac{3}{4}$ grains of the mass, represent 4 grains of compound extract of colocynth, 3 of extract of jalap and calomel each, and $\frac{3}{4}$ grain of gamboge.

ELATERIUM.

Elaterium is a substance deposited by the JUICE of the FRUIT of Momordica Elaterium, Ecbalium agreste, or Squirting Cucumber (*Nat. Ord.* Cucurbitaceæ), an annual vine of the south of Europe now cultivated in England. The fruit has the shape of a small oval cucumber, and, when fully ripe, separates from the peduncle, and throws out its juice and seeds with considerable force, through an opening in the base. Pure elaterium is obtained by slicing the fruit, and allowing the juice to drain through a sieve. The juice deposits a *sediment,* which dries in very light, thin, nearly flat, pulverulent, greenish-gray cakes, and is the genuine elaterium. It is almost inodorous, and has a bitter, acrid taste. The commercial elaterium, which is obtained chiefly from England, is made by expression. The drug is to be considered inferior when it is dark-coloured, much curled, and hard. Elaterium yields its virtues to alcohol and not to water. Its active principle is called *elaterin,* which crystallizes in colourless, shining, rhombic, six-sided tables, without smell, but of a bitter, sharp taste, insoluble in water, but readily soluble in alcohol ($C_{20}H_{28}O_5$); it proves powerfully cathartic in doses of $\frac{1}{20}$ to $\frac{1}{12}$ of a grain.

Effects and Uses.—Elaterium is a hydragogue cathartic of great violence of operation, and in overdoses has frequently proved fatal. It has also a diuretic action. It is a very efficient remedy in the treatment of dropsies, and is also a useful revulsive in cerebral affections; but, in administering it, considerable caution is required. Dose of the *pure* drug (termed *Clutterbuck's elaterium*), gr. $\frac{1}{8}$; of the drug of the shops, gr. j to gr. ij; but it is most safely given in divided doses.

OLEUM TIGLII—CROTON OIL.

Croton oil is a FIXED OIL obtained from the SEEDS of Croton Tiglium (*Nat. Ord.* Euphorbiaceæ), a small tree of the East Indies. The Croton seeds resemble the Castor seeds in shape and size, and consist of a blackish shell, sometimes covered with a yellowish-brown epidermis, and enclosing a yellowish oily kernel. They are highly irritant and cathartic, but are not imported into this country. They contain a volatile oil, a FIXED OIL, resin, acetic, butyric, and valerianic acids, together with a peculiar acid termed *tiglic* ($H_2C_5H_7O_2$). The CROTON OIL of the shops is obtained by expression, and is a mixture of the fixed oil proper, the resin, and tiglic acid. A principle termed *crotonol* is said to produce the peculiar inflammation of the skin. The oil is made both in India and England, the Indian oil being of a pale straw-colour, and the English reddish-brown; the latter is the variety now found in the shops. It has a viscid consistence, which is increased by age, a faint peculiar odour, and an extremely acrid, pungent taste; it is soluble in ether and the volatile and fixed oils, and partially so in alcohol.

Physiological Effects.—Croton oil, taken internally, is a powerful hydragogue purgative, occasionally increasing also the secretions from the kidneys. One or two drops are usually sufficient to produce active catharsis, but sometimes as much as eight or ten drops may bė taken without affecting the bowels. It operates very speedily, often causing evacuations in half an hour, and is apt to produce considerable depression of the vascular system. In overdoses it has frequently proved fatal. *Rubbed on the skin,* croton oil causes rubefaction and a pustular or vesicular eruption; and, rubbed over the abdomen, it will sometimes purge.

Medicinal Uses.—Croton oil, from the smallness of the dose required, and the speediness of its action, is an extremely valuable purgative in obstinate constipation, and in cerebral disorders, particularly coma. As a *counter-irritant*, it is extensively employed in pulmonary and laryngeal affections, diseases of the joints, &c. Dose, one or two drops made into pill, with bread-crumb. For *external use*, it may be diluted with one or two parts of olive oil or oil of turpentine.

MERCURIAL CATHARTICS.

The preparations of mercury, employed as cathartics, are *calomel*, *blue pill*, and *mercury with chalk*. Their purgative effects depend partly on the increased flow of bile which they occasion, and partly on the stimulus which they give to secretion from the mucous follicles of the intestinal canal, and from the pancreas. They are rarely employed alone, owing to the slowness and uncertainty of their action; but are usually combined with, or followed by other cathartics (as jalap, senna, rhubarb, compound extract of colocynth, or some of the saline preparations). The mercurial cathartics are usually administered with a view of combining a purgative action with an effect on the secretions, particularly that of the liver; also, as anthelmintics; and as revulsives in cerebral and other affections. They are well adapted to infantile cases, from the facility of their administration, and are especially beneficial in the ephemeral febrile attacks to which children are subject; they, moreover, rarely produce salivation in children.

HYDRARGYRI CHLORIDUM MITE (*Mild Chloride of Mercury, or Calomel*). (Noticed at length under the head of *Alteratives*.) Dose, as a *cathartic*, gr. vi to xij, in pill or in powder, with syrup or molasses; to be followed, in from four to six hours, by some other cathartic. Sometimes, when it is exhibited with a view to a full action on the liver, gr. j or ij may be given every hour or two until the whole purgative dose is taken: or, it may be administered at bedtime, with an aperient draught the next morning. For children, larger doses are required in proportion than for adults: gr. iij–vj may be given to a child from three to six years old. Calomel occasionally causes griping pain in the bowels, with bilious vomiting; this is attributable, not to any irritable qualities in the medicine, but to the acrid character of the bile secreted. Calomel is an ingredient of the *Compound Cathartic Pills.*

PILULÆ HYDRARGYRI (*Pills of Mercury*) commonly called *Blue Pills* (see *Alteratives*), are analogous in their cathartic action to calomel, but milder. They are given in about the same doses, and in the same combinations, &c.

HYDRARGYRUM CUM CRETA (*Mercury with Chalk*), (see *Alteratives*), combines antacid with mercurial effects. It is a very mild preparation—weaker than even blue pill. It is used as a laxative, in bowel-complaints and other affections of children. Dose, gr. v–xx for adults; for children, gr. ij or iij to viij or x, in *powder*, and not in pill.

ENEMATA.

In cases of irritability of the stomach—or with the view of hastening the action of cathartics taken by the mouth—or to remove feculent accumulations in the lower bowels—or to relieve tympanites—or for the purpose of revulsion, *cathartic enemata* are frequently administered.

When it is desired simply to open the bowels mechanically, tepid water, flaxseed tea, or other demulcent infusion may be employed. The common *laxative enema* consists of a tablespoonful of common salt, molasses, and lard or olive oil, each in two-thirds of a pint of warm water; castor oil, or Epsom salt may be added to increase the cathartic effect. Senna tea, or some other cathartic infusion is often employed. To relieve flatulency, oil of turpentine (f℥ss to f℥j, in emulsion), or milk of assafetida (f℥ij to f℥iv), may be given. The latter is an excellent preparation in infantile cases.

ORDER III.—DIAPHORETICS.

Diaphoretics (from διαφορεω, *I transpire*), called also *sudorifics*, are medicines which promote transpiration from the skin. The action of the cutaneous exhalants may be increased by various means. The mere introduction of a large quantity of fluid into the system will produce sweating, if the skin be kept warm. Exercise and a warm temperature, by determining a flow of blood to the cutaneous vessels, act in the same way. Nauseants occasion diaphoresis, by relaxing the orifices of the cutaneous vessels; stimulants, by exciting them to increased secretion. Diaphoretics are employed therapeutically, for their evacuant, revulsive, and alterative effects, and to promote absorption. Different classes of diaphoretics are required for different morbid conditions.

1. *Nauseating Diaphoretics.*—Most of the *emetics*, in nauseating doses, produce a powerful relaxing diaphoretic action, and are much employed, with this view, in inflammatory cases, when not contraindicated by the presence of gastric irritability. The PREPARATIONS OF ANTIMONY (see p. 210), and IPECACUANHA (see p. 229), are chiefly resorted to as nauseating diaphoretics. Ipecacuanha is often given as a diaphoretic, in combination with opium, in the form of *Dover's Powder* (see p 58).

2. *Refrigerant Diaphoretics.*—The saline and ethereal preparations classed as *refrigerants* (see p. 216), produce a gentle relaxing diaphoretic action, unattended with nausea. They are used to allay febrile excitement, and reduce the temperature of the body.

3. *Stimulating Diaphoretics.*—This group includes the diffusible stimulants, aromatic substances generally, of every class, and many narcotics, particularly opium and camphor. They are contraindicated in high inflammation, but are very serviceable in rheumatic and pulmonary affections, after vascular excitement has been reduced, and in all diseases where the surface of the body is cold. *Opium*, in the form of *Dover's Powder*, may be employed in inflammatory cases, where other stimulating diaphoretics are inadmissible, and is given with advantage in an early stage of acute rheumatism, dysentery, and catarrh, unless the action of the pulse be very strong, when this should be previously moderated. The operation of

the diaphoretic stimulants is promoted by the free use of warm diluent drinks, and warm covering to the body.

4. *Alterative Diaphoretics.*—Under this head are comprised a class of diaphoretic medicines, which produce a gradual and nearly insensible increase of the cutaneous secretion, and are supposed to promote the elimination of noxious matters from the blood, through the vessels of the skin. They are employed chiefly in chronic rheumatic and cutaneous affections, and in secondary syphilis.

ALTERATIVE DIAPHORETICS.

SARSAPARILLA.

The name Sarsaparilla is applied to the ROOTS of Smilax officinalis and other species of Smilax (*Nat. Ord.* Smilaceæ), twining, prickly shrubs of Mexico, Guatemala, and the warm countries of South America. The roots consist of numerous wrinkled, slender pieces, of the average thickness of a writing quill, several feet long, springing from a common head or rhizome, and are frequently found in the shops with portions of the stems attached. Several varieties are known: 1. *Honduras Sarsaparilla,* the most common variety in the United States, comes in bundles two or three feet long, composed of several long, thin roots, folded lengthwise, of a dirty grayish or reddish-brown colour. 2. *Jamaica Sarsaparilla,* which is probably derived also from Central America, comes in shorter bundles, and is known by the red colour of the epidermis. 3. *Vera Cruz Sarsaparilla* comes in large, loose bales, bound with cords or leather thongs, containing the roots folded on themselves, consisting of a head with numerous long radicals. 4. *Brazilian* or *Rio Negro Sarsaparilla* comes in cylindrical bundles, each of which is closely wrapped by a flexible stem, with fewer rootlets than the Honduras variety; it is distinguished by the amylaceous character of its interior structure. 5. *Guatemala Sarsaparilla* resembles the Brazilian.

Sarsaparilla roots are several feet in length, about the

thickness of a goose-quill, cylindrical, more or less wrinkled longitudinally, and consist of a whitish-brown or pink cortical portion, covered with a thin gray, brown, or red epidermis, and inclosing a layer of whitish ligneous fibre, and a central pith. The *cortical portion* is more active than the interior portions; the central medulla contains a good deal of starch. Sarsaparilla, in the dried state, is nearly inodorous, but its decoction has a strong smell. It has a mucilaginous, slightly bitter taste, and, when chewed for some time, produces a persistent acrid impression on the mouth; this acridity of taste is the criterion of good sarsaparilla. Water and diluted alcohol extract its virtues, but they are impaired by long boiling. It contains an active principle, called *similacin* or *sarsaparillin*, starch, resin, extractive, &c.

Effects and Uses.—The physiological effects of sarsaparilla, beyond a slight diaphoretic action, are not very obvious; in large doses, it occasionally produces nausea and vomiting. Its efficacy, however, in eradicating various morbid symptoms is well established, and its mode of action, though obscure, is generally attributed to a purifying influence on the blood, through the function of the skin. It is employed in secondary syphilis, particularly where the disease resists or is aggravated by the use of mercury; also in chronic rheumatism, skin diseases, and cachectic conditions of the system generally.

Administration.—Dose, of the *powder*, ʒss, three or four times a day—not much used, however, in this form. The *compound decoction* is made by boiling six troyounces of sarsaparilla, a troyounce of bark of sassafras root, guaiacum wood, and liquorice root, each, and 180 grains of mezereon, in 4 pints of water for 15 minutes, then digesting for 2 hours at 200°, and, after straining, adding water enough to make the decoction measure 4 pints—dose, f℥iv–vi, three times a day. The *compound syrup* (which contains also guaiacum wood, pale rose, senna, liquorice root, and the oils of sassasfras, anise, and gaultheria), is a favourite preparation: corrosive sublimate should not be given with it, as it is decomposed into calomel. Dose, f℥ss, three times a day. Of the *fluid extract*, the dose is f℥ss. The *compound fluid extract* contains the ingredients of the compound decoction, except the guaiacum—dose, f℥j, three or four times a day.

ARALIA NUDICAULIS—FALSE SARSAPARILLA.

The ROOT of Aralia Nudicaulis, False Sarsaparilla, or Small Spikenard (*Nat. Ord.* Araliaceæ), a small, indigenous, perennial plant, possesses alterative diaphoretic properties similar to those of sarsaparilla, and is employed as a substitute for it, in the same manner and doses.

The ROOT of *A. racemosa* or *American Spikenard*, and the BARK of *A. spinosa*, or *Angelica-tree*, are also employed as alterative diaphoretics.

GUAIACI LIGNUM—GUAIACUM WOOD.

GUAIACI RESINA—GUAIAC.

Guaiacum Wood, or *Lignum Vitæ*, and Guaiac, are products of Guaiacum officinale (*Nat. Ord.* Zygophyllaceæ), a large evergreen tree of South America and the West Indies. The WOOD, which is remarkable for its hardness and density, is imported in logs or billets, covered with a thick gray bark; the outer portion or sapwood is of a pale yellow colour, the inner, of an olive-brown. The *heart-wood* is the officinal portion: it is usually kept in the shops in the state of shavings or raspings; they are inodorous, unless heated, and, when chewed for some time, they have a bitterish, pungent taste. Guaiacum wood yields its virtues to alcohol, and partially to water; they depend on the guaiac contained in the wood.

Guaiac is a peculiar *resin*, obtained from Guaiacum officinale, by spontaneous exudation, by incision, by dry-heat, or by decoction of the comminuted wood. It comes in large, irregular, semi-transparent, brittle pieces, of varying size—externally, of a deep green or olive colour, and internally, red. It has a slight, balsamic odour, which is rendered stronger by heat, and, though at first nearly tasteless, leaves a hot, acrid sensation in the mouth and throat. Water dissolves it partially, alcohol completely. It is probably a mixture of several substances, among which are *guiaretinic acid* ($C_{20}H_{26}O_4$) and *guiacin*, a glucoside; most oxidizing agents, as nitric and chromic acids, &c., produce a blue, then green, and finally a brown colour with tincture of guaiacum.

Effects and Uses.—Guaiacum wood and guaiac are stimulant diaphoretics, and in large doses cathartic. They are principally used for their alterative virtues in chronic rheumatism, secondary syphilis, and skin diseases; guaiac has been used as a laxative. They are considered also to possess emmenagogue properties, and are employed in amenorrhœa and dysmenorrhœa.

Administration.—*Guaiacum wood* is used only as an ingredient in the compound decoction and syrup of sarsaparilla. Dose of *guaiac*, gr. x to gr. xxx, in pill or emulsion, sometimes combined with alkalies. The *tincture* (six troyounces to alcohol Oij), and *ammoniated tincture* (six troyounces to ar. sp. of ammonia Ojj), are much used in chronic rheumatism; the former is given also in amenorrhœa; dose, f℥j, three or four times a day. They are decomposed by water, and should be administered in mucilage, syrup, or milk.

MEZEREUM—MEZEREON.

Mezereon is the BARK of Daphne Mezereum and Daphne Gnidium (*Nat. Ord.* Thymelaceæ), European shrubs, which grow to the height of four or five feet. The root-bark is the part employed in Great Britain, but the bark of our shops, which is brought from Germany, is the STEM-BARK. It comes in strips, from two to four feet long, and an inch or less in breadth, folded in bundles, or wrapped in the shape of balls. It has a thin, grayish, or reddish-brown, wrinkled epidermis, and a tough, pliable, whitish inner bark. When fresh, it has a faint nauseous smell, but, when dry, it is nearly inodorous. Its taste is at first sweetish, afterwards highly acrid. It yields its virtues to water and alcohol, and contains a peculiar crystalline principle called *daphnin*, and a *resin*, to which it owes its acridity.

Effects and Uses.—The topical action of mezereon is irritant and vesicant. When swallowed in large quantities, it is highly acrid; in medicinal doses, it promotes the action of the secreting and exhaling organs, particularly the skin and kidneys. It is chiefly employed in conjunction with sarsaparilla (in the compound decoction, &c.), as an alterative diaphoretic, in rheumatic, syphilitic, and cutaneous affections. As a *masticatory*, it has been chewed for the relief of paralysis of the muscles of deglutition. The *fluid extract* is the only preparation for internal administration; dose, 10 minims; the *ointment* (made by mixing 4 fluidounces of fluid extract with 14 troyounces of lard, and 2 troyounces of yellow wax, previously melted together), is used as a stimulating application to blistered surfaces and indolent ulcers.

SASSAFRAS.

This is the BARK of the ROOT of Sassafras officinale (*Nat. Ord.* Lauraceæ), an indigenous tree of middling size. The bark is found in the shops in small irregular pieces of a cinnamon colour, sometimes invested with a brownish epidermis. It has a highly fragrant odour, and a sweetish aromatic taste. Its virtues are extracted by water and alcohol, and it contains a little tannic acid, and a *volatile oil* (*oleum sassafras*). The oil is said to act as a physiological antidote against tobacco.

Effects and Uses.—Sassafras bark is a mild stimulant alterative diaphoretic, used chiefly in combination with sarsaparilla. Its principal virtues are probably aromatic. Dose of the *oil*, two to ten drops. (For *Sassafras Pith*, see *Demulcents*.)

STILLINGIA.

The ROOT of Stillingia sylvatica (*Nat. Ord.* Euphorbiaceæ), commonly called *Queen's Delight*, a perennial plant, growing to the height of two feet in our south Atlantic States, is highly esteemed by Southern physicians, as an alterative diaphoretic in secondary syphilis, scrofula, cutaneous affections, and chronic rheumatism. Dose of the powder 15 to 30 grains; the *fluid extract* is officinal and may be given in the dose of f℥ss; a decoction and tincture are extemporaneously prepared.

ORDER IV.—DIURETICS.

Diuretics (from δια, *thoroughly*, and ουρεω, *I make water*), are medicines which excite the secretion of urine. The flow of urine may be promoted *indirectly*, by increasing the quantity of fluid taken into the stomach, or by the removal of causes which check its secretion, or by mental emotion, a cool temperature, &c It is promoted *directly* by the use of medicinal agents which specifically affect the kidneys; they are termed diuretics. A large proportion of diuretic medicines are found among the agents which influence other secretions, particularly *diaphoretics*. The functions of transpiration and urination are to some extent vicarious, and the same articles will prove diaphoretic or diuretic, as their action may be directed to the skin or kidneys. External warmth and warm drinks determine the action of such medicines to the skin; and, on the other hand, if the skin be kept cool, and cool diluents freely administered, the secretion from the kidneys is promoted.

Blenorrhetics, or medicines which have a special action on the mucous membranes, exert also a diuretic influence—probably the result of the stimulating impression which they make on the mucous membrane of the urinary passages. When the action of the kidneys is obstructed by disease of the heart, *sedatives* prove diuretic, by their tranquillizing influence on the action of the heart. In cases of obstruction of the portal system, *mercurials* increase the efficacy of the diuretics proper; and also *cathartics*, by stimulating the flow of bile and the pancreatic juice.

The principal *therapeutic* employment of diuretics is *to pro-*

mote the absorption of dropsical effusions. They are also useful in nephritic disorders attended with obstructed secretion; to wash out calculi from the pelvis of the kidneys, ureters, and bladder; in gravel, with the view of rendering the urine more dilute; and they may be resorted to as evacuants, to reduce inflammation.

As diuretics act by becoming absorbed, they should be administered in a very diluted state to prevent a cathartic effect.

The following groups of medicines, noticed under other heads, are employed also as diuretics:

1. *The Saline and Ethereal Refrigerants* (see p. 216).
2. *The Alkaline Carbonates* (see *Antacids*); and the *Alkaline Salts, which contain a vegetable acid*, as the acetates, citrates, and tartrates. The acid tartrate of potassium, or CREAM OF TARTAR (see p. 245), is a very active diuretic.

POTASSII ACETAS (*Acetate of Potassium*). This salt ($KC_2H_3O_2$), formerly termed *sal diureticus*, from its decided diuretic action, is made by saturating acetic acid with bicarbonate of potassium. It occurs, when pure, as a white, foliaceous, satiny mass, of a warm, pungent taste, very deliquescent, and wholly soluble in water and alcohol. In small doses, it is diuretic; and, in larger doses, gently cathartic. It is a good deal employed as a diuretic in dropsies, as an antacid in acute rheumatism, as a preventive of the formation of uric acid calculi, and it has also been found useful as an alterative in cutaneous affections. As is the case with all the alkaline salts containing vegetable acids, the acid of this salt is decomposed in the system into carbonic acid. Although increasing the flow of urine, the acetate of potassium diminishes the amount both of uric acid and of urea in the secretion. Hence it is valuable in gout, and, like colchicum, it may perhaps check the actual formation of uric acid in the system. Dose, ℈j to ʒj, three or four times a day.

SODII ACETAS (*Acetate of Sodium*), is prepared from crude pyroligneous acid, which is saturated with cream of lime, and the solution of acetate of calcium thus formed is decomposed by sulphate of sodium; repeated solution and recrystallization, with fusion, furnish a pure salt in the form of white or colourless striated prisms ($NaC_2H_3O_2,3H_2O$), which effloresce in dry air, are wholly soluble in water, tolerably soluble in alcohol, and have a sharp, bitterish, not disagreeable taste. Its effects and uses are analogous to those of acetate of potassium, over which it has the advantage of not being deliquescent. Dose, ℈i to ʒi.

3. *Sedatives* (see p. 204), particularly DIGITALIS (see p. 204), which is very much employed in *cardiac* dropsies, in combination with squill.

4. *Blennorrhetics* (see p. 283), particularly the OLEORESINS.

5. Most of the *Stimulating Diaphoretics*.

6. Among *Astringents*, UVA URSI (p. 169), and PIPSISSEWA (p. 171).

SPECIAL DIURETICS.

SCILLA—SQUILL.

Squill is the BULB of Scilla maritima (*Nat. Ord.* Liliaceæ), a perennial plant, which grows on the shores of the Mediterranean. It has fibrous roots, attached to a roundish-ovate bulb, from which both the leaves and flower-stem spring directly, the latter appearing first; the leaves are broad-lanceolate, and from twelve to eighteen inches long; the stem is about two feet high, and bears pale, yellowish-green flowers.

The fresh bulb is pyriform, of the size of the fist to that of a child's head, and consists of thick, fleshy, concentric scales, attenuated at their edges, and attached to a rudimentary stem; the outer scales are very thin and papery. Two kinds of squill bulbs are met with, the *white* and the *red*, which differ only in the colour of their scales, and are identical in medicinal virtues. Both abound in a viscid, acrid juice, which is very much diminished by drying, with little loss of medicinal power. For importation, squill is usually sliced and dried, and is found in the shops in white or yellowish-white pieces, which, when dry, are brittle, but, when moist, flexible. They absorb moisture readily, and should be kept in well-stoppered bottles. They have a feeble odour, a bitter, nauseous, acrid taste, and yield their virtues to water, alcohol, and vinegar. Two active principles have been found in squill: one an acrid, poisonous, resinoid substance, soluble in alcohol and not in ether, the other a bitter yellow principle, soluble in water and alcohol; the bitter principle is much the less powerful.

Physiological Effects.—In small doses, squill promotes secretion from the mucous membranes and the kidneys—its diuretic effect being much the most marked and constant. In larger doses, it excites nausea, vomiting, and occasionally purging; and, in excessive doses, it acts as an acro-narcotic poison—gr. xxiv having proved fatal. The symptoms are violent vomiting and purging, abdominal pains, bloody or suppressed urine, reduction of the pulse, with collapse, or death may be preceded by convulsions; after evacuation of the stomach, opiates and demulcents are to be administered, and, if syncope or collapse occur, alcoholic stimuli.

Medicinal Uses.—Squill is employed principally in the treatment of dropsy; it should not be used, however, in cases complicated with degeneration of the kidneys or inflammation of the bladder. Digitalis is much prescribed in combination with squill in the treatment of cardiac dropsies, and calomel is often added with a view to its action on the absorbents. As a *blennorhetic expectorant*, squill is an excellent remedy in chronic and subacute bronchial affections; it is, however, improper in the early stages of inflammatory cases. As an *emetic*, squill is too dangerous for general use; but it forms an ingredient in some emetic preparations administered in croup.

Administration.—Dose, as a *diuretic* or *expectorant*, gr. j, repeated and gradually increased till nausea supervenes. Gr. vj to gr. xij will vomit. Of the *vinegar* (*acetum scillæ*), (four troyounces to diluted acetic acid Oij), the dose is ♏xxx to f℥ij; of the *fluid extract*, ♏j; of the *syrup*, made by dissolving 24 troyounces of sugar in a pint of *vinegar of squill*, at a gentle heat, f℥j; of the *compound syrup*, known as *hive syrup* (which is prepared by percolation, by first making a solution of seneka and squill, in diluted alcohol and water, converting it into a syrup, and dissolving in it tartar emetic, one grain of which is contained in every ounce of the syrup), 10 drops to f℥j, according to the age; of the *tincture* (four troyounces to diluted alcohol Oij), 20 to 40 drops. The *compound pills of squill* contain also ginger, ammoniac, and soap, and are used as a stimulant expectorant; dose, one pill, three or four times a day, each pill containing half a grain of squill and one grain of ammoniac.

COLCHICUM.

Colchici Radix, Colchicum Root; Colchici Semen, Colchicum Seed.

Colchicum autumnale, or Meadow-Saffron (*Nat. Ord.* Melanthaceæ), is a small, biennial, bulbous plant, which grows wild, in moist meadows, in England and other temperate parts of Europe. The bulb, or corm, as it is botanically termed, appears in midsummer as the lateral offset from the corm of the preceding year, and sends up the flower-stem in the autumn—the leaves and fruit following in the succeeding spring. The leaves are broadly lanceolate, about five inches long; the flowers of a lilac or light-purple colour; and the fruit oblong, elliptical, and three-celled.

The CORMS and SEEDS are the portions used medicinally. The corms are gathered in July, just before the sprouting of the flower from the young corm. They are somewhat like tulip-bulbs in appearance, but solid and not composed of scales. They are covered by an external brown membrane, and an inner reddish-yellow one, and are an inch and a half to two and a half inches in length, with a longitudinal groove. Internally, they are white, fleshy, and solid, and contain an acrid, bitter, milky juice. As found in the shops, they are in the dried state, sometimes whole, but usually cut into transverse slices, about an eighth of an inch thick, with a notch on one side, and deprived of the outer brown membrane. They have a hircine odour, and a bitter, hot, and acrid taste. The seeds are brown, about the size of black mustard-seeds, inodorous, and have a bitter, acrid taste; they are less apt to be injured by drying than the corms.

Colchicum corms and seeds yield their virtues to vinegar and alcohol; they both contain a peculiar non-crystallizable, alkaloid active principle; soluble in water, readily so in alcohol, but insoluble in ether, termed *colchicia*, ($C_{34}H_{19}NO_{10}$), which is a powerful poison; colchicia, in the saline form, is converted into another isomeric principle, termed colchiceine, and resin, but not probably with loss of medicinal effect. Colchicia makes with concentrated nitric acid a violet solution, becoming yellow, by dilution with water; with concentrated sulphuric acid, it produces an intensely yellow colour.

Physiological Effects.—Colchicum is a local irritant. Taken internally, in small doses, it stimulates the secretions generally; in larger doses, it produces nausea, vomiting, and purging, and commonly a reduction of the frequency of the pulse; in excessive doses, it is an acro-narcotic poison, producing death by a sedative action on the heart, the cerebral functions being usually unaffected. Tannic acid is a partial antidote; opiates, demulcents, and stimulants are to be given. Although placed among the diuretics, colchicum does not evince a more decided action on the kidneys than on other secretions, as those of the skin, liver, and mucous membranes.

Medicinal Uses.—Colchicum has long enjoyed a high reputation in the treatment of gout; and, although its *modus medendi* is rather obscure, it is universally admitted to possess a more decided control over the disease than any other remedy. Its efficacy has been attributed to a combined sedative, anodyne, and eccritic action; but, as it has a marked effect in diminishing the amount of uric acid, excreted in the urine, it probably arrests the formation of this acid in the blood, and in this way produces its anti-arthritic influence. It is usually administered in repeated doses, till an effect is produced on the bowels, though purging does not promote its curative effect. Epsom salt and magnesia are often combined with it as in the celebrated *Scudamore's draught* (*magnesia*, gr. xv to xx; *sulphate of magnesium*, ʒj to ʒij; *wine of colchicum seed*, fʒj to fʒij, in any pleasant vehicle). An excellent combination in the treatment of gout, is colchicum (*wine of the seed*, fʒi), with iodide of potassium (ʒij), dissolved in cinnamon water (fʒviij),—dose, fʒss, three times a day, until purgation is produced. Quinine and digitalis are also often given advantageously, with colchicum, in gout.* When it is desired to act on the kidneys and skin rather than the bowels, opiates are sometimes added. In rheumatism, it is also employed, but it has little control over this disease. It has been occasionally resorted to as a diuretic in dropsy, as a sedative in febrile and inflammatory diseases, as an anthelmintic, as an expectorant, and in some nervous affections.

Administration.—Dose of the corm or seeds, in *powder*, gr. ij to gr. viij; the seeds are to be preferred. The liquid preparations, which are more generally used than the powder, are: The *wine of the root* (*vinum colchici radicis*), (twelve troyounces to Sherry wine Oij), dose, ♏x to f℥ss; *wine of the seed* (*vinum colchici seminis*), (four troyounces to wine Oij), dose, f℥ss–j; *tincture* (four troyounces *of the seed* to diluted alcohol Oij), dose, f℥ss to f℥i. An *acetic extract of the root* is also employed—dose, gr. i–ij; and a *fluid extract of the seed*, and also *of the root*—doses, 4 to 12 drops.

ERIGERON.

Three varieties of *Erigeron* are officinal: E. Canadense, or Canada Fleabane, E. heterophyllum, or Various-leaved Fleabane, and E. Philadelphicum, or Philadelphia Fleabane (*Nat. Ord.* Asteraceæ). They are herbaceous indigenous plants, two or three feet high, with ovate or lanceolate toothed leaves, and white, blue, or purple flowers. The LEAVES and TOPS are officinal. *Canada Erigeron*, which is found in the Northern and Middle States, has an agreeable odour, and a bitter, acrid, somewhat astringent taste. It contains bitter extractive, tannic and gallic acids, and volatile oil; and is diuretic, tonic, and astringent. The *oil of Canada Erigeron* possesses hæmostatic properties, and has been used in hemorrhagic dysentery and uterine hemorrhage—dose, 5 to 10 drops; a *fluid extract of Canada Erigeron* may be given in the dose of f℥i–iv. *Various-leaved* and *Philadelphia Fleabane*, popularly known as *scabious*,

* Lartigue's celebrated gout-pills are, acetic extract of colchicum root, 2 grains, extract of digitalis, 1 grain, compound extract of colocynth, 20 grains, to be mixed and divided into 5 pills—one to be taken at night.

common plants all over the United States, have an aromatic odour, and a slightly bitterish taste. Their most striking medicinal action is diuretic, and they have long been favourite remedies in dropsical and nephritic affections. An *infusion* or *decoction* to the amount of a pint (containing a troyounce of the herb), may be taken daily.

APOCYNUM CANNABINUM—INDIAN HEMP.

This is an indigenous herbaceous plant (*Nat. Ord.* Apocynaceæ), growing to the height of two or three feet, with oblong-

Fig. 24

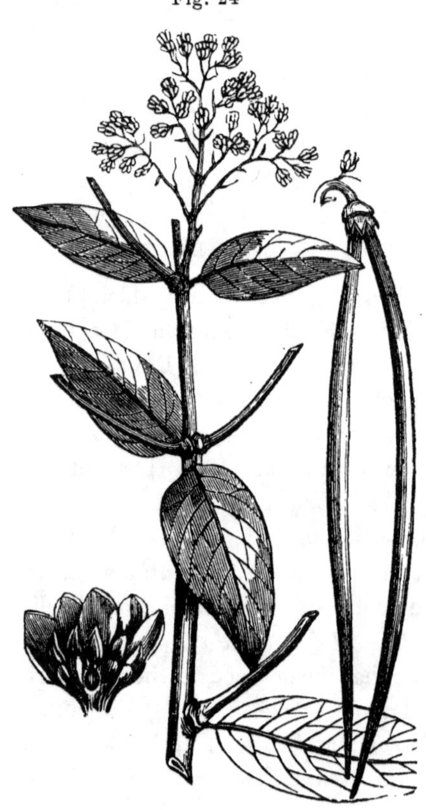

ovate leaves, and small, greenish, campanulate flowers. The ROOT is the officinal portion; it is of a yellowish-brown colour when young, and of a dark-chestnut when old, has a strong odour, and a nauseous, acrid, bitter taste. The fresh root, when wounded, pours out a milky juice; it yields its virtues to water and alcohol, and contains tannic and gallic acids, gum, resin, a bitter principle, &c., and a peculiar active principle termed *apocynin*. A. androsæmifolium, or Dogsbane, is possessed of much the same properties.

Effects and Uses.—Indian Hemp (which is not to be confounded with Cannabis Indica, p. 79), is an emeto-cathartic, diuretic, diaphoretic, and sedative. It is chiefly employed in the treatment of dropsy in the form of *decoction* (half a troy-ounce to water Ojss, boiled to Oj), of which f℥i–ij may be taken two or three times a day.

TARAXACUM—DANDELION.

Taraxacum Dens-leonis, or Dandelion (*Nat. Ord.* Cichoraceæ), is a small herbaceous, perennial plant, common to most parts

Fig. 25.

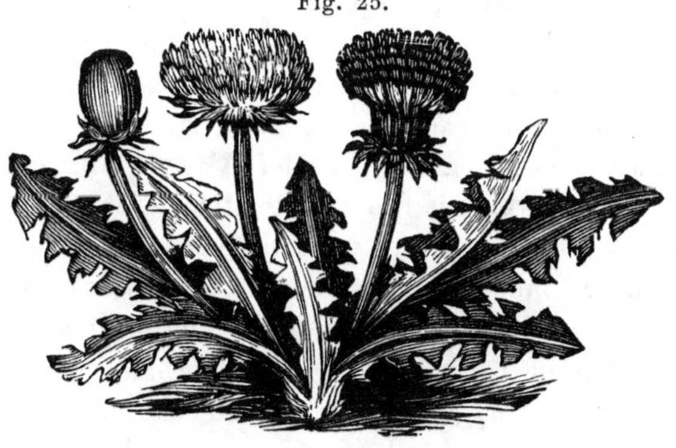

of the world, and found abundantly throughout the United States. It has a fusiform root, which sends up numerous long, sinuated, bright-green leaves, and flower-stems, about six inches high, bearing golden-yellow flowers. The ROOT is the officinal portion, and *should be gathered in the autumn.* In the fresh state, it is several inches long, branched, fleshy, of a light-brown colour externally, whitish within, and abounds in a milky juice; the *fresh* root is preferable for use. When dried, it is shrunken, wrinkled, and brittle. It is without smell, but has a bitter taste. Boiling water extracts its virtues, which depend on a peculiar bitter crystallizable principle termed *taraxacin*, soluble in boiling water, alcohol, and ether.

Effects and Uses.—Taraxacum is diuretic and slightly aperient, with some tonic action, and a special determination to the liver. It is a valuable remedy in hepatic dropsies, and is also employed in dyspepsia, accompanied by derangement of the liver. It is given in the form of *infusion* (two troyounces to boiling water Oj),—dose f℥ij, three times a day; *extract* (an inspissated juice, which should not be kept above a year),—dose ℈j to ʒj three times a day; and *fluid extract*,—dose, fʒi–ij, three times a day.

JUNIPERUS—JUNIPER.

The FRUIT, or berries, of Juniperus communis, (*Nat. Ord.* Pinaceæ), an evergreen European shrub, naturalized in the United States, are used as adjuvants to the more active diuretics. When dried, they are about the size of a pea, of a blackish-purple colour, and a sweetish, terebinthinate aromatic taste; they are given in *infusion* (a troyounce to boiling water Oj). Their virtues depend on a *volatile oil* (OLEUM JUNIPERI) ($C_{10}H_{16}$), the dose of which is from five to fifteen drops, two or three times a day. The *compound spirit* (a fluidrachm and a half of the oil, with 10 minims each of the oils of caraway and fennel, dissolved in 5 pints of alcohol and 3 pints of water), is a pleasant addition to stimulating diuretic and blennorrhetic combinations, and a good stomachic and carminative,—dose, f℥i–ij. The *spirit* is made by dissolving a fluidounce of the *oil* in 3 pints of stronger alcohol,—dose, f℥i–ij.

CAROTA—CARROT SEED.

Daucus Carota, or Wild Carrot (*Nat. Ord.* Apiaceæ), is a very common indigenous plant, which is found also wild in Europe. It has a biennial spindle-shaped root, an erect branching stem two or three feet high, tripinnate leaves with narrow, pointed leaflets, and small white flowers, arranged in umbels. The FRUIT or SEEDS, which are the officinal portion, are light, of a brownish colour, an oval shape, convex and bristly on one side, and flat on the other. They have an aromatic odour, a warm, pungent, bitterish taste, and contain a volatile oil, on which their virtues depend.

Effects and Uses.—Carrot-seeds are aromatic and diuretic, and are a good deal employed in dropsical and nephritic affections, agreeing well with the stomach, from their aromatic oil. The infusion is a popular remedy for the relief of strangury from blisters. Dose, ʒss to ʒj, or an *infusion* (half a troyounce to water Oj), *ad libitum.*

The ROOT of this plant possesses the same properties as the seeds. The ROOT of the cultivated plant, the well-known garden carrot, is employed as an application to sloughing ulcers.

SCOPARIUS—BROOM.

Sarothamnus Scoparius, or Broom (*Nat. Ord.* Fabaceæ), is a common European shrub, cultivated in the United States, from three to five feet high, with numerous bright-yellow flowers. The TOPS of the branches are the officinal portion, but the *seeds* are also used. The twigs are pentangular (with small, oblong, downy leaves), of a bright-green colour, a strong, peculiar odour, when bruised, and a bitter, nauseous taste. Two principles are found in broom-tops, *scoparin,* a neutral, crystallizable body, supposed to be the diuretic constituent, and a volatile alkaloid, *sparteia* ($C_{15}H_{26}N$), said to be narcotic.

Effects and Uses.—Broom is an efficient diuretic, in large doses producing free purging. It is a valuable and reliable remedy in dropsy, best given in decoction, half an ounce to a pint of water, boiled down to half a pint, of which an ounce may be given every hour or two, till the bowels are disturbed. A fluid extract (not officinal) is used in doses of fʒss–i.

CANTHARIS—CANTHARIDES.

The properties, &c., of *cantharides* will be noted fully under the head of *Irritants* (subdivision *Epispastics*). Taken internally, they sometimes prove diuretic, and generally excite irritation of the genito-urinary passages, as strangury, priapism, &c.; and, in overdoses, act as an acro-narcotic poison. They are employed in atonic dropsies, incontinence of urine, amenorrhœa, seminal weakness, impotence, &c. Dose, gr. i–ij, twice a day, in pill. They are most commonly administered in *tincture* (a troyounce to diluted alcohol Oij),—dose, gtt. x, or more, three or four times a day, till strangury supervenes.

The following medicines, though less frequently resorted to than the foregoing, possess very decided diuretic properties, and may be employed with advantage in the treatment of dropsical and nephritic affections:

The ROOT of HYDRASTIS CANADENSIS, or YELLOW ROOT (*Nat. Ord.* Ranunculaceæ), a small indigenous plant, with yellow, fugacious flowers, and a red fruit resembling raspberries, contains the alkaloid, *berberina* (previously noticed), and another alkaloid, *hydrastia*. It is contorted, rugose, of a bright-yellow colour, and has a strong, somewhat narcotic odour, and a bitter taste. It is tonic as well as diuretic, and is a very efficacious diuretic in promoting the discharge of calculi from the kidneys; the *fluid extract* may be given in doses of f℥ij–iv.

The SEED of DELPHINIUM CONSOLIDA, or LARKSPUR (*Nat. Ord.* Ranunculaceæ), a European plant, cultivated in our gardens, and to some extent naturalized. It contains an alkaloid, *delphinia,* and is a good diuretic, though in large doses producing vomiting and purging. The tincture (an ounce to a pint of diluted alcohol) is given in doses of from 10 to 20 drops, three times a day.

The ROOT of PETROSELINUM SATIVUM, or PARSLEY (*Nat. Ord.* Apiaceæ), a European plant, cultivated in our vegetable gardens for its leaves. Parsley contains a peculiar principle termed *apiol*, a yellowish oily liquid, which has been used in amenorrhœa and dysmenorrhœa, in the dose of four grains, morning and evening.

The ROOT of COCHLEARIA ARMORACIA, or HORSE-RADISH (*Nat. Ord.* Brassicaceæ), a European plant, cultivated here for its root, which is used as a condiment.*

ORDER V.—BLENNORRHETICS.

Blennorrhetics (from *βλεννα*, *mucus*, and *ρεω*, *I flow*), are medicines which promote the secretion of the mucous membranes. They are employed therapeutically in morbid conditions of these membranes, with a view to the restoration of healthy action, in cases of deficient, abnormal, or excessive secretion.

When administered with the object of stimulating the secretion of mucus from the bronchial or laryngeal membrane, this class of agents is termed *expectorants*. They are prescribed in the subacute and chronic forms of bronchitis and laryngitis, and in the declining stages of the acute forms of these affections and pneumonia. In the early or inflammatory stages of acute bronchitis and laryngitis, the stimulating expectorants are inadmissible, until expectoration has been established.

The blennorrhetics are less employed in gastro-enteric affections than in those of other mucous membranes, owing to their tendency to produce catharsis. Several of the oleoresins are, however, used with advantage in certain forms of chronic diarrhœa, and the oil of turpentine is highly esteemed in the treatment of the diarrhœa of typhoid fever.

The oleoresinous articles of this group are extensively employed in diseases of the urino-genital mucous membranes,—

* Under the name of *cider mixture*, a compound infusion is used in dropsy, of which the following is the formula: Juniper berries, mustard seed, and ginger, each half an ounce, horse-radish, parsley-root, each an ounce, cider, two pints—dose, a wineglassful, two or three times a day.

gonorrhœa, gleet, leucorrhœa, incontinence of urine, cystitis, &c.

The following are the articles chiefly resorted to for their influence on the mucous membranes:

SENEGA—SENEKA.

Polygala Senega, or Seneka Snakeroot (*Nat. Ord.* Polygalaceæ), is a small indigenous plant, found in all parts of the United States, but most abundantly in the South and West.

Fig. 26.

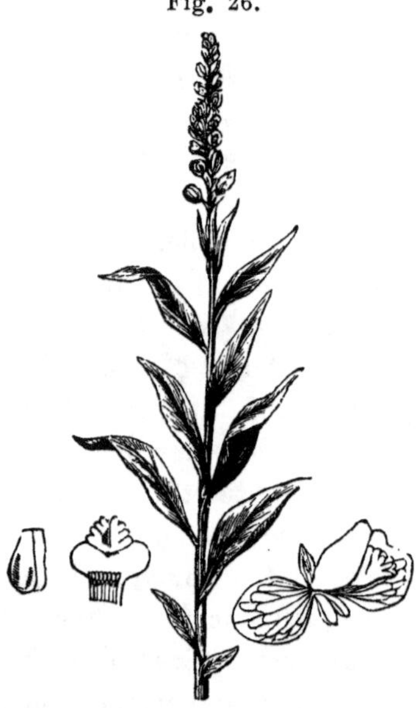

It has a perennial, branching root, several erect annual stems, about a foot in height, alternate lanceolate leaves, and small, whitish flowers, arranged in a terminal spike. The ROOT is the officinal portion. It occurs in the shops in twisted pieces, varying in thickness from the size of a quill to that of the little finger, attached to a knotty head, and marked with a ridge along their whole length and numerous annular protuberances. The cortical portion is hard, resinous, of a yellowish-brown colour, and *contains the active qualities of the root.* The central ligneous portion is white and inert. The odour of seneka is peculiar and disagreeable, but faint in the dried root; the taste is at first mucilaginous and sweetish, but afterwards becomes acrid and very irritating.

The virtues of seneka are extracted by cold and hot water and alcohol. It contains a peculiar acrid acid principle called *polygalic acid*, on which its activity chiefly depends; this is thought to be a glucoside derivative of *saponin*, a glucoside found in Soapwort and other plants.

Effects and Uses.—Seneka, in small doses, is an active excitant of the mucous membranes and secretions generally, and in large doses proves emetic and cathartic. It is chiefly prescribed as a stimulating expectorant in chronic and subacute bronchial affections, and in the latter stages of acute bronchitis, pneumonia, &c. As an ingredient in the *compound syrup of squill*, it is much employed in the treatment of croup, but, except in some such combination with tartar emetic or other emetic nauseant, it is scarcely admissible in the early stages of this disease. Seneka is also thought to possess emmenagogue properties, and is highly extolled by many practitioners in the treatment of amenorrhœa. It has been occasionally used as a diuretic in dropsies, and, in emeto-cathartic doses, has been found useful in rheumatism.

Administration.—Dose, in *powder*, gr. x to ℈j; but it is chiefly given in *decoction* (a troyounce boiled for fifteen minutes in water enough to make the decoction measure Oj), dose, f℥ij, three or four times a day. An *extract* (*alcoholic*), is given in the dose of from one to three grains; a *fluid extract*, in the dose of ♏x–xx; and a *syrup* is also used, in the dose of f℥i–ij, (made by percolating four troyounces of seneka with two pints of diluted alcohol, evaporating to half a pint, and dissolving in this tincture fifteen troyounces of sugar by a gentle heat).

CIMICIFUGA.

Cimicifuga racemosa, Black Snakeroot, or Cohosh (*Nat. Ord.* Ranunculaceæ), is a very common indigenous perennial plant,

Fig. 27.

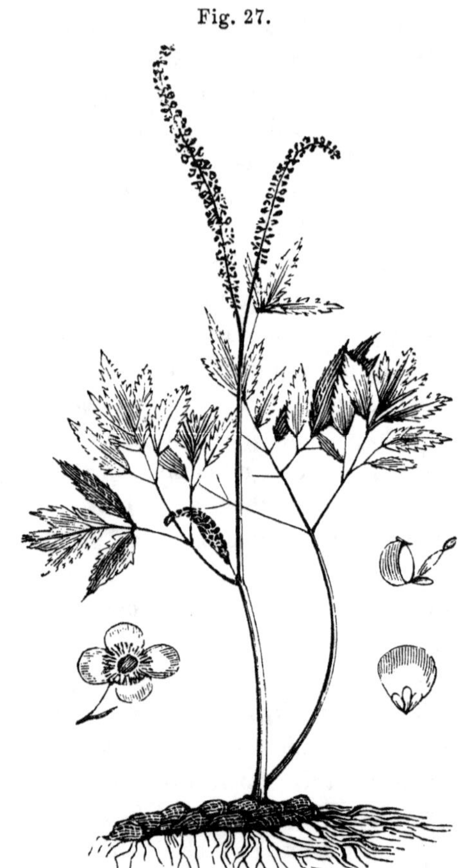

growing to the height of from four to eight feet, with ternate leaves, oblong-ovate, incised, and toothed leaflets, and small, white flowers, disposed in a long raceme. The ROOT is the part employed. It consists of a rugged, blackish-brown caudex, from a third of an inch to an inch in thickness, often several inches in length, furnished with numerous slender radicles.

Internally, its colour is whitish; it has a peculiar, faint, disagreeable odour, and a bitter, somewhat astringent taste. It imparts its virtues to boiling water, and contains gum, starch, two resins, tannic and gallic acids, salts, and a volatile oil, which is probably an active constituent, as the root deteriorates by keeping.

Effects and Uses.—The effects of cimicifuga are not very accurately known, but it is undoubtedly an active stimulant of the secretions, particularly those of the mucous membrances, skin, and kidneys, with, probably, in large doses, a sedative and antispasmodic action. It is believed, also, to act on the uterus like ergot. It has been employed with great advantage as an expectorant in chronic bronchial affections, and even phthisis pulmonalis, and has been also used as a diaphoretic in rheumatism, and as a diuretic in dropsies. As an antispasmodic in chorea, it enjoys a high reputation, and it is also recommended in the spasmodic forms of hysteria, particularly when connected with amenorrhœa. It is employed too, occasionally, to promote the expulsion of the placenta after delivery, in the relief of after-pains, and in menorrhagia. A saturated alcoholic solution has been used, with good effect, as an application to the eyelids in ophthalmia.

Administration.—Dose, in *powder*, ℈j to ʒj; a *decoction* (not officinal) is employed. Of the *fluid extract*, the dose is fʒss–j.

ALLIUM—GARLIC.

Allium sativum (*Nat. Ord.* Liliaceæ), is a small, perennial, bulbous plant, which grows wild in the south of Europe, and is cultivated in all parts of the world. The BULB is the portion used. As found in the shops, it is somewhat spherical in form, about an inch in diameter, with a portion of the stem attached, covered with a white, membranous envelope, and consists of five or six smaller bulbs, of a curved, oblong shape, called *cloves* of garlic. They have a strong, irritating, characteristic odour, and a bitter, acrid taste. Water, alcohol, and vinegar extract their virtues, which depend on an *essential oil*, which is of a yellow colour, very volatile and irritating; it is a sulphide of a peculiar radical, termed *allyl*, $(C_3H_5)_2S$.

Effects and Uses.—Garlic is a local irritant and rubefacient, and, taken internally, quickens the circulation and stimulates the secretions generally. It is a good deal employed as an expectorant in chronic and subacute catarrhal affections, particularly in infantile cases, and, occasionally, as a stomachic in flatulence, and as a diuretic in atonic dropsies. *Externally*, it is used as a revulsive rubefacient to the feet, as a resolvent of indolent tumours, and as a liniment in infantile convulsions.

Administration.—A clove may be swallowed entire, or cut into small pieces. Dose of the *fresh bulbs*, ʒi–ij, in pill; of the *juice*, fʒss, mixed with sugar; of the *syrup* (made by macerating 6 troyounces of garlic in 10 fluidounces of diluted acetic acid, expressing, mixing the residue with 6 fluidounces more of diluted acetic acid, expressing, and dissolving in the expressed liquid 24 troyounces of sugar), fʒj, for children.

SCILLA—SQUILL.

Squill, already noticed among diuretics, is one of the most powerful and valuable stimulating expectorants in the Materia Medica. (For properties, doses, preparations, &c., see p. 273).

TEREBINTHINA—TURPENTINE.

The term *turpentine* is applied to liquid or concrete vegetable juices, consisting of resin combined with a peculiar essential oil, called *oil of turpentine*. Two kinds of turpentine are recognized by the U. S. Pharmacopœia: 1. The *common American white turpentine*, which is procured chiefly from Pinus palustris (*Nat. Ord.* Pinaceæ), a large indigenous evergreen tree of our Southern States, where it is called *Long-leaved Pine*, *Yellow Pine*, and *Pitch Pine*, and in part also from Pinus Tæda, found in Virginia, and other species of Pinus. 2. *Canada turpentine* (*Terebinthina Canadensis*), kept in the shops under the name of *Canada balsam* or *balsam of fir*, the product of Abies balsamea, the American Silver Fir, or Balm of Gilead Tree (*Nat. Ord.* Pinaceæ), a handsome tree about 40 feet in height, inhabiting the northern portions of North America. Many other varieties of turpentine are known in commerce, as *Bordeaux turpentine*, *Venice turpentine*, *Chian turpentine*, &c.

White turpentine comes from North Carolina and other Southern States, and is collected from excavations made in the trunks of the trees, into which the turpentine runs in the mild weather. It is yellowish-white, and somewhat translucent, semi-fluid in summer, firm and hard in winter, but becoming permanently hard by exposure to the air, and has a peculiar aromatic odour, and a warm, pungent, bitterish taste. *Canada turpentine* comes from Canada and Maine. It is procured by breaking the vesicles, which are found between the bark and wood of the trees, and collecting the liquid contents in a bottle. When fresh, it has the consistence of honey, but gradually solidifies by age. It is yellow, transparent, tenacious, of a peculiar, pleasant terebinthinate odour, and a slightly bitter, acrid taste.

Chemical Constituents.—The turpentines yield, by distillation, a *volatile oil*, known as *oil of turpentine*, and leave a residue consisting exclusively of *resin*. Both the *oil* and *resin* are officinal. The turpentines are inflammable, nearly insoluble in water, but almost wholly soluble in alcohol and ether.

Physiological Effects.—The local operation of the terebinthinates is irritant. When applied to the skin, they produce a rubefacient effect, and, when swallowed, *in large doses*, promote the peristaltic motion of the intestines. Taken internally, in small doses, they are absorbed, and prove excitant to the vascular system and the secretions generally, especially the mucous membranes; they communicate a violet odour to the urine. The activity of the terebinthinates depends on their *volatile oil*.

Medicinal Uses.—Turpentine is employed chiefly in diseases of the various mucous membranes, as gonorrhœa, gleet, leucorrhœa, cystorrhœa, chronic bronchitis, and chronic mucous diarrhœa. It is also used in rheumatic complaints; and in cathartic doses, in cases of ascarides, constipation, and colic.

Administration.—Dose, as a *blennorrhetic*, ℈j to ʒj, in *pill*, *emulsion*, or *electuary;* as an *anthelmintic* or *cathartic*, half a troyounce to an ounce, in emulsion. The *white turpentine* is generally used in this country.

Oleum Terebinthinæ (*Oil of Turpentine*) ($C_{10}H_{16}$), commonly called *Spirit of Turpentine*, is the active principle of turpentine, obtained by distillation. It is a limpid, colourless, volatile, and inflammable liquid, of a strong, penetrating, peculiar odour, and a hot, pungent, bitterish taste; very slightly soluble in water, less soluble in alcohol than the volatile oils generally, and wholly soluble in ether; exposed to the air, it absorbs oxygen, with the formation of resin. This oil has been already noticed under the head of aromatic stimulants (p. 196). Its effects and medicinal uses are the same as those of turpentine, for which it is usually substituted in practice. Locally, it acts as a rubefacient. When swallowed in large doses, as fʒi–ij, it commonly passes off by the bowels; and, taken in small doses, it is absorbed, and stimulates the circulation and the secretions of the mucous membranes, kidneys, and skin. It often produces strangury and considerable irritation of the urinary-genital passages. Poisonous effects from the oil of turpentine are rare, as it generally passes off by the bowels; it may, however, produce severe vomiting and purging, bloody or suppressed urine, intense irritation of the urino-genital organs, unconsciousness with dilated pupils, and even death. In *large doses*, it is employed as an anthelmintic and cathartic, and is much used as a clyster for the relief of tympanites. In *small doses*, it is greatly prescribed in chronic discharges and hemorrhages from the various mucous membranes; in the latter stages of typhoid fever as a combined stimulant and blenorrhetic; as a diaphoretic in rheumatism and neuralgia; in infantile diabetes, nephritic disorders, dropsy, &c. As a *rubefacient*, it is a valuable counter-irritant in numerous diseases; turpentine stupes are highly efficacious in catarrhal affections.

Dose, gtt. v–xxx, repeated, as a *blennorrhetic stimulant;* f℥ss–f℥j, as a *cathartic enema*, or *anthelmintic*, in emulsion. *Linimentum terebinthinæ* (oil of turpentine Oss, melted with resin cerate twelve troyounces), is used as an application to burns and scalds.

Pix Liquida (*Tar*) is an impure turpentine, procured by burning, from the wood of Pinus palustris, and other species of Pinus. It is a brownish-black, viscid, semi-liquid substance, of a peculiar empyreumatic odour, and a bitterish, resinous, somewhat acid taste—soluble in alcohol, ether, and the volatile and fixed oils. It consists of resin, united with acetic acid, oil of turpentine, and various volatile, empyreumatic products. By distillation, it yiëlds *pyroligneous acid* and *oil of tar*—the residuum being pitch.

The *oil of tar* contains, besides oil of turpentine, *creasote* (see p. 174), and other principles.

Effects and Uses.—Tar resembles the turpentines in its effects, and is employed in chronic catarrhal affections and other diseases of the mucous membranes. Its vapour has been employed in bronchitis; and, externally, it is an excellent application in tinea capitis, psoriasis, and other cutaneous affections. Dose, ℨss to ℨj, several times a day, in pill or electuary; or the *infusion* (infusum picis liquidæ), (made by digesting tar Oj with water Oiv), may be taken in the quantity of Oi–ij, daily. *Glycerite of tar* (*glyceritum picis liquidæ*), is made by rubbing a troyounce of tar first with two troyounces of carbonate of magnesium, and then with six fluidounces of a mixture of four fluidounces of glycerin, two of alcohol, and ten of water; the residue is to be rubbed with half of the remaining liquid, and the process again repeated with the remaining liquid; the residue is to be percolated with the expressed liquids previously mixed, and afterwards water enough is added to make the whole measure a pint; a fluidounce contains 30 grains of tar. The *syrup* (though not officinal) is a good preparation, and may be made by dissolving 40 parts of sugar in 21 parts of the infusion. The *ointment* (*unguentum picis liquidæ*), is made by mixing equal parts of tar and melted suet.

Resina (*Resin*), commonly called *rosin*, is the residue after the distillation of the oil from turpentine. It is a yellowish-brown, semi-transparent, solid, brittle substance, with a slight terebinthinate odour and taste—insoluble in water, soluble in ether, alcohol, and the essential oils, readily uniting by fusion with wax and the fixed oils, and forming soluble soaps with alkalies. When agitated with water, in a state of fusion, it becomes opaque and *white*. It is not used *internally*, but is extensively employed in the formation of *plasters* and *ointments*, to which it communicates great adhesiveness and slightly stimulant properties.

Ceratum Resinæ (*Resin Cerate*), commonly called *basilicon ointment*, is made by melting resin (5 parts), lard (8 parts), and yellow wax (2 parts), together: it is an excellent mild stimulant application to burns, blistered surfaces, &c. *Compound Resin Cerate*, made by melting 12 troyounces of resin, suet, and yellow wax, each, with 6 troyounces of turpentine, and 7 troyounces of flaxseed oil, is a good stimulant cerate, very popular under the name of *Deshler's Salve*. *Emplastrum Resinæ* (*Resin Plaster*), made by melting one part of resin with six parts of lead plaster, is the well-known *adhesive plaster*, used to retain the edges of wounds in contact, to produce extension in the treatment of fractures, to protect excoriated surfaces, to promote absorption, &c.

COPAIBA.

Copaiba is an OLEO-RESIN obtained from several species of Copaifera (*Nat. Ord.* Amyridaceæ), large trees peculiar to South America. C. multijuga, a native of Brazil, is now recognized as the principal source of copaiba, and most of the copaiba of commerce is probably derived from the province of Para, in Brazil; Central America also yields copaiba. The juice is obtained from incisions in the stems of the trees; as it at first exudes, it is clear, colourless, and very thin, but it soon acquires a thicker consistence and a yellowish hue. As found in the shops, it is a clear, transparent liquid, of the consistence of olive oil, of a pale-yellow colour, a peculiar agreeable smell, and a pungent, nauseous, acrid taste. By exposure to the air, it acquires a deeper colour and denser consistence.

Copaiba is insoluble in water, but soluble in alcohol, ether, and the volatile and fixed oils; with alkalies and alkaline earths, it forms a soap. It is chemically, an *oleo-resin*, with a minute portion of acetic acid; the VOLATILE OIL is officinal; the *resin* possesses acid properties, and is called *copaivic acid.* By exposure to the air, copaiba gradually becomes darker and thicker, and finally hard and brittle, owing to the volatilization and oxidation of its oil. Copaiba was formerly called a *balsam*, but this title is incorrect, as it contains no *benzoic* or *cinnamic acid.*

Effects and Uses.—The effects of copaiba are very analogous to those of the terebinthinates. In large doses, it proves cathartic, and occasionally emetic, and, in small doses, it is absorbed, communicating its peculiar odour to the secretions and exhalations, and stimulating the secretions from the mucous membranes and kidneys; it is also a gentle excitant to the circulatory system. The urine of persons, who have taken copaiba for some time, yields a precipitate with nitric acid, like albuminous urine, by the action of the acid on the resin. Copaiba is employed in diseases of the mucous membranes, particularly those of a chronic character, as chronic bronchitis, chronic diarrhœa, leucorrhœa, gonorrhœa, gleet, catarrh, and irritation of the bladder, &c. As a remedy in gonorrhœa, it has long enjoyed great popularity, and is given with advantage even in the earliest stages of the disorder.

Administration.—Dose, gtt. xx to f℥j, three times a day in *emulsion*, with some aromatic water,* or in pills (*pills of copaiba*), made by mixing 2 troyounces of copaiba with 60 grains of magnesia, and dividing the mass after it concretes into 200 pills, or inclosed in *capsules* of gelatin; the pills are absorbed

* *Chapman's Copaiba Mixture* is, Copaiba and Spirit of Nitrous Ether, each half a fluidounce, powdered Gum Arabic and Sugar, each a drachm, Cd. Spirit of Lavender, 2 fluidrachms, Tincture of Opium, a fluidrachm, distilled water, 4 fluidounces—dose, a tablespoonful 3 times a day.

with difficulty. It is also administered as a clyster, in *emulsion*. Cubeb is frequently prescribed with copaiba, in the treatment of gonorrhœa.

Oleum Copaibæ (*Oil of Copaiba*), ($C_{15}H_{24}$), obtained by distillation from copaiba, is usually colourless, with the odour and taste of copaiba, and produces the same effects on the system. Dose, gtt. x–xv, in *emulsion*, or dropped on sugar.

CUBEBA—CUBEB.

Cubeb is the unripe fruit of Piper Cubeba, or Cubeba Officinalis (*Nat. Ord.* Piperaceæ), a climbing, perennial plant of Java and other parts of the East Indies. The berries are gathered for use when unripe, and are dried. They are about the size of a small pea, of a blackish or grayish-brown colour, a reticulated surface, and furnished with a stalk two or three lines long. The shell is hard, and contains a blackish seed, which is white and oily within. The odour of cubeb is aromatic; the taste warm, acrid, and camphoraceous. The berries deteriorate by age, most rapidly in powder, owing to the escape of their volatile oil. Their most interesting constituents are a volatile oil (which is officinal), ($C_{15}H_{24}$), a principle called *cubebin*, and *resinous* matter; the resinous matter consists of both a hard and soft resin, the former insoluble in ether, the latter soluble in ether, of acid reaction, and termed *cubebic acid*. The *oil* is carminative and stimulant, and the blenorrhetic and diuretic properties of cubeb reside chiefly in the *resin;* cubebin is inert.

Effects and Uses.—In large doses, cubeb, like the other oleo-resins, produces more or less gastro-enteric disturbance. In small doses, it produces a stomachic effect like that of black pepper; after its absorption, it acts as a gentle excitant to the vascular system, with a very decided stimulant action on the mucous surfaces, particularly those of the urino-genital apparatus; it also frequently proves diuretic. It is eliminated chiefly by the urine, increasing the excretion of uric acid, and under its use, the urine yields a precipitate with nitric acid.

An eruption, like urticaria, sometimes follows the administration of both copaiba and cubeb. It is used chiefly in the treatment of gonorrhœa, and should be given in the early stage of the disease. In other mucous discharges, as chronic catarrh with profuse secretion, leucorrhœa, gleet, cystitis, &c., cubeb has also been employed with advantage.

Administration.—Dose of the *powder*, ʒi–iij, three times a day, in gonorrhœa; in chronic mucous disorders, smaller doses are given. The OIL is often employed, but it does not possess the full virtues of cubeb—dose, gtt. x–xij, to be repeated and gradually increased; it may be taken in emulsion, or dropped on sugar, or made into gelatinous capsules with oil of copaiba. The *oleo-resin* contains both the volatile oil and resin, with a portion of cubebin, and is an excellent preparation—dose ♏ v–xxx, suspended in water; of the *tincture* (four troyounces to diluted alcohol Oij), the dose is fʒi–ij, three times a day; of the *fluid extract*, the dose is fʒss–i. *Troches of cubeb* are made with half a fluidounce of the oleo-resin, a fluidrachm of oil of sassafras, 4 troyounces of liquorice, 3 troyounces of sugar, 2 troyounces of gum Arabic, mixed with enough syrup of Tolu to form a mass, and divided into 480 troches.

MATICO.

This name is given to the LEAVES of Artanthe elongata (*Nat. Ord.* Piperaceæ), a shrub of Peru. They are two or three inches long, by about an inch in breadth, oval-lanceolate and acuminate in shape, crenate, strongly veined or reticulated, bright green on the upper surface, paler beneath, of a pleasant, aromatic odour, and a strong spicy taste. They contain chlorophyll, resin, volatile oil, and a peculiar bitter principle, soluble in water and alcohol, termed *maticin*.

Effects and Uses.—Matico is a pleasant, aromatic tonic, with a special determination to the mucous membranes. It is used as an alterative stimulant in the entire circle of diseased mucous membranes, especially those of the urinary passages. It is also used internally as a hemostatic, and locally as a styptic.

Dose, of the *powder*, ʒss–j, three times a day. An *infusion* (not officinal) may be made by dissolving a troyounce in a pint of boiling water—dose, a wineglassful; of the *fluid extract*, the dose is fʒss–j.

PAREIRA—PAREIRA BRAVA.

Pareira Brava is stated by the U. S. Pharmacopœia to be the ROOT of Cissampelos Pareira (*Nat. Ord.* Menispermaceæ), a climbing plant of the West Indies and South America; but it is more probably the ROOT of Chondodendron tomentosum or Cocculus chondodendron, a native of Brazil. It comes to us in large, wrinkled, twisted, or forked, cylindrical pieces, of variable thickness and length, covered with a thin, grayish-brown bark. The interior is ligneous, yellowish, porous, inodorous, and of a sweetish, nauseous, bitter taste. It imparts its virtues to water, and contains a bitter alkaline principle, termed *cissampelina* ($C_{18}H_{21}NO_3$), resin, fecula, &c.

Effects and Uses.—Pareira Brava is an excellent remedy in chronic diseases of the urinary passages, particularly chronic inflammation or irritation of the bladder, with morbid secretion. It is thought to be also tonic, aperient, and diuretic. Dose, in substance, ʒss to ʒj. But it is more conveniently given in *infusion* (a troyounce to boiling water Oj), dose, f℥i–ij; the *fluid extract* is much used—dose from half a fluidrachm to a fluidrachm.*

BUCHU.

This is the name given to the LEAVES of Barosma crenata and other species of Barosma (*Nat. Ord.* Rutaceæ), shrubby plants, growing at the Cape of Good Hope. As found in the shops, buchu leaves are from three-quarters of an inch to an inch and a half long, from three to five lines broad, elliptical, lanceolate-ovate, or obovate, sometimes pointed, sometimes

* A good prescription, in irritable bladder, is Fluid Ex. Pareira Brava, f℥i, Cd. Spirit of Juniper, f℥ij, Benzoic Acid, ʒi, Sulphate of Morphia, gr. i—dose, a teaspoonful three times a day.

blunt, notched and glandular at the edges, and of a green colour, paler on the under surface. Three varieties are known, viz.: *short* or *round* buchu (derived from B. crenata), *medium-sized* (from B. crenulata), and *long* buchu (from B. serratifolia). They have a strong, aromatic odour, and a bitterish taste, like that of mint. Water and alcohol extract their virtues, which depend on a *volatile oil* and *bitter extractive*.

Effects and Uses.—Buchu is a gentle stimulant to the secretions generally, particularly to the kidneys and urinary mucous membranes; it may be made to act also as a diaphoretic. It is employed in chronic catarrh of the urethra and bladder, nephritic complaints, retention or incontinence of urine—as a diuretic, in dropsies—and as a diaphoretic, in rheumatic and cutaneous complaints. Dose, of the *powder*, gr. xx–xxx; of the *infusion* (a troyounce to boiling water Oj), f℥i–iv; of the *fluid extract* (f℥ss–f℥j).

MYRRHA—MYRRH.

Myrrh is a GUM-RESINOUS EXUDATION from Balsamodendron Myrrha (*Nat. Ord.* Amyridaceæ), a small shrubby tree of Arabia Felix and Africa; B. Ehrenbergianum is thought to be also a source of myrrh, and most of the myrrh of commerce is probably derived from the eastern coast of Africa. The juice exudes spontaneously and concretes upon the bark. It is imported from Bombay, and occurs in small, semi-transparent, reddish-yellow fragments or tears—sometimes agglutinated together in large masses—of irregular shape and size, an agreeable, peculiar odour, and a bitter, aromatic taste. It is bitter and pulverizable, has a resinous fracture, and makes a light-yellowish powder. Inferior kinds of myrrh are darker and less translucent and odorous. Myrrh is a gum-resin (the resin being termed *myrrhic acid*), containing also a little volatile oil. It forms with water an emulsion, and is soluble in alcohol and ether.

Effects and Uses.—Myrrh is a stimulant expectorant and emmenagogue. It is prescribed in chronic catarrhal and asthmatic affections, in which a combined corroborant and expectorant effect is desirable; and also in chlorosis, amenorrhœa, &c. Chalybeates and aloes are frequently united with it in uterine affections. Locally, it is a good application to spongy gums, aphthous sore mouth, &c.

Administration.—Dose, gr. x to ʒss, in powder or pill, or suspended in water, as in *Mistura Ferri Composita* (see p. 141). The *tincture* (three troyounces to alcohol Oij), is chiefly employed externally—dose, internally, fʒss to fʒj. *Pills of Aloes and Myrrh*, *Compound Galbanum Pills*, and *Compound Iron Pills*, are officinal emmenagogue preparations of myrrh.

BENZOINUM—BENZOIN.

Benzoin is a SOLID BALSAM obtained from Styrax Benzoin, or Benjamin Tree (*Nat. Ord.* Styraceæ), a tall tree of Sumatra, Java, Borneo, and Siam. It is obtained by incisions in the bark, from which it readily exudes, afterwards hardening by exposure to the sun and air. Two kinds are known, the more valuable consisting chiefly of whitish *tears*, united by a reddish-brown connecting medium, and called *benzöe amygdaloides*, the other of brown or blackish *lumps*, without tears, known as *benzöe in sortis* (*benzoin in sorts*). Benzoin is volatile, has a fragrant odour, a feeble, slightly aromatic taste, is soluble in alcohol and ether, and is precipitated from its alcoholic solution by water. Its chief constituents are *resin* and BENZOIC ACID, which places it among the BALSAMS; it contains also a trace of extractive and of volatile oil; and sometimes cinnamic acid.

Effects and Uses.—Benzoin is a topical irritant, and, after absorption, stimulates the mucous passages, especially the aërian membranes. It resembles myrrh in its effects, but is rather more acrid and stimulating. It is adapted to chronic bronchial affections, but is seldom employed alone. As a fumigation in chronic laryngitis, it has been recommended by Trousseau and Pidoux. Dose, gr. x to ʒss. The *tincture of benzoin* (6 troyounces to alcohol 2 pints), and the *compound tincture* (containing benzoin 3 troyounces, aloes half a troyounce, storax 2 troyounces, balsam of Tolu a troyounce, dissolved in alcohol 2 pints), are used as stimulating expectorants and in bowel complaints—dose, f℥ss to f℥ij. *Ointment of benzoin* is made by adding 2 fluidounces of the tincture to 16 troyounces of melted lard, and evaporating off the alcohol; as benzoin has the property of obviating the rancidity to which lard is liable, this is a very useful vehicle for medicated ointments. Benzoin is much used in fumigating pastilles.

Acidum Benzoicum (*Benzoic Acid*) ($HC_7H_5O_2$), is obtained from benzoin by sublimation, or by the action of alkalies; it is also made in Germany from hippuric acid. As obtained by sublimation, it occurs in white, soft, feathery, hexagonal crystals, of a silky lustre, and not pulverulent. It has more or less of the agreeable odour of the balsam, a warm, acrid, and acidulous taste, is inflammable, sparingly soluble in cold water, rather soluble in boiling water, but perfectly soluble in alcohol, alkaline solutions, and fixed oils. It is a constituent of *the balsams.*

Effects and Uses.—Benzoic acid is a local irritant, acting on the general system as a stimulant, with a particular direction to the mucous surfaces. Dose, gr. x. In its passage through the system, it abstracts nitrogen from the elements of urea, and passes out with the urine in the form of hippuric acid; hence its use in uræmic poisoning.

Ammonii Benzoas (*Benzoate of Ammonium*) ($NH_4C_7H_5O_2$), is made by adding water of ammonia to an aqueous solution of benzoic acid, and occurs in the form of minute, white, shining, thin, four-sided, laminar crystals, with a slight odour of benzoic acid, and a bitterish saline, somewhat balsamic taste, and slightly acrid, but persistent aftertaste. It is soluble in water and alcohol, and, when heated, sublimes without residue. It is incompatible with the ferric salts. This salt, when taken internally, is probably decomposed by the gastric acids, and produces the constitutional effects of benzoic acid, for which it may be substituted; the ammonia renders it stimulant and antacid, and acceptable to irritable stomachs,—dose, 10 to 20 grains.

STYRAX—STORAX.

Storax is a BALSAM, prepared from the BARK of Liquidambar orientale (*Nat. Ord.* Styraceæ), a native of Asia Minor. It is obtained by steaming the bruised bark and then expressing it, and occurs in yellowish or brownish lumps, light and friable, yet more or less tenacious, of a fragrant odour and a warm taste. It contains volatile oil, termed *styrol* (C_8H_8), resin, with cinnamic acid, and is therefore a balsam. Alcohol and ether are its proper solvents. It is almost always more or less adulterated.

Effects and Uses.—It is used as a stimulant expectorant, chiefly in the compound tincture of benzoin,—dose, gr. x–xx.

BALSAMUM PERUVIANUM—BALSAM OF PERU.

Balsam of Peru is an EMPYREUMATIC LIQUID BALSAM, obtained from Myrospermum Peruiferum (*Nat. Ord.* Leguminosæ), a tree of Central America. Myroxolon Pereiræ has more recently been described as the source of this balsam. It is obtained from incisions in the bark, and is collected on rags inserted in the openings, which are afterwards boiled in water, when the balsam settles at the bottom, and the water is poured off. A *white* balsam, obtained from the fruit of this tree by expression, and a tincture of the fruit in rum, are also known in Central America. Balsam of Peru has the consistence of honey, a dark, reddish-brown colour, a pleasant smell, a warm, bitterish, acrid taste, and is soluble in alcohol, and partially so in boiling water. It is heavier than water. Its constituents are *resin, essential oil,* and *cinnamic acid.*

Effects and Uses.—It is a stimulating blennorrhetic and tonic, occasionally employed in chronic catarrhs, asthma, gonorrhœa, leucorrhœa, &c., but not much used in this country. Externally, it is applied to indolent ulcers. Dose, f℥ss, in emulsion.

BALSAMUM TOLUTANUM—BALSAM OF TOLU.

Balsam of Tolu is a SEMI-LIQUID BALSAM obtained from Myrospermum Toluiferum (*Nat. Ord.* Leguminosæ), a tree of the neighbourhood of Carthagena. It is procured from incisions in the trunk of the tree, and concretes in the vessels in which it is received. It has a soft, tenacious consistence, varying with the temperature, and by age becomes hard and resin-like. It is shining, translucent, of a reddish-brown colour, a fragrant odour, and a warm, sweetish, pungent taste. It is inflammable, entirely soluble in alcohol and essential oils, and, like the other balsams, yields its acid to boiling water. Its ingredients are *resin*, *volatile oil*, and *cinnamic acid.*

Effects and Uses.—It is a stimulant blennorrhetic and tonic, useful in chronic catarrhal affections, and, from its agreeable flavour, much employed as an ingredient of cough mixtures. The vapour of an ethereal solution of this balsam is inhaled with advantage for the relief of cough. Dose, gr. x–xxx, in emulsion, frequently repeated. The *tincture* (*tinctura Tolutana*), (three troyounces to alcohol Oij) is added to cough mixtures; dose, f℥i–ij. The *syrup* (*syrupus Tolutanus*), (made by rubbing 2 fluidounces of tincture of Tolu with 120 grains of carbonate of magnesium, 2 troyounces of sugar, and a pint of water, filtering, and in the filtered liquid dissolving 24 troyounces of sugar at a gentle heat), is used as a vehicle for other medicines. Balsam of Tolu is an ingredient of the *compound tincture of benzoin.*

The following GUM-RESINS, previously noticed among *anti-spasmodics*, are employed as *expectorants.*

ASSAFŒTIDA (*Assafetida*). (See p. 100.)

AMMONIACUM (*Ammoniac*). (See p. 103.)

GALBANUM. (See p. 102.)

ORDER VI.—EMMENAGOGUES.

Emmenagogues (from ἐμμήνια, the *catamenia*, and ἀγωγος, *exciting*) are medicines which promote the menstrual discharge. This discharge may be suppressed from various causes, and hence very opposite classes of remedies are employed to restore it. Thus, when amenorrhœa depends on *anœmia*, the PREPARATIONS OF IRON are the most effectual emmenagogues ; on the other hand, when it occurs in connection with *plethora*, BLOOD-LETTING and EVACUANTS are resorted to. There are probably no articles which exert any specific influence upon the catamenia, as the discharge from the uterus is not one of the excretions through which medicinal agents pass out of the system. Medicines, however, which excite the pelvic circulation, and stimulate the organs in the neighbourhood of the uterus, have a tendency to increase or excite the menstrual discharge. They are—

1. The *drastic cathartics*, as ALOES (p. 249), BLACK HELLEBORE (p. 259), &c.
2. Many of the *stimulating diuretics*, particularly CANTHARIDES (p. 282).
3. Some of the *blennorrhetics*, particularly SENEKA (p. 284).
4. GUAIACUM (p. 268), usually classed with the *diaphoretics*.

Indirectly, the menstrual discharge is frequently promoted by—

1. *Chalybeates*, which are the best emmenagogues in chlorotic and anæmic cases.
2. *Mercurials*, which prove emmenagogue from their influence in exciting the secretions generally.

The following articles are employed exclusively as emmenagogues :

SABINA—SAVINE.

Savine is the TOPS of Juniperus Sabina (*Nat. Ord.* Pinaceæ), a small, evergreen, bushy shrub of the South of Europe. They resemble closely the tops of *Juniperus Virginiana*, the indigenous *Red Cedar*, which are sometimes substituted for savine in the shops. The latter has a greenish colour, a strong, peculiar, heavy odour, and a bitter, nauseous, resinous taste. Its virtues depends on a *volatile oil*, which is officinal.

Physiological Effects.—Savine is a local irritant. Taken internally, in medicinal doses, it stimulates the circulation and secretions, with a very decided action on the uterus. In large doses, it will cause vomiting, purging, abdominal pain, suppressed or bloody urine, with symptoms of nervous depression, as shown in unconsciousness, stertorous breathing, perhaps convulsions, and death, usually from collapse; fatal results have sometimes occurred from its use to provoke premature labour.

Medicinal Uses.—Savine is employed *internally*, almost exclusively as an emmenagogue, and is considered one of the best medicines that can be used to stimulate the action of the uterine vessels. Pereira pronounces it "the most certain and powerful emmenagogue of the whole Materia Medica." It has also been recommended in chronic rheumatism, and as an anthelmintic. *Topically*, it is used to keep up the discharge from blisters, to destroy warts, &c. Dose, in powder, gr. v–x; but it loses much of its oil by drying; of the *fluid extract*, the dose is ♏v–x. *Ceratum Sabinæ* (three parts of fluid extract added to twelve parts of resin cerate) is used to make perpetual blisters.

Oleum Sabinæ (*Oil of Savine*) ($C_{10}H_{16}$), is the preparation principally used internally. Dose, gtt. v–x.

Ruta (*Rue*). The leaves of Ruta graveolens (*Nat. Ord.* Rutaceæ) a perennial European plant, are ranked among emmenagogues, and are used, popularly, to provoke abortion. Their action is similar to that of savine, than which, however, they are less powerful. Dose, gr. xv–xxx, two or three times a day. Of the *oil* (*oleum rutæ*), the dose is gtt. ij–v.

Rubia (*Madder*). The root of Rubia tinctorum, or *Dyer's Madder* (*Nat. Ord.* Rubiaceæ), a European plant, is occasionally employed as an emmenagogue. Dose, ʒss, three or four times a day.

CLASS III.—HÆMATICS.

ORDER I.—HÆMATINICS.

This order (from αιματινα, the *red colouring matter of the blood*), includes only the PREPARATIONS OF IRON, or CHALYBEATES. The chalybeates increase the number of blood-corpuscles, or the amount of hæmatin in the blood, and are employed therapeutically in diseases dependent on a deficiency of these elements. They belong eminently to *hæmatics* (or medicines which occasion changes in the condition of the blood); but, as they possess also general and local tonic effects, independent of their action on the blood, they have been classed and treated of among the *mineral tonics* (see p. 139).

ORDER II.—ALTERATIVES.

Alteratives may be defined to be medicines, which produce such a modification of the nutritive processes, as enables the vital principle to restore healthy action, in morbid conditions of the system. Their effects are chiefly owing to a correcting influence on the quality of the circulating fluid. Thus, in inflammations, they diminish the abnormal quantity of fibrin in the blood, render its red corpuscles less disposed to aggregation, and decrease the number and adhesiveness of its white globules. In part, also, their curative operation is of a *substitutive* character, by setting up an *antagonistic* action, which takes the place of diseased action in the system.

Under the influence of alteratives, the secretions and exhalations are increased, the textures softened, inflammatory action is arrested, and morbid growths and deposits are absorbed. The exudation of plastic or coagulable lymph is checked, and, as a consequence, also the formation of false membranes. Visceral and glandular enlargements and indurations are diminished and often disappear, and phlegmonous inflammation, of every kind, is opposed.

If pushed too far, the alteratives soften and even destroy

the textures, impoverish the blood so as to interfere with the functions of nutrition, and produce a condition of marasmus and cachexia.

Their principal therapeutic employment is as *antiphlogistics* or *resolvents*. The *mercurials* are chiefly employed in *acute* inflammations,—the preparations of *iodine* in *chronic* inflammations. In the treatment of acute inflammatory affections, mercurials are among the most important of our resources—especially in such as have a tendency to terminate in effusions of coagulable lymph. The iodic and bromic preparations are adapted to inflammations of a chronic character—and are particularly serviceable in indurations or enlargements of glands and organs, and in affections of the bones and fibrous tissues.

By their *substitutive* or *antagonistic* action, alteratives are highly efficacious in the treatment of many diseases. In this way, syphilis is cured by the use of mercury, and intermittent fever by the use of arsenious acid.

Owing to the injurious results which follow the prolonged exhibition of alteratives, they are to be administered with caution, and their effects closely watched.

HYDRARGYRI PRÆPARATA—PREPARATIONS OF MERCURY.

Metallic mercury or quicksilver is obtained principally from the sulphuret (*native cinnabar*). The chief supply of quicksilver was long derived from Spain and Austria, but the markets of the United States are now furnished from New Almaden, in California. Mercury is an odourless, tasteless, volatile liquid metal, of a whitish colour. Its equivalent number is 200; its symbol is Hg.

While it retains the liquid metallic state, mercury is inert; but, when taken internally, it sometimes combines with oxygen in the alimentary canal, and thus becomes active. In the state of vapour, it frequently proves injurious—in some instances exciting salivation, ulceration of the mouth, &c.; in others, inducing a peculiar affection of the nervous system, termed *shaking palsy* (*tremor mercurialis*), which is often attended with loss of memory, vertigo, and other evidence of cerebral disturbance, and sometimes terminates fatally. Workmen in quicksilver are liable to this affection. It is supposed by some chemists, that the activity of mercurial emanations is owing to the oxidation of the metal, before it is inhaled; by others, that, in the finely-divided state, in which it exists as a vapour, it is in itself poisonous.

All the compounds of mercury possess activity. Some of them are violent caustic poisons; all of them are more or less irritant. When the mercurials are taken internally, their effects vary with the quantity administered. In *small* and *repeated* doses, their influence is first shown in an increase of the activity of the secernents and exhalants. The cutaneous, mucous, biliary, salivary, urinary, and probably also, the pancreatic secretions, are all increased in amount, and at the same time the absorbent system becomes more active, so that accumulations of fluids, morbid enlargements, indurations, &c., will often disappear.

Lately, the cholagogue action of mercurials has been denied, from the results of experiments upon animals, in whom, after the establishment of external fistulous orifices connecting with the gall-bladder, the administration of mercurials has been found not to increase the amount of the biliary secretion. Such experiments, however, involving the severance of numerous nerve-branches, leading to and from the liver, can settle nothing as to an action upon the biliary secretion, which, like all other secretory operations, is dependent upon proper innervation.

When mercury is given in *larger doses*, these effects are more intense. The mucous membrane of the mouth and the salivary glands not only take on increased secretory action, but become irritated and inflamed. The gums first show the mercurial influence, and are tender and tumefied; the whole mouth soon becomes sore; the tongue is swollen; and the saliva and buccal mucus flow abundantly, sometimes to the extent of several pints a day. At the same time, the breath acquires a peculiar fetidity, and the patient perceives a metallic taste in the mouth. The *resolvent* action of mercury is now still more obvious than when its impression is milder, and considerable emaciation usually ensues, from the absorption of fat. These effects, which are termed *sialagogue* (from the excessive flow of saliva), are commonly produced for the cure of diseases, and, as a general rule, gradually subside, leaving the health unimpaired. When, however, the use of mercury is pushed too far, or it is administered to persons peculiarly susceptible of its action, a train of very serious symptoms ensues—as excessive salivation, ulceration of the mouth, sloughing of the gums, loosening of the teeth, and, occasionally, necrosis of the alveolar processes. A peculiar febrile condition, called *mercurial fever*, diarrhœa, skin-diseases, neuralgia, rheumatism, disorder of the nervous system, and marasmus, are other symptoms which are frequently noticed after the abuse of mercury.

After its absorption, mercury produces several important changes in the quality of the blood. Immediately upon the establishment of salivation, the blood exhibits an inflammatory crust; but, at a later period, it loses colour, consistence, and coagulability, and the proportion of fibrin to serum becomes diminished. This *antiplastic* action on the blood renders mercurials valuable as antiphlogistic remedies.

Medicinal Uses.—Liquid metallic mercury was formerly administered to remove mechanical obstructions of the bowels, but its use has been abandoned. The preparations of mercury are employed therapeutically with various objects.

1. As *indirect tonics* and *cholagogues*,—with a view to their action on the secretions,—in dyspepsia and constipation, accompanied with torpor of the liver, in gout, rheumatism, chronic skin diseases, &c. Blue pill, mercury with chalk, and calomel, are employed with this view; the two former are preferred as least irritating.

2. As *sialagogues.* The chief value of mercurials is shown when a full impression is made on the system, as evidenced by salivation. This condition is usually established by the *internal* exhibition of mercurials, but it may also be produced by *fric-*

tion or by *fumigation.* In putting the system under the influence of mercury, it is not necessary to excite a high degree of ptyalism, though in chronic diseases, it is often proper to keep up the effect for some time. During the maintenance of ptyalism, the patient should use warm clothing, avoid exposure to cold, and take light and nourishing food. If excessive discharge or ulceration occur, astringent gargles, as brandy and water, solutions of chlorinated soda or lime, alum, &c., may be employed. In cases of sloughing sores, nitrate of silver or the mineral acids should be applied. Gastro-enteric irritation is to be treated with laxatives and opiates. The mercurial cachexia requires change of air, generous diet, tonics, &c. When the system is contaminated with mercury, it may be eliminated by the use of iodide of potassium, which forms soluble compounds with the mercury retained in the economy.

As sialagogues, mercurials are chiefly employed in inflammations, dysentery, cholera, dropsies, and syphilis. It is in *inflammations* that the value of mercurials is most conspicuous. After depletion, the mercurial preparations, from their antiplastic action on the blood, are probably the most efficacious means at our command for the relief of internal inflammations. They are *most* useful in inflammations of *serous* tissues, especially where these are connected with the exudation of coagulable lymph, and also where there is a tendency to the formation of false membrane, as in *plastic* croup; in iritis, a mercurial impression is considered indispensable by oculists. In scrofulous, malignant, or gangrenous inflammations, mercury is objectionable. In *dysentery* and *cholera*, mercurials are highly valuable remedies, and enter into nearly all the varieties of treatment adopted in these diseases. In *syphilitic* diseases, mercury has long been regarded as the only reliable antisyphilitic agent. It has no direct curative influence on the primary symptoms; but, after the system has been contaminated with the syphilitic virus, mercury is the most certain and rapid means of destroying it. Wherever the hard chancre, with distinct induration (which is always indicative of constitutional taint), is present, mercurials should invariably be administered. In hepatic and inflammatory *dropsies*, mercurials are employed with advantage, with a view to their action both on the secretions and absorbents. Where much debility exists, however, and in granular disease of the kidneys, mercurials are objectionable. The preparations of mercury have been exhibited as sialagogues in many other diseases, as paralysis, colica pictonum, rheumatism, chronic visceral diseases, particularly of the lungs and liver, &c. They must be always considered as contra-indicated in scrofulous or tuberculous subjects, in cases of malignant disease, in extensive suppuration, marasmus, Bright's disease of the kidneys, &c.

Blue pill and calomel are the sialagogues principally resorted to; but other preparations, as the iodides, are employed in syphilis. In administering mercurials, for their sialagogue action, we sometimes observe a *cumulative* effect: they may be exhibited, particularly to children, for some time without result, when suddenly the most violent symptoms of mercurial saturation will be developed.

3. As *purgatives*. The employment of calomel, blue pill, and mercury with chalk, as cathartics and anthelmintics, has been previously noticed (see p. 263).

The following are the preparations of mercury which are employed medicinally:

1. Metallic Mercury. When intimately mixed with pulverulent or fatty bodies, mercury loses its liquid character—is said to be *killed*, *extinguished*, or *mortified*—and acquires medicinal activity. Its activity is probably owing to its reduction to a state of minute division, which enables it to enter into combinations in the stomach. The officinal preparations of metallic mercury are: *Pilulæ Hydrargyri* (*Pills of Mercury*), *Unguentum Hydrargyri* (*Mercurial Ointment*), *Emplastrum Hydrargyri* (*Mercurial Plaster*), *Hydrargyrum cum Cretâ* (*Mercury with Chalk*).

2. Oxides.—*Hydrargyri Oxidum Nigrum* (*Black Oxide of Mercury*), *Hydrargyri Oxidum Flavum* (*Yellow Oxide of Mercury*), *Hydrargyri Oxidum Rubrum* (*Red Oxide of Mercury*).

3. CHLORIDES.—*Hydrargyri Chloridum Mite* (*Mild Chloride of Mercury, or Calomel*), *Hydrargyri Chloridum Corrosivum* (*Corrosive Chloride of Mercury*, or *Corrosive Sublimate*).

4. IODIDES.—*Hydrargyri Iodidum Viride* (*Green Iodide of Mercury*), *Hydrargyri Iodidum Rubrum* (*Red Iodide of Mercury*).

5. *Hydrargyri Cyanidum* (*Cyanide of Mercury*).

6. *Hydrargyrum Ammoniatum* (*Ammoniated Mercury*).

7. *Hydrargyri Sulphas Flava* (*Yellow Sulphate of Mercury*).

8. *Hydrargyri Sulphuretum Rubrum* (*Red Sulphuret of Mercury*).

9. NITRATES.—*Unguentum Hydrargyri Nitratis* (*Ointment of Nitrate of Mercury*), *Liquor Hydrargyri Nitratis* (*Solution of Nitrate of Mercury*).

PILULÆ HYDRARGYRI (*Pills of Mercury*). This preparation, generally known as *Blue Pills*, is made by rubbing mercury (384 grains), with confection of rose (576 grains), till all the globules disappear; then adding powdered liquorice root (192 grains), beating the whole into a mass, and dividing into 384 pills. The trituration is now generally effected by machinery—usually by steam power. It is a soft, dark blue mass, of a convenient consistence for making into pills. The mercury is in a state of minute division, and is chemically unaltered, though, perhaps, a very small portion of it is in a state of oxidation. Each pill contains three grains of the pilular mass and one grain of mercury. The preparation changes colour from being kept, becoming of an olive and even reddish tint, in consequence of the further oxidation of the metal. As it is often adulterated, it is important that it should be purchased of a reliable house.

Effects and Uses.—In full doses (gr. v–xv), blue pill acts as a *laxative;* when given for this purpose, it is usually followed in a few hours by a saline cathartic. In doses of gr. i–ij–iij, repeated at proper intervals, it is employed as an *alterative* or *sialagogue*, and is the favourite preparation for exciting salivation in chronic affections. When it moves the bowels, opium is combined with it. It may be pleasantly given suspended in mucilage or syrup.

UNGUENTUM HYDRARGYRI (*Mercurial Ointment*) (called also *Blue Ointment*), is made by rubbing two parts of mercury with one part of suet and lard each, until the globules disappear. It is an unctuous, fatty body, of a bluish-gray colour, consisting of equal weights of *fatty matter* and finely divided *mercury*. A very small portion of protoxide is, perhaps, present, and, as the ointment becomes darker by age, a further oxidation of the mercury probably takes place.

Effects and Uses.—Mercurial ointment, when either swallowed or rubbed into the integuments, produces the constitutional effects of mercury; locally, it has but little irritant effect. It is scarcely ever used *internally* in the United States or Great Britain, though, in France, it is highly esteemed as a sialagogue, in the dose of gr. ij, repeated. *Externally*, it is used to mercurialize the system by friction, or applied to blistered surfaces; to disperse non-malignant tumors; as a dressing to syphilitic sores; to destroy pediculi; and to prevent suppuration and pitting in small-pox.

EMPLASTRUM HYDRARGYRI (*Mercurial Plaster*), is made by rubbing 6 troyounces of mercury with 2 troyounces of olive oil and resin each, previously melted together, till the globules disappear; and then adding 12 troyounces of melted lead plaster. It is used as a discutient of venereal and other enlargements, to prevent pitting in small-pox, &c., and is applied to the side in chronic hepatitis; it may induce salivation. The *plaster of ammoniac with mercury* (*emplastrum ammoniaci cum hydrargyro*), is made by mixing with heat 60 grains of olive oil with 8 grains of sublimed sulphur, then adding 3 troyounces of mercury, and to this mixture adding 12 troyounces of ammoniac, previously boiled with a little water, and strained; it is more stimulating than the foregoing.

HYDRARGYRUM CUM CRETA (*Mercury with Chalk*) (called also *Gray Powder*), is prepared by rubbing three parts of mercury with five parts of *prepared chalk*, till all the globules disappear. It is a grayish powder, containing mercury chiefly in a state of minute division. In full doses, it is a gentle laxative, milder even than blue pill; in smaller doses, it is an excellent alterative; and the chalk renders it antacid. It is chiefly employed as an alterative in infantile cases. Dose, for adults, gr. v–xx; for children, gr. ij or iij to gr. viij or x, in *powder*, and not in pills, as in the latter form the mercury becomes squeezed out of the chalk. The chlorides and nitro-muriatic acid are incompatible with all the metallic preparations of mercury.

HYDRARGYRI OXIDUM NIGRUM (*Black Oxide of Mercury*). This preparation, although discarded from the Pharmacopœia, has still claims to notice. It is obtained by agitating calomel (mercurous chloride) in a solution of potassa; chloride of potassium is formed in solution, and mercurous oxide (Hg_2O) precipitates. As first prepared, it is a greenish-black powder; but, on exposure to light or heat, it is converted into a mixture of metallic mercury and mercuric oxide, and becomes olive-coloured. It is odourless, tasteless, insoluble in water, but soluble in nitric and acetic acids. Its effects are alterative, sialagogue, and purgative, and it is one of the least irritating of the mercurial preparations—but it is little used internally, on account of the uncertainty of its composition. Dose, gr. $\frac{1}{4}$ to gr. i–ij, in pill. Externally, it has been employed as a fumigating agent; also, as an application to chancres and other sores, suspended in a weak solution of chloride of calcium, under the name of *black wash* (made extemporaneously by adding calomel ʒj to solution of lime Oj).

HYDRARGYRI OXIDUM RUBRUM (*Red Oxide of Mercury*). This is mercuric oxide (HgO). It is usually made by dissolving mercury in diluted nitric acid, with a gentle heat, by which mercuric nitrate is formed; and the nitric acid is afterwards decomposed and driven off by calcination. The red oxide of mercury, which is commouly called *red precipitate*, occurs in small, shining scales, of a brilliant red colour, with a shade of orange. It has an acrid taste, and is nearly insoluble in water. Its effects are those of a powerful irritant, and, when taken internally, even in small doses, it excites vomiting and purging—in large doses, gastro-enteritis. It is rarely or never used internally, (dose, gr. $\frac{1}{16}$–$\frac{1}{8}$); externally, it is applied as an escharotic, either in powder or ointment, to chancres, indolent ulcers, &c. *Unguentum hydrargyri oxidi rubri* (*ointment of red oxide of mercury*), consists of one part of red oxide mixed with seven parts of *ointment:* it is a very useful stimulating ointment in indolent ulcers, porrigo, ophthalmia, &c.

HYDRARGYRI OXIDUM FLAVUM (*Yellow Oxide of Mercury*), is made by mixing a solution of corrosive sublimate with solution of potassa; chloride of calcium is formed in solution and mercuric oxide (HgO) is precipitated as an orange-yellow powder, which, on being heated, assumes a red colour. It is without odour, of an acrid taste, is very slightly soluble in water, and is insoluble in cold alcohol and ether. This preparation has been recently introduced into the Pharmacopœia, and is now preferred for some purposes to the *red oxide*, owing to its greater purity, and, especially, to its occurring in the form of *a completely amorphous powder*, exhibiting no evidence of crystalline particles, even under the microscope. This gives it a superiority, as a local application to the conjunctiva in diseases of the eye, over the *red oxide*, which, from the *crystalline* character of its particles, causes more or less irritation. *Unguentum hydrargyri oxidi flavi* (*ointment of yellow oxide of mercury*), consists of one part of yellow oxide mixed with seven parts of *ointment.* *Yellow wash* (a favourite application to phagedœnic venereal ulcers), consists of the yellow oxide of mercury suspended in a weak solution of chloride of calcium, and is made by adding half a drachm of corrosive sublimate to a pint of solution of lime.

HYDRARGYRI CHLORIDUM MITE (*Mild Chloride of Mercury*). This preparation (mercurous chloride), well known as *Calomel*, (HgCl) is made by subliming a mixture of mercurous sulphate and chloride of sodium (common salt); a double decomposition takes place, by which mercurous chloride and sulphate of sodium are formed. The mercurous sulphate is previously obtained by boiling mercury in sulphuric acid, and afterwards triturating the resulting mercuric sulphate with mercury. *Calomel*, as thus procured in mass, is liable to contain a little corrosive sublimate. It should be reduced to powder, and washed repeatedly with boiling distilled water, until the absence of a white precipitate with ammonia shows that the corrosive sublimate has been removed. With a view of obtaining calomel in a state of very minute division, its vapour is condensed in a receiving vessel filled with steam, whereby it takes the form of a very fine powder, and is perfectly free from corrosive sublimate. The calomel thus prepared (known as *Jewell's* or *Howard's* calomel) is finer and more active than can be obtained by levigation and elutriation.

Calomel, as usually manufactured by sublimation, is in the form of white, fibrous, crystalline cakes. It may be obtained in the shape of quadrangular, prismatic crystals. As found in the shops, it is a light-buff or ivory-coloured powder, tasteless, inodorous, insoluble in water, alcohol, and ether, unalterable in the air, but blackening by long exposure to light. It should be kept in bottles painted black or covered with black paper. *Jewell's* calomel is a perfectly white powder. *When pure*, calomel is completely vaporizable by heat; it strikes a black colour free from reddish tinge, with solutions of the fixed alkalies; and should not, when digested with water, form a white precipitate with ammonia, unless it contain corrosive sublimate.

Incompatibles.—The alkalies, alkaline earths, alkaline carbonates, soaps, and hydrosulphates, are *incompatible* with calomel. Nitro-muriatic acid should not be prescribed with it, for fear of generating corrosive sublimate. Preparations containing hydrocyanic acid, the chlorides of ammonium, sodium, and potassium, produce the same change. It is asserted that calomel is converted into corrosive sublimate in the stomach by the muriatic acid which it encounters, but there are many reasons for rejecting this hypothesis.

Effects and Uses.—Calomel produces the effects of the mercurials already described, and, in purgative doses, proves also a valuable anthelmintic. From the certainty and mildness of its operation, it is more employed than any of the other preparations of mercury, although blue pill, which, if less certain, is milder, is preferred under some circumstances. Calomel has been frequently taken in very large doses, without any bad effects; but cases are recorded in which, in excessive quantity, it has acted as an irritant poison. As a *purgative*, it is employed in doses of gr. vi–xij, in fevers, hepatitis, colica pictonum, dysentery, and many other affections; as an *anthelmintic*, in the same doses; and, in both cases, it is to be followed in a few hours by a saline draught, castor oil, or senna. Calomel is often given in combination with other cathartics, as jalap, rhubarb, aloes, scammony, colocynth, and gamboge. As an *antiphlogistic*, in inflammatory cases, calomel is given in doses of gr. $\frac{1}{2}$ to gr. j, every one, two, or three hours; as an *eccritic*, in these doses, twice or thrice a day. In the dose of gr. j, frequently repeated, it is one of the best means of checking obstinate vomiting. It is frequently added to other medicines, to increase their action on the secretions, as diuretics, antimonials, &c. To children, calomel may be given in proportionally larger doses than to adults, and it rarely salivates them. In infantile diarrhœa, very minute doses of calomel, as gr. $\frac{1}{16}$, $\frac{1}{12}$, $\frac{1}{8}$, every hour or two, are highly efficacious. *Externally*, calomel is applied in powder, as an errhine, in amaurosis; and, made into an ointment (a drachm to a troyounce of lard), it is an excellent application in a variety of cutaneous affections.

HYDRARGYRI CHLORIDUM CORROSIVUM (*Corrosive Chloride of Mercury*). This is mercuric chloride, commonly called *Corrosive Sublimate* ($HgCl_2$). It is made by subliming a mixture of chloride of sodium and mercuric sulphate (which is previously obtained by boiling mercury with sulphuric acid); double decomposition takes place, resulting in the formation of mercuric chloride and sulphate of sodium. Corrosive sublimate occurs in the form of white, semi-transparent, crystalline masses, permanent in the air, inodorous, and of an acrid, styptic taste. It is soluble in 16 parts of cold water and 3 parts of boiling water, more soluble in alcohol, and still more so in ether. The aqueous solution, when exposed to light, is decomposed, with the precipitation of calomel and evolution of hydrochloric acid. It is *incompatible* with many of the metals, the alkalies and their carbonates, soap, lime-solution, tartar emetic, nitrate of silver, the acetates of lead, the sulphides and iodides of potassium and sodium, the sulphides generally, syrup of sarsaparilla, and with many vegetable substances (as the bitters) and albuminous liquids (as milk, &c.). The *tests* for detecting corrosive sublimate in solution are: 1. A solution of potassa, soda, or lime throws down a yellow precipitate; 2. Carbonate of potassium, a brick-red precipitate; 3. Ammonia, white ammoniated mercury; 4. Iodide of potassium, a bright scarlet-red iodide of mercury, readily soluble in excess of the precipitant; 5. Protochloride of tin, in small amount, a white precipitate of calomel—in excess, a dark-gray precipitate of metallic mercury; 6. Sulphuretted hydrogen, or a sulphide, in minute amount, produces a whitish or gray precipitate, and, in large amount, a black sulphide; 7. If the solution is acidulated with hydrochloric acid, and bright *copper*-foil, wire, or gauze is plunged into it, the copper becomes coated with a silvery-white deposit of mercury—or a slip of *gold*-foil, wound round a slip of zinc-foil, may be introduced into the liquid, when it will become covered with a silvery film of metallic mercury, and, in both cases, the metal may be afterwards obtained by sublimation in the form of globules.

Physiological Effects.—In medicinal doses as gr. $\frac{1}{16}$–$\frac{1}{8}$, corrosive sublimate occasions a beneficial alterative effect, without any obvious activity. Its continued use may cause salivation, but it has less tendency to produce this result than any other preparation of mercury. Medicinal doses, if too large or too long continued, frequently produce gastro-enteric symptoms and the constitutional effects of mercury. In excessive doses, corrosive sublimate is a violent *caustic poison*, from its affinity for albumen, fibrin, and other constituents of the tissues. It acts very rapidly, producing the most intense gastro-enteritis, with violent vomiting and purging, abdominal pain and tenderness, bloody stools, with death, from collapse, or, after a time, with convulsions and coma. The best *antidote* is *albumen* (in the form of white of eggs); or, if this is not attainable, *gluten* (in wheat flour), or *casein* (in milk), may be substituted. The *protosulphide of iron* (if given immediately), and a mixture of *iron filings* (two parts) with *gold dust* (one part), also decompose corrosive sublimate. In case of poisoning, the stomach must be evacuated as soon as possible, and the after treatment consists in the free use of demulcents, opiates, and topical depletion.

Medicinal Uses.—Corrosive sublimate is chiefly used as an alterative in secondary syphilis, both by the stomach and by hypodermic injection; also in cutaneous and rheumatic affections, and as a sorbefacient in old dropsies; it is a good remedy, too, in chronic diarrhœa and dysentery with slimy and bloody discharges. Dose, gr. $\frac{1}{16}$–$\frac{1}{8}$, three or four times a day, in pill or solution. It has been used in secondary syphilis hypodermically: dose, gr. $\frac{1}{30}$. *Externally*, it may be used as a caustic; a weak solution (gr. $\frac{1}{2}$–i–ij to water f℥j) is much employed as a wash to ulcers, an injection in gleet, a collyrium, &c. An ointment (gr. $\frac{1}{2}$–i–ij to lard ℥j), is a good application in porrigo, tinea, eczema, pityriasis, and skin-diseases generally of parasitic origin. There is danger from the external application of corrosive sublimate to a large surface.

Hydrargyri Iodidum Viride (*Green Iodide of Mercury*), is made by rubbing mercury and iodine together, with the addition of a little alcohol. It is mercurous iodide (HgI), and is a greenish-yellow powder, insoluble in water and alcohol, but soluble in ether. By exposure to light it is partially decomposed, and becomes of a dark-olive colour.

Effects and Uses.—This mercurial exercises a specific influence over the lymphatic and glandular systems, and is employed in syphilis and scrofula occurring in the same individual. Dose, gr. j, gradually increased to gr. iij or iv; it should not be given with iodide of potassium, which decomposes it into red iodide and metallic mercury. *Externally*, it is applied, in the form of ointment, to syphilitic ulcers, &c.

Hydrargyri Iodidum Rubrum (*Red Iodide of Mercury*), is mercuric iodide (HgI_2). It is made by mixing solutions of iodide of potassium and mercuric chloride, from which a double decomposition ensues, resulting in the formation of chloride of potassium in solution, and red iodide of mercury is precipitated. It is a scarlet-red powder, which becomes yellow when heated, insoluble in water, but soluble in boiling alcohol and solutions of iodide of potassium, chloride of sodium, &c. It is a powerful irritant and caustic, and is employed in the same cases as the green iodide, though much more energetic. It is useful in rheumatism, especially of a syphilitic origin. Dose, gr. $\frac{1}{16}$, gradually increased to gr. $\frac{1}{4}$, in pill or alcoholic solution; or, still better, dissolved in a solution of iodide of potassium. *Externally*, it is much used in the form of *ointment* (*unguentum hydrargyri iodidi rubri*), (16 grains mixed with a troyounce of *ointment*).

Hydrargyri Cyanidum (*Cyanide of Mercury*). This salt is made by adding a solution of ferrocyanide of potassium to sulphuric acid, by which hydrocyanic acid is produced, and this, being received in a vessel containing water and red oxide of mercury, generates water and mercuric cyanide ($HgCy_2$). It is usually found in the form of permanent, prismatic, white, and opaque crystals, of a disagreeable styptic taste, soluble in water, but not in alcohol. It is an active poison, and is used as an antisyphilitic remedy, as a substitute for corrosive sublimate, over which it has the advantage of not producing epigastric pain, and not being decomposed by alkalies and organic substances. Dose, gr. $\frac{1}{16}$ to $\frac{1}{8}$.

Hydrargyrum Ammoniatum (*Ammoniated Mercury*). This preparation, commonly called *White Precipitate*, is made by precipitating a solution of corrosive chloride of mercury by ammonia; chloride of ammonium is formed in solution, and ammoniated mercury is thrown down. It is the chloride of mercuric ammonium. In symbols the reaction may be thus expressed: $HgCl_2+2NH_4HO=NH_2Hg''Cl+NH_4Cl+2H_2O$. It is a perfectly white powder, insoluble in water and alcohol, decomposed by boiling water, inodorous, and has an earthy, afterwards metallic taste. It is largely adulterated, chiefly with sulphate of calcium. Its *effects* are poisonous, but it is *used* only as an external application, in the form of *ointment* (*unguentum hydrargyri ammoniati*, one part of ammoniated mercury to twelve parts of *ointment*), to cutaneous eruptions, and to destroy pediculi. Four grains, mixed with half an ounce of powdered sugar, make a good snuff-powder in ozœna.

HYDRARGYRI SULPHAS FLAVA (*Yellow Sulphate of Mercury*). This salt, commonly called *Turpeth Mineral*, from its resemblance to the root of *Ipomœa turpethum*, is made by throwing mercuric sulphate (as obtained from the action of sulphuric acid on mercury), into *boiling water;* the mercuric sulphate is instantly decomposed into a soluble acid salt and the insoluble yellow oxysulphate—*Turpeth Mineral*—which is precipitated ($Hg_3O_2SO_4$). It is an inodorous, lemon-yellow powder, entirely dissipated by heat, of a rather acrid taste, and sparingly soluble in water. It has been employed as an *alterative*, in doses of gr. $\frac{1}{4}$–$\frac{1}{2}$; as an *emetic*, in croup and chronic enlargement of the testis, in doses of gr. ij–v; and as an *errhine*, in chronic ophthalmia and diseases of the head. In an overdose, it is poisonous, forty grains having proved fatal.

HYDRARGYRI SULPHURETUM RUBRUM (*Red Sulphuret of Mercury*), or *Cinnabar* (which is found as a *native* combination), is manufactured by subliming a mixture of one part of sublimed sulphur and five parts of mercury. It is mercuric sulphide (HgS), and occurs in the form of heavy, brilliant, deep-red, crystalline masses, which are inodorous, tasteless, entirely volatilizable by heat, and insoluble in water and alcohol. It is not employed internally, but is used in the way of *fumigation*, in venereal ulcers of the throat and nose; ʒss may be thrown on a red-hot iron and inhaled; but the *black oxide* is a better substance for mercurial fumigation. Cinnabar is used as a paint, under the name of *vermilion*.

UNGUENTUM HYDRARGYRI NITRATIS (*Ointment of Nitrate of*

Mercury.) The *Nitrate of Mercury* is employed chiefly in the form of ointment. This preparation, known as *Citrine Ointment*, is made by dissolving a troyounce and a half of mercury in 3½ troyounces of nitric acid, and adding the solution to 16 troyounces of lard melted at 200°, stirring until effervescence ceases. The chemical changes which result here are not precisely known; but a mercuric oxynitrate ($Hg_6O_4 4NO_3$), is probably formed, with fatty acids and elaïdin. Citrine ointment has a fine yellow colour and unctuous consistence; but, if not very carefully made, it becomes greenish, hard, and friable. It is an excellent stimulant and alterative application, much employed in porrigo, psoriasis, crusta lactea, impetigo, psorophthalmia, and a wide range of ulcerated and eruptive affections. It is best to dilute it, at first, with lard.

LIQUOR HYDRARGYRI NITRATIS (*Solution of Nitrate of Mercury*) (*mercuric nitrate*) ($Hg2NO_3$), is made by dissolving 3 troyounces of mercury in 5 troyounces of nitric acid, mixed with 6 fluidrachms of distilled water; and, when reddish vapours cease to arise, evaporating the liquid to 7½ troyounces; it is now also prepared by dissolving 3 troyounces and 120 grains of red oxide of mercury in a mixture of 3 troyounces and 300 grains of nitric acid in 6 fluidrachms of distilled water. It is a dense, transparent, nearly colourless liquid (sp. gr. 2.165), of a strongly acid taste, and is employed as a caustic application in hospital gangrene, venereal and malignant ulcers, and, diluted, in cutaneous affections.

IODINIUM—IODINE.

Iodine is an elementary, non-metallic substance, found in the vegetable, animal, and mineral kingdoms of nature,—as marine plants, oysters, sponges, mineral springs, &c. It is chiefly manufactured from the residuum of *kelp* (the impure soda obtained from the incineration of sea-weeds), in which it exists as an iodide of sodium, by the action of sulphuric acid and black oxide of manganese. It occurs in crystalline scales, of a bluish-black colour and metallic lustre, of a strong, peculiar odour, and a hot, acrid taste. It is very volatile—evaporating even at common temperatures—is freely soluble in glycerin, alcohol, and ether, and but very slightly soluble in water (1 part in 7000 parts of water). Its solubility in water is very much increased by the addition of certain salts, as the iodide of potassium, chloride of sodium, &c. When heated, its vapour has a rich violet colour, whence its name (from ιώδης, violet). Iodine may be detected in very minute quantity by starch, which produces with it a deep-blue colour; if in combination, the iodine must be first freed with a little nitric acid, or still better with *chromic acid* (which may be evolved by the addition of a single drop of very dilute solution of bichromate of potassium, when starch and nitric acid have been employed ineffectually). Chloroform has also been proposed as a test.

Physiological Effects.—Iodine acts *locally* as an irritant; when applied to the skin it stains it yellow, and causes itching, redness, and desquamation; and, when inhaled in the form of vapour, it excites cough and heat in the air-passages. Taken internally, in *medicinal doses*, it usually at first excites the appetite and strengthens the digestion, though it soon irritates the stomach. It is probably absorbed in the upper part of the small intestines, by being dissolved in the alkaline fluids of this canal, and, after absorption, it frequently produces a remedial alterative and resolvent effect, without any obvious disturbance of the functions. Usually, patients become thin under its use, though sometimes its alterative action on the nutrition produces embonpoint. It excites the secretions generally, increasing the flow of urine, slightly relaxing the bowels, often producing a marked irritant effect on the respiratory mucous membrane and salivary glands, and is readily and rapidly eliminated from the blood, chiefly in the urine. If administered in too large doses, or to persons of irritable stomach, it produces subacute gastro-enteritis; and, when continued for a long time, it will produce gastro-enteric symptoms—headache, giddiness, and other evidences of cerebro-spinal disturbance—marasmus—sometimes discoloration of the skin—occasionally salivation—and frequently a *wasting of the mammæ and testicles.* This train of symptoms is termed *iodism.* In excessive doses, it may act as an irritant poison, and has even produced death: but such a result is rare. Enormous quantities have been taken with very slight effects. The antidote is starch. The absorption of iodine is shown by its presence in the blood and various secretions.

Medicinal Uses.—Iodine is a most valuable *resolvent* remedy, in chronic visceral and glandular enlargements, indurations, thickening of membranes, tumours, &c. It is chiefly employed in *bronchocele* and *scrofula,* but it is useful in every variety of chronic tumour and enlargement; also as an alterative in secondary syphilis and other chronic affections; and as an emmenagogue. Its *vapour* has been inhaled with benefit in chronic bronchitis and phthisis. It is a valuable *topical* remedy and is applied in the form of tincture, with the greatest advantage to enlarged glands (especially when scrofulous), in the various cutaneous affections, lupus, erysipelas, rheumatism, gout, phlegmons, carbuncles, wounds, diseases of joints, poisoned parts, to prevent pitting in smallpox, as a counter-irritant to the chest in phthisis, chronic bronchitis, and pleurisy, as an *injection* in hydrocele, in encysted bronchocele, and even into the pleural cavity in chronic pleurisy, &c., &c. Iodine ranks also among the best of the disinfectants, being very available from the ease of its application as well as its ready portability.

Administration.—Iodine is rarely exhibited alone, but usually in conjunction with iodide of potassium (see p. 324). To avoid gastric irritation, it is best given after a meal, particularly when amylaceous substances have been taken, as it forms with them iodide of starch. Dose, gr. $\frac{1}{4}$–$\frac{1}{2}$, two or three times daily. *Liquor Iodinii Compositus—Compound Solution of Iodine*—sometimes known as *Lugol's Solution*—(Iodine ʒvj, iodide of potassium a troyounce and a half, distilled water Oj), is the usual preparation in which iodine is administered internally; dose, six drops, three times a day, in sweetened water, and gradually increased. The *tincture* (*tinctura iodinii*), (a troyounce to alcohol Oj), is of a deep-brown colour, and undergoes a gradual change, when kept long; water precipitates the iodine from it, hence it is little employed internally; dose, gtt. x–xx, repeated and increased. *Externally*, it is extensively applied to erysipelatous and poisoned parts, chilblains, in cutaneous affections, &c., &c. The *compound tincture* (*tinctura iodinii composita*), (iodine half a troyounce, iodide of potassium a troyounce, alcohol Oj), has the advantage over the tincture, that it may be diluted with water without decomposition; dose, gtt. xv–xxx. *Iodine ointment* (*unguentum iodinii*) (made with iodine ℈j, iodide of potassium gr. iv, water ♏vj, and lard a troyounce), is employed as a local application in goitre, scrofulous tumefactions, &c.; it does not keep well. The *compound iodine ointment* (*unguentum iodinii compositum*), (iodine 15 grains, iodide of potassium 30 grains, water 30 minims, lard a troyounce), is used for the same purpose, as the preceding; they both impart an orange colour to the skin. *Iodine baths* have been employed, with iodine and iodide of potassium dissolved in water, in a *wooden* bath-tub, in the proportion of iodine gr. iij, and iodide gr. vj, to a gallon of water.

Iodine is employed in medicine, in various chemical combinations. The *iodides of iron*, *lead*, and *mercury*, have been noticed. The *iodide of starch* is highly recommended; dose, a teaspoonful, three times a day, to be increased. The *iodide of zinc* (see p. 152), is employed as a tonic and astringent. The *iodide of sulphur* (*sulphuris iodidum*) is prepared by heating together 4 parts of iodine and 1 part of sublimed sulphur; it is a grayish-black solid substance, of a radiated crystalline appearance, having the smell and taste of iodine, decomposed upon exposure to the air and by boiling water and alcohol, insoluble in water, but soluble in 60 parts of glycerin; it is used internally in scrofulous and cutaneous affections, in doses of gr. ½–i, and, externally, in tinea capitis, lupus, lepra, acne, &c., in the form of *ointment* (*unguentum sulphuris iodidi*), (30 grains to a troyounce of lard).

POTASSII IODIDUM—IODIDE OF POTASSIUM.

This salt is prepared by treating an aqueous solution of potassa with iodine in slight excess. By this process, a mixture of iodide of potassium and iodate of potassium is obtained, and the iodate is afterwards deoxidized and converted into iodide by heat and mixture with powdered charcoal. Iodide of potassium (KI), occurs in semi-opaque, white, or transparent, anhydrous crystals, permanent in a dry air, rather deliquescent in a moist one, of an acrid, saline taste, somewhat like that of common salt. It is wholly soluble in water and alcohol, and its aqueous solution dissolves iodine, forming *ioduretted iodide of potassium.* It is frequently adulterated with other salts. It is incompatible with ammonium salts, sulphate, nitrate, phosphate, and borate of sodium, sulphates of potassium and magnesium, sp. nitrous ether, soluble lead salts, and the mercurials generally; with chlorate of potassium, if a mineral acid be added, a poisonous iodate of potassium is produced.

Effects and Uses.—The effects of iodide of potassium are analogous to those of iodine, but less energetic. *Locally,* it acts as an irritant, and, in large doses, sometimes occasions nausea, vomiting, heat of stomach, and purging; but it may be given in larger doses, and for a longer period, than iodine, without causing gastro-enteric derangement. It stimulates the secretions, particularly those from mucous membranes, and very often produces coryza. Its constitutional effects are powerfully *alterative* and *resolvent,* and it is employed in *bronchocele, scrofula, secondary syphilis,* and other chronic diseases, particularly those accompanied with enlargements or indurations. It is a most valuable anti-syphilitic remedy, when the bones and fibrous tissues are affected. In chronic rheumatism and gout, particularly where the fibrous tissues are attacked, it is of great efficacy. As a diuretic in dropsy, it has been found useful; and in spasmodic asthma it often gives great relief. As an eliminative antidote, in mercurial and saturnine poisoning, its action has been already noticed. It has been recommended in hydrocephalus; and has recently been found to exercise a beneficial operation in the treatment of aneurism.

Administration.—Dose, gr. v–xv, or even more, three times a day, in solution. An *ointment* (ʒj to lard ʒvij, with boiling water fʒss) is employed for the same purposes as iodine ointment, and does not discolour the skin; it is, however, of feebler efficacy.

Ammonii Iodidum—Iodide of Ammonium (NH_4I) is made by the double decomposition of iodide of potassium and sulphate of ammonium in hot aqueo-alcoholic solution. It occurs as a white, granular, very deliquescent salt, becoming yellowish-brown by exposure, very soluble in water and alcohol, of a taste like that of iodide of potassium, but a little sharper. It has been used in the same way as the latter salt.

Sodii Iodidum—Iodide of Sodium (NaI) may be made by the double decomposition of iodide of iron and carbonate of sodium. It is a soluble, white, crystalline salt, used to fulfil the same indications as iodide of potassium, than which it is said to be better borne. It is not officinal.

IODOFORMUM—IODOFORM.

Iodoform is obtained by the action of chlorinated lime upon a heated alcoholic solution of iodide of potassium, which yields iodate of calcium and iodoform, the latter being separated by the solvent action of boiling alcohol. It is a teriodide of formyl (CHI_3), and occurs in the form of small scaly, yellow crystals, having a saffron-like odour and sweet taste, insoluble in water, but soluble in alcohol, ether, chloroform, and the fixed and volatile oils. It is devoid of irritant action, and produces the constitutional effects of iodine, besides an anodyne influence. Large doses produce tetanic convulsions in animals. Dose, 1 to 3 grains, three times a day in pill. In the form of *vapour*, it is said to possess anæsthetic properties, but inferior to those of chloroform. *Externally*, it acts as a powerful local anæsthetic, and has been found a good application to chancres and irritable ulcers, as bed sores; it is used also to relieve the pain of cancerous sores, and, for these purposes, it may be dusted over the ulcerated surface, which is then to be dressed with glycerin spread upon lint; a saturated solution of iodoform in chloroform is serviceable in relieving the pain of neuralgia and gout; an iodoform suppository is also useful in painful diseases of the rectum and bladder.

BROMINIUM—BROMINE.

Bromine is an elementary body, bearing close chemical and medicinal affinities to iodine. It is a constituent of sea-water and of many mineral springs. In Europe, it is obtained principally from the mother liquors of the salt mines of Stassfurt, in Germany; in this country, from saline springs in western Pennsylvania, Ohio, and West Virginia, in which it exists as a bromide of magnesium. It is a volatile, dark-red liquid (sp. gr. 3), of a caustic taste, and a strong, disagreeable smell, sparingly soluble in water, more soluble in alcohol, and still more so in ether. Its *effects on the system* have been thought to be analogous to those of iodine, and it has been employed as an alterative resolvent in bronchocele, scrofulous tumors, skin-diseases, &c., particularly in cases in which iodine does not answer, or has lost its activity; but bromine and the bromides are now known to exert a powerfully tranquillizing influence in various forms of irritable action of the nervous centres, as spasmodic diseases, especially epilepsy, wakefulness, nymphomania, &c. It is given in *aqueous solution* (1 part to 40 parts of distilled water), dose, six drops, several times a day; but it is exhibited internally chiefly in the form of the bromides. It is a good application in hospital gangrene, and, properly diluted, it is used as a wash for ulcers. In overdoses, bromine is an irritant poison, and has proved fatal; ammonia is said to be an *antidote*.

POTASSII BROMIDUM (*Bromide of Potassium*) (KBr), is prepared by adding a solution of pure carbonate of potassium to a solution of bromide of iron. The iron is precipitated, and bromide of potassium remains in solution, from which it is obtained by evaporation. It occurs as a permanent, colourless, anhydrous, crystalline salt, of a pungent, saline taste, very soluble in water, and slightly soluble in alcohol. Bromide of potassium has been used as a substitute for the iodide, in bronchocele, scrofula, chronic cutaneous affections, secondary syphilis, fibroid tumours of the uterus, &c., but it is inferior in these diseases to the iodic salt. It has, however, proved a very efficacious remedy in diseases of the nervous centres, as whooping-cough, infantile convulsions, hysteria, laryngismus stridulus, and especially epilepsy, over which it is believed to exert more control than any other article of the Materia Medica. As an anti-tetanic remedy, it now ranks at the head of our resources, in cerebro-spinal meningitis, in strychnia-poisoning, and in tetanus. In the insomnia of mania and of mania-a-potu, it is often efficacious; and it has been found to be the most efficient remedy which we possess in allaying venereal excitement, and hence its employment in nymphomania, chordee, &c., and as a preventive of masturbation in prisons, barracks, &c. Given with or before opium, it often prevents the unpleasant effects of that article, and is useful in the vomiting of pregnancy. It is used, too, to obtund the sensibility of the fauces, before the exhibition of the laryngoscope. Dose, from fifteen to twenty, and even thirty grains, several times a day; in tetanus, much larger amounts. No fatal case of poisoning from this salt is on record.

AMMONII BROMIDUM (BROMIDE OF AMMONIUM) (NH_4Br), is prepared by dissolving bromine in water of ammonia, or by acting on bromide of iron with carbonate of ammonium. It occurs in colourless crystals, which, on exposure to the air, gradually become yellowish (in consequence of the liberation of hydrobromic acid), has a saline, pungent taste, is very soluble in water, and moderately soluble in alcohol. Its effects, uses, and doses are analogous to those of bromide of potassium, but rather larger doses are required. It is also highly recommended in doses of ten or fifteen grains, every two or three hours, in acute rheumatism.

The BROMIDE OF SODIUM (NaBr) has lately been employed

in preference to the bromide of potassium, as having more bromine; and still more recently, the BROMIDE OF LITHIUM (LBr) has been recommended as the most efficacious of the bromides. In bromide of potassium there is about 66 per cent. of bromine; in bromide of sodium, 78 per cent.; and in bromide of lithium, nearly 92 per cent. *Bromide of Magnesium* sits well on the stomach. Bromides of iron and mercury have been also employed.

OLEUM MORRHUÆ—COD-LIVER OIL.

This is a FIXED OIL, obtained from the LIVER of Gadus Morrhua, or the *common cod*,—a well-known fish of the Northern Atlantic,—and probably, also, from the livers of several other species of Gadus. It is prepared by subjecting the livers to heat, either in boilers with water, or by means of steam externally applied, and afterwards draining off the liquid portion, from which the oil separates on standing. It is said to be sometimes procured also by expression. Three varieties are known, the *white* or *pale-yellow*, the *brownish-yellow*, and the *dark-brown*. They differ chiefly in the mode of preparation—the *pale* being prepared from fresh livers, the *dark-brown* from those which are collected at sea and have undergone putrefactive decomposition, and the *brownish-yellow* from those in which putrefaction has only partially commenced. The pale oil is the purest; the dark oil is the most offensive to the taste and smell, and the least acceptable to the stomach.

Cod-liver oil is of the consistence of lamp-oil, and has a peculiar odour and taste, resembling that of shoe-leather, which is usually prepared in the United States with this oil. These sensible properties are probably the best test of the genuineness of the oil, and it should be rejected, if the smell and taste of shoe-leather are wanting, or if those of lamp-oil or fish-oil are very perceptible. The sp. gr. of the best oil is about 0.917. The oil undergoes a gradual change from exposure to the air, and should therefore be kept in full and well-stoppered bottles. It is scarcely soluble in water, somewhat so in alcohol, readily soluble in ether, chloroform, and glycerin. It contains a great variety of *chemical constituents*, the most important of which are *fatty acids*, several *biliary principles*, a peculiar brown substance called *gaduin* (which is not, however, supposed to be the *active* ingredient), *iodine*, *chlorine*, and traces of *bromine*.

Cod-liver oil may be distinguished from other oils by the agency of sulphuric acid, a drop of which, when added to fresh cod-liver oil, on a porcelain plate, causes a centrifugal movement in the oil, and gives rise to a fine violet colour, soon passing into yellowish or brownish-red. This reaction is attributable, however, to the bile contained in the oil. By reaction with ammonia, in distillation, the peculiar volatile principle, *prophylamia* (the odorous principle of pickled herring), is developed.

Physiological Effects.—Cod-liver oil, like all fats, is appropriated in the small intestine, and not in the stomach. Its prolonged use, in doses which allow it to be retained by the stomach, produces very marked beneficial effects in a wide range of chronic diseases, dependent on a vitiated condition of the functions of digestion, assimilation, and nutrition. Its modus medendi is not well understood: some therapeutists believing it to act merely as a nutritive agent, valuable from the readiness with which it is assimilated—others attributing its curative powers to an alterative action from the iodine and bromine, or other principles which it contains. Its effects are, however, probably due merely to its nutrient action, in supplying a sufficiency of molecular base for interstitial growth. The biliary principles which it contains promote its absorption and appropriation by the system. The most striking feature of its action on the economy is *increase of weight*; and, usually, where it fails to increase the weight, it is of little service. It is believed, also, to diminish the formation of uric acid in the system, and hence may be useful in gout. In *large doses*, cod-liver oil produces nausea and diarrhœa, and these effects occasionally follow the use of medicinal doses.

Medicinal Uses.—Cod-liver oil has long been known as a remedy in rheumatic diseases; and within the last twenty-five years it has come into extensive use, as an alterative in tuberculous and scrofulous affections. In the treatment of phthisis pulmonalis, it is now looked upon, in Great Britain and the United States, as superior to any other agent, and as possessing an undoubted power of arresting the progress of both the general and the local symptoms in this disease. Although efficacious in all the stages of phthisis, its value is most conspicuous in the earlier stages, especially before the formation of true tubercles. Over the different forms of scrofula, it exercises also a very decided control—particularly glandular enlargements, ulcers, diseases of the joints and spine, ophthalmia, &c. In the various cutaneous affections, tertiary syphilis, chronic rheumatism and gout, and the entire circle of chronic disorders, in which there is a tendency to marasmus, and where the nutrition is defective, cod-liver oil is employed with benefit. Its good effects are most conspicuous, in proportion to the youth of the patient.

Administration.—Dose, a tablespoonful two or three times a day; though, if unacceptable to the stomach, it is best to begin with smaller, as teaspoonful doses. The addition of a little ether (as from 12 to 20 drops to a teaspoonful of oil) promotes its digestion. It must be persevered with for a long time before its good effects appear. It is best given in some aromatic water, or a little ardent spirit, or the froth of porter; and it may be rendered more agreeable to the stomach by combination with one of the mineral acids. The union of the oil with lime-water, just enough to form a soap, often renders it acceptable to delicate stomachs, and it may be flavoured with oil of bitter almonds. If it produce diarrhœa, astringents should be administered with it. It is used as a *clyster*, in cases of ascarides and lumbricoides; and, *externally*, in cutaneous affections and opacity of the cornea.

ARSENICI PRÆPARATA—PREPARATIONS OF ARSENIC.

Metallic arsenic is inert, though, when swallowed, it may prove powerfully poisonous, by becoming oxidized and converted into arsenious acid. It is not used in medicine.

ACIDUM ARSENIOSUM (*Arsenious Acid*), (As_2O_3), sometimes called *White Arsenic*, *Oxide of Arsenic*, or *Arsenic*, is obtained principally as a secondary product in the roasting of cobalt ores (the arseniurets of cobalt) in Saxony and Bohemia. It is afterwards purified by sublimation; and, when recently prepared, occurs in glassy, colourless, transparent masses, of a vitreous fracture, which gradually become white and opaque, progressively from the surface inwards. It is sometimes kept in the shops in the form of a fine white powder; but, in this state, it is liable to adulteration with chalk or sulphate of calcium, and it should therefore be always purchased in masses. It is entirely volatilized by heat, at a temperature not exceeding 400°, has no smell, and little or no taste; is soluble in water (more readily, when *transparent* than opaque), and also in alcohol and oils; *cold* water dissolves from $\frac{1}{1000}$th to $\frac{1}{500}$th part of its weight of arsenious acid, or about half a grain to a fluidounce; if boiled for a short time with water, about $\frac{1}{80}$th part will be dissolved; if boiled for an hour, $\frac{1}{40}$th part will be dissolved, or about 12 grains to the ounce.

Tests.—Owing to the frequent use of arsenious acid as a poison, a knowledge of the means of detecting its presence is of great importance. In the *solid* state, it may be recognized in the first place by its *volatility* (heated over a spirit-lamp, it passes off as white, inodorous vapour, and is deposited on a cool surface as an amorphous powder or in octohedral crystals); secondly, when thrown on burning charcoal, it is deoxidized, and gives out the *garlicky odour* of metallic arsenic; and, thirdly, if heated in a glass tube with charcoal or black flux, it sublimes and condenses in the form of a brilliant, steel-gray ring or mirror. In *aqueous solution*, arsenious acid may be detected by the following reagents; *sulphuretted hydrogen* or *sulphide of ammonium* produces a *lemon* or *sulphur-yellow* sulphide of arsenic; the addition first of *ammonia* and then of *nitrate of silver*, produces a *canary-yellow* arsenite of silver; and the addition of *potassa* and then of *sulphate of copper*, produces an *apple* or *grass-green* arsenite of copper; 100 grains, boiled with dilute muriatic acid, and then treated with sulphuretted hydrogen, yield a deposit of sulphide of arsenic, weighing 124 grains. The sulphide of arsenic may be *reduced*, and made to yield metallic arsenic, if heated with soda-flux or potash-flux. The most delicate test, however, of arsenious acid in solution is that of *nascent hydrogen*, termed *Marsh's test.* When the acid is submitted to the action of nascent hydrogen (evolved by the action of diluted sulphuric acid on pure zinc), it is deoxdized, and unites with the hydrogen to form arseniuretted hydrogen gas. This gas has a garlicky odour, and is recognized by its burning with a bluish-white flame, which deposits on a plate of cold glass or porcelain, held over the jet, a lustrous steel-gray or brownish-black spot or mirror of metallic arsenic, surrounded by a faint white ring of arsenious acid; the metallic spot deposited is distinguishable from antimony, obtained by a similar process, by the addition of a drop or two of fuming nitric acid, with heat, which dissolves both metals, the solutions yielding on evaporation white residues, but the arsenical residue, touched with a drop of strong solution of nitrate of silver, assumes a brick-red colour, while the antimonial residue remains unchanged; and also the arsenic can be dissolved by a solution of hypochlorite of sodium or calcium, which does not affect antimony. Another test is that of *Reinsch*, and consists in boiling a solution of the acid with muriatic acid and copper-foil or wire, when the latter acquires a steel-gray coating of metallic arsenic, passing as it increases into black. *When arsenious acid is dissolved with liquid organic substances*, it should first be separated from insoluble matters by filtration, and the metallic arsenic may be then obtained by *Reinsch's process;* and the liquid or subliming tests afterwards applied. If the poison be mixed with *solid organic substances*, they should be cut up and boiled with water, acidulated with muriatic acid, and the solution afterwards filtered, and again boiled, &c.

Physiological Effects.—Arsenious acid acts *locally* as an escharotic, by destroying the vitality of the parts to which it is applied. In medicinal doses, it stimulates the digestive and nutritive functions, as is shown by the well-known results of arsenic eating among the peasantry of Austria. Its physiological effects are not, at first, very obvious. When continued for some time, it generally produces more or less heat and dryness of the throat and stomach, with nausea, increased secretion from the bowels and kidneys, irritation of the conjunctiva, and a peculiar swelling of the face termed *œdema arsenicalis;* after the latter symptom appears, the medicine should be suspended. In *too long-continued* or *too large medicinal doses*, arsenious acid sometimes produces a sort of chronic poisoning, characterized by disorder of the digestive apparatus, conjunctivitis, œdema, salivation, a cutaneous eruption, loss of the hair and nails, paralysis, convulsions, and, if its use be persevered in, coma and delirium may result, terminating in death. In *excessive doses*, arsenious acid is a violent poison, usually destroying life by gastro-enteritis, in from one to two or three days. When very large quantities are taken, it sometimes acts on the cerebro-spinal system, producing death by narcotism, in a few hours. Occasionally, gastro-enteric and cerebro-spinal symptoms both occur. Two grains of arsenious acid have proved fatal, though much larger amounts have been taken with impunity; very large quantities often cause emesis, which removes the poison from the stomach.

Dissections, in cases of poisoning from this agent, reveal redness (sometimes accompanied with extravasations of blood), ulceration, softening, effusion of lymph, and even gangrene, in the alimentary canal. The blood is often fluid and dark-coloured. The absorption of arsenious acid into the system, after its administration, is shown by its presence in the blood, viscera, bile, urine, &c. It is rapidly eliminated by the urine, and also by the bile, and even the skin and saliva.

Antidotes and Treatment in cases of Poisoning.—The evacuation of the contents of the stomach, by the stomach-pump or emetics, should be the first object in these cases. Demulcent drinks are to be also freely given. The HYDRATED OXIDE OF IRON should be administered, as soon as it can be procured, in the state of *pulp* or *magma*. It is prepared by the action of an alkaline solution on a ferric salt; *water of ammonia* is directed by the U. S. Pharmacopœia, to be added to a *solution of the tersulphate of iron* (see p. 142). The hydrated oxide of iron is a soft, moist, reddish-brown magma, which acts as an *antidote* to arsenious acid, by forming with it an insoluble, inert, ferrous arseniate ($Fe_3 2AsO_4$). The dose is about twelve times the supposed amount of poison taken, and it should be given in the *fresh* and *pulpy* state, as it gradually loses its antidotical virtues when kept. The *subcarbonate of iron* also acts as an antidote, but this is much less powerful than the pulpy hydrate. *Light magnesia* (which has not been too strongly calcined), and freshly-precipitated *gelatinous magnesia*, may be also used as antidotes. The after treatment consists in the use of demulcents, opiates, and, if necessary, stimulants.

Medicinal Uses.—Arsenious acid is a very valuable alterative remedy, but it must be exhibited with caution. It is employed with the greatest success in the treatment of *miasmatic affections*, as *intermittent fevers*, especially such as have resisted the use of cinchona, or have frequently reappeared; in *chronic cutaneous affections*, particularly the scaly diseases (lepra, eczema squamosum, psoriasis, and pityriasis); also in *certain affections of the nervous system*, chorea in particular, over which it exercises a marked control; in chronic rheumatism, in phthisis, in the tertiary forms of syphilis, in irritable dyspepsia, gastric ulcer, diarrhœa, bronchitis, and as a tonic generally. As an *external application*, arsenious acid has been applied to indolent sinuses, lupus, onychia maligna, &c., either pure or mixed with several parts of sulphur; its use is, however, attended with danger of constitutional effects. It is an ingredient of various empirical compounds, employed in the treatment of cancer.

Administration.—Dose, gr. $\frac{1}{16}$ to $\frac{1}{12}$, in pills with bread-crumb, three times a day, to be reduced when conjunctivitis appears, and suspended after the establishment of the *œdema arsenicalis;* and, after being taken a fortnight, it should always be intermitted for a day or two. It is less apt to occasion gastric irritability, when given immediately after a meal. The usual and safer form of exhibiting this remedy, is that of solution with potash.

LIQUOR POTASSII ARSENITIS (*Solution of Arsenite of Potassium*), or *Fowler's Solution.* This is prepared by boiling 64 grains of arsenious acid and bicarbonate of potassium, each, in half a fluidounce of distilled water, then adding 12 fluidounces more of distilled water, half a fluidounce of compound spirit of lavender, and afterwards water enough to make the solution measure a pint. It is a transparent liquid, of an alkaline reaction, and has the colour, taste, and smell of spirit of lavender. It is a solution of the arsenite of potassium (KH_2AsO_3), and is decomposed by the reagents which act upon arsenic, and is *incompatible* with infusions and decoctions of cinchona. Its *effects and uses* are analogous to those of arsenious acid, though some practitioners have denied their therapeutic identity. The *antidote* is ferric subacetate ($Fe_23C_2H_3O_2$), which renders inert all the salts of the acids of arsenic. Dose, gtt. v to gtt. x, and even gtt. xx, three times a day. Each fluidrachm contains half a grain of arsenious acid.

SODII ARSENIAS (*Arseniate of Sodium*), is made by melting together arsenious acid, nitrate of sodium, and carbonate of sodium, then dissolving the fused salt in boiling water, and afterwards crystallizing. In this process, the arsenious acid is oxidized into arsenic acid by the nitric acid of the sodium nitrate, and then combines with the soda of both salts, to form colourless, transparent, prismatic crystals ($Na_2HAsO_4,7H_2O$), slightly efflorescent, very soluble in water, of a somewhat saline, slightly acrimonious taste. This salt is employed to fulfil the therapeutic indications of the other arsenical preparations, and has the advantage of a somewhat milder local action. Dose, gr. $\frac{1}{12}$–$\frac{1}{8}$. It is sometimes prescribed externally in the form of baths, in chronic nodose rheumatism and gout, ʒss–ʒij or ʒiij, in each bath. It is generally used internally in the form of

LIQUOR SODII ARSENIATIS (*Solution of Arseniate of Sodium*), made by dissolving 64 grains of arseniate of sodium (rendered anhydrous at a heat not exceeding 300°), in a pint of distilled water; dose, gtt. x–xx. Cigarettes, made of paper saturated with a solution, two or three times the officinal strength, are smoked in asthma.

LIQUOR ARSENICI CHLORIDI (*Solution of Chloride of Arsenic*) ($AsCl_3$), is made by boiling 64 grains of arsenious acid with 2 fluidrachms of muriatic acid and 4 fluidounces of distilled water, until the acid is dissolved, and adding to the solution, when cold, water enough to make it measure a pint. This is a recently introduced preparation, and is believed to be especially valuable in lepra and chorea, and generally where the arsenicals are indicated; dose, the same as that of Fowler's Solution, than which it is thought to be less apt to disturb the stomach.

ARSENICI IODIDUM (*Iodide of Arsenic*) (AsI_3), made by rubbing 5 parts of iodine and 1 part of arsenic together, is an orange-red, crystalline, volatilizable solid, wholly soluble in water, and has been used both *internally* and *externally* in skin diseases. Dose, gr. $\frac{1}{8}$, three times a day; for external use, gr. iij to lard ℥j.

LIQUOR ARSENICI ET HYDRARGYRI IODIDI (*Solution af Iodide of Arsenic and Mercury*). This solution, known as *Donovan's Solution*, is prepared by dissolving 35 grains of iodide of arsenic and red iodide of mercury, each, in half a pint of distilled water. It is merely an aqueous solution of the two iodides (AsI_3 and HgI_2). It has a pale-yellow colour, a slightly styptic taste, and is *incompatible* with the salts of morphia.

Effects and Uses.—This is a highly valuable alterative preparation, in the various forms of popular and scaly cutaneous affections, and in obstinate syphilis. It was introduced by Mr. Donovan, of Dublin, in 1839, and has been a good deal employed in the United States. Dose, gtt. v to gtt. xx or more, three times a day.

CALCII PHOSPHAS PRÆCIPITATA—PRECIPITATED PHOSPHATE OF CALCIUM.

This salt is made by reacting upon bone-ash with muriatic acid, which dissolves the phosphate of calcium in the bones, and gives it up again, on the addition of water of ammonia. It is a white, inodorous, tasteless, insoluble powder, sometimes called the *Bone Phosphate of Calcium* ($Ca_3 2PO_4$). It is an important and valuable medicine, not only in diseases of deficient ossification, as ununited fracture, caries of the bones, rickets, &c., but in all conditions of defective cell-growth and mal-nutrition, from its undoubted influence in promoting natural cell-growth and nutrition. Thus, it is employed (often in connection with other phosphates, as those of iron, sodium, and potassium), in scrofula, phthisis, anæmia, diarrhœa, chronic bronchitis, abscesses, and wasting diseases of every kind. Dose, five to ten grains, and it may be well given dusted in a little milk. A better (because more soluble) preparation is the *Lacto-phosphate of Calcium*, made by the action of lactic acid upon the phosphate of calcium. An emulsion, containing 50 per cent. of cod-liver oil and 2 grains of lacto-phosphate to the drachm, is an excellent preparation—dose, a teaspoonful to a tablespoonful.

CALCII HYPOPHOSPHIS—HYPOPHOSPHITE OF CALCIUM.

This salt is prepared by boiling phosphorus in a mixture of hydrate of calcium in boiling water; phosphuretted hydrogen escapes, and phosphate and hypophosphite of calcium are formed in the liquid, from which the insoluble phosphate and residuary lime are separated by filtration, and the hypophosphite is afterwards crystallized out, in the form of white, pearly crystals, of a nauseous, bitter taste, soluble in 6 parts of water, and insoluble in alcohol. All the soluble sulphates and carbonates produce precipitates with this salt ($Ca2PH_2O_2$).

POTASSII HYPOPHOSPHIS—HYPOPHOSPHITE OF POTASSIUM ($K2PH_2O_2$), is prepared by mixing solutions of hypophosphite of calcium and carbonate of potassium. It occurs in white, opaque, confused, crystalline masses, having a disagreeable, bitter taste, very deliquescent, and very soluble in water and alcohol, but insoluble in ether.

SODII HYPOPHOSPHIS—HYPOPHOSPHITE OF SODIUM, ($Na\,2PH_2O_2$), is prepared by mixing solutions of hypophosphite of calcium and crystallized carbonate of sodium, and crystallizes in white tables, of a pearly lustre, very deliquescent (but less so than the potassium hypophosphite), very soluble in water and alcohol, and insoluble in ether.

The hypophosphites have been lately introduced in the treatment of phthisis, under an impression that they prove useful by furnishing phosphorus to the tissues. They more probably act by stimulating cell-growth and nutrition, and may be given to fulfil the same indications as the precipitated phosphate of calcium. The soluble salts of mercury and silver are incompatible with them. Dose, 10 to 30 grains, three times a day. The hypophosphite of calcium is the most eligible salt, but they are often given together, in the form of syrup. The *hypophosphite of iron* was noticed with *chalybeates* (see p. 146). The *hypophosphite of ammonium* is also used.*

AMMONII CHLORIDUM—CHLORIDE OF AMMONIUM.

This salt, formerly termed muriate of ammonia, and often known as *Sal Ammoniac*, is obtained from the *gas-liquor* of coal gas works (usually by neutralizing the ammonia with muriatic acid), and also in the preparation of animal charcoal from bones. It is brought in the *crude* state from Calcutta, for use in the arts, and in the *refined* state, for medicinal employment, from England. It occurs in white, translucent, tough, fibrous, hemispherical, convex-concave cakes (NH_4Cl), about two inches

**Syrup of Hypophosphites:* Dissolve 96 grains of hypophosphite of iron in hypophosphorous acid, then in 6 fluidounces of water dissolve 256 grains of hypophosphite of calcium, 192 grains of hypophosphite of sodium, and 128 grains of hypophosphite of potassium, mix and add water enough to make 9 fluidounces; in this dissolve 12 troyounces of sugar and half a fluidounce of fluid extract of vanilla. Each fluidrachm contains about 5 grains of the hypophosphites.

thick, difficult to powder, inodorous, of a pungent, saline taste, slightly deliquescent, very soluble in water, and less so in alcohol.

The Pharmacopœia directs that the imported salt should be *purified* for medicinal use by the addition of 5 fluidrachms of water of ammonia to a solution of 20 troyounces of chloride dissolved in 2 pints of water. *Purified chloride of ammonium* (*Ammonii chloridum purificatum*), occurs as a snow-white, crystalline powder, soluble in 2½ parts of cold, and in its own weight of boiling water, and soluble also in alcohol.

Effects and Uses.—The local action of chloride of ammonium is that of an irritant. In large doses it purges. In small doses, after absorption, it proves a powerful resolvent alterative, diminishing the solid constituents of the blood, with an increased flow of the secretions generally; it has an especial action upon the mucous membranes, promoting nutritive changes and epithelial exfoliation. Under its use, the solids of the urine are increased, except uric acid, which is slightly diminished. Even in very large amounts, it is not considered poisonous. It is not much employed in Great Britain or the United States, but it is extensively used in Germany—as a refrigerant in mild fevers attended with stoppage of the secretions—as a resolvent in organic enlargements—in amenorrhœa—and in catarrhs, urethritis, &c. Of late, this salt has been used with advantage in muscular rheumatism and in neuralgia; and its resolvent powers are highly spoken of in fibroid tumours of the uterus. Dose, gr. v–xxx, every two or three hours, in powder or mucilaginous solution. *Externally*, it is used in solution (immediately upon being dissolved), as a refrigerant lotion (℥i to half a pint of water), in cutaneous affections and indolent ulcers (ʒi to half a pint of water), and also a discutient and vulnerary.

AMMONII PHOSPHAS—PHOSPHATE OF AMMONIUM.

Although not officinal, this salt enjoys considerable reputation as an alterative. It is made by adding Stronger Water of

Ammonia to Diluted Phosphoric Acid, evaporating and crystallizing ($2NH_4PO_4$). It occurs in transparent colourless crystals, having the form of six-sided tables, of an alkaline, somewhat saline taste, soluble in water, and insoluble in alcohol. As usually found in the shops, it is a mixture of the neutral and of the acid phosphate of ammonium.

Effects and Uses.—It has been used in this country as a remedy in gout and rheumatism, and is highly esteemed. In combination with carbonate of ammonium and aromatic spirit of ammonia, it has been also lately used with advantage in diabetes. Dose, ten to forty grains, three or four times a day, dissolved in an aromatic water.

POTASSII CHLORAS—CHLORATE OF POTASSIUM.

This salt is prepared by various processes: a good one is by reacting upon solution of caustic potassa, mixed with lime, with a stream of chlorine—the chlorine is converted into chloric acid by oxygen from the lime, and the acid combines with the potassa to form chlorate of potassium ($KCLO_3$). It is a white anhydrous salt, crystallizing in rhomboidal plates of a pearly lustre, and is inodorous, and of a cool, saline taste. It is but little changed by exposure to the air, is soluble in 16 parts of cold water and 2 parts of boiling water. It is said to be soluble in all the animal fluids without decomposing them, or undergoing change itself.

Effect and Uses.—Chlorate of potassium, when taken internally, gives a bright arterial tinge to the venous blood, reduces the volume and frequency of the pulse, and largely increases the secretion of urine, by which it passes out of the system unchanged. The appetite is improved under its use, and salivation is an occasional effect. Large doses may be taken with impunity, but excessive quantities are said to have produced fatal gastro-enteric inflammation. Lately, a fatal case of poisoning from this salt has been reported, in which death was produced by a tablespoonful, apparently from blood-poisoning, the heart and large vessels having been found filled with coagula. As it contains a large supply of oxygen, it was at first employed, with a view to its oxidizing influence in contaminated conditions of the blood, as in malignant fevers, syphilis, &c.; and, whatever the modus medendi, it is still considered a valuable alterative in typhus, scarlatina, &c. Probably, its most positive remedial effects are seen in various forms of stomatitis, follicular, mercurial, and gangrenous. It is also used in diphtheria, croup, cyanosis, asthma, and even neuralgia. *Externally* in solution, it is an admirable wash or gargle in stomatitis, ozœna, the sore throat of scarlatina, subacute and chronic pharyngitis, diphtheria, and fetid ulcerated surfaces generally; mixed with sugar, the powder is an excellent application in the aphthous sore mouth of children. Dose, *internally*, fifteen to thirty grains, every three or four hours, in some pleasant vehicle. *Troches of Chlorate of Potassium* (*trochisci potassii chloratis*), are made by rubbing together 5 troyounces of chlorate of potassium, 18 troyounces of sugar, 2 troyounces of tragacanth, and 30 grains of vanilla, and with water forming a mass, to be divided into 480 troches, each containing 5 grains of chlorate of potassium. For *external* use, ʒij–iv may be dissolved in half a pint of water.

POTASSII BICHROMAS—BICHROMATE OF POTASSIUM.

The chief ore from which salts containing chromium are obtained is chrome ironstone, found in Sweden and in southeastern Pennsylvania; by roasting the powdered ore with carbonate of potassium and nitre, the yellow chromate of potassium is obtained, and by acidulating a solution of this with sulphuric acid, the red or bichromate, is formed (K_2CrO_4,CrO_3); it separates in orange-red, anhydrous, tabular crystals, soluble in water, insoluble in alcohol, and of a cooling, bitter taste.

Effects and Uses.—It is an irritant caustic, acting in overdoses as a corrosive poison, for which the proper antidotes are magnesia, soap, and the alkaline carbonates. In small doses, it is alterative, and has been used in syphilis, with encouraging results. In larger doses, it is emetic. Externally, it is a good application, in powder, or in saturated solution, to syphilitic warts, excrescences, &c. Dose, as an *alterative*, gr. $\frac{1}{8}$ daily, in pill, with some bitter extract; as an *emetic*, gr. $\frac{3}{4}$.

POTASSII PERMANGANAS—PERMANGANATE OF POTASSIUM.

This salt is made by mixing together equal parts of black oxide of manganese and chlorate of potassium with a slight excess of caustic potassa, dissolving in a little water, evaporating to dryness, and exposing to a nearly red heat; chlorate of potassium yields oxygen, which converts the black oxide of manganese into permanganic acid, and this combines with the potassa to form permanganate of potassium ($K_2Mn_2O_8$). It occurs in the form of slender prismatic crystals, of a deep-purple colour, inodorous, and of a sweetish astringent taste. It dissolves readily in water, making a beautiful lilac solution, which is readily decolorized by Fowler's arsenical solution.

Effects and Uses.—There is little experience, as regards the action of this salt, when administered internally, although alterative effects are attributed to it (and probably with reason), in poisoned conditions of the blood, as in malignant fevers, diphtheria, pyæmia, &c. It is as a powerful *disinfectant*, that it at present claims chief attention, and it now ranks at the head of this class of agents, in destroying fetid odours, and poisonous organic emanations. Its power in this respect is due to the evolution of oxyen, in its more active form, *ozone*. It is used externally, in dressing foul and fetid or gangrenous ulcers, particularly in hospital gangrene, as an application to carbuncles, as a gargle in diphtheria, &c. It may be sprinkled in powder on gangrenous surfaces, or applied in solution, of the strength of half an ounce, an ounce, or two ounces to a pint of water. As a *disinfectant* and *deodorizer*, a solution of from one to ten grains to an ounce of water, may be exposed in saucers, or sprinkled on the floor, or thrown into the air in spray by the atomizer. One to three grains may be given *internally* in solution, through the day. *Solution of Perman-*

ganate of Potassium (*liquor potassii permanganatis*) contains 64 grains of the salt in a pint of distilled water—half a fluidounce contains 2 grains. *Condy's Fluid* is of half this strength.

AQUA CHLORINII—CHLORINE WATER.

This is an aqueous solution of *Chlorine*, which is generated by heating 3 troyounces of muriatic acid, diluted with 2 fluidounces of water, with half a troyounce of black oxide of manganese. The chlorine is conducted by suitable tubes, through 2 fluidounces of water, into a bottle containing 20 fluidounces of distilled water, with which it is agitated, and the *chlorine water* is afterwards transferred to a well-stoppered bottle, made impervious to light. It should be kept in a cool place, protected from the light, but it is soon decomposed. It occurs as a greenish-yellow liquid, having an astringent taste and the suffocating odour of the gas. Its employment internally is chiefly in essential malignant fevers, as scarlatina and typhus, also in syphilis and diseases of the liver, and as an antidote for hydrocyanic acid. Dose, f℥i–iv, diluted. Externally, it is used, diluted, as a wash in skin diseases, as an antiseptic, and by inhalation in bronchial affections. Chlorine acts as a disinfectant and deodorizer, chiefly by its affinity for the hydrogen of moisture and the liberation of oxygen; its gaseous form gives it advantages in this respect. Solutions containing chlorine and other antiseptics are useful applications to suppurating surfaces, by preventing the decomposition of pus and thereby pyæmia. In case of poisoning by chlorine, albumen is the best antidote.

CALX CHLORINATA—CHLORINATED LIME.

This preparation, often called *Chloride of Lime*, is prepared by passing chlorine over hydrate of calcium till saturation is effected, and is said to be a mixture of hypochlorite and chloride of calcium ($CaCl_2O_2$ and $CaCl_2$); it occurs as a loose, grayish-white powder, or friable lumps, dry or but slightly moist, readily soluble in water, of a bitter, caustic taste, and a faint odour of chlorine. Exposed to air and moisture, it slowly yields hypochlorous acid ($HClO$), and this soon breaks up into water, chloric acid ($HClO_3$) and free chlorine, and the chloric acid again yields chlorine; 25 per cent. of chlorine should be furnished by good chlorinated lime. It has been used as an alterative, in typhus, malignant scarlatina, syphilis, &c., in doses of from one to five grains, in solution, several times a day; and as a wash, *externally*, one part dissolved in a hundred parts of water—or as a paste. It is chiefly, however, as a *disinfectant*, that it is employed. Its effects are essentially those of chlorine, like which it decomposes hydrosulphuric and hydrocyanic acids, and should not be given with mercurials.

Liquor Sodæ Chlorinatæ (*Solution of Chlorinated Soda*) ($NaCl,NaClO$), sometimes termed *Labarraque's Disinfecting Liquid*, is made by decomposing a solution of carbonate of sodium by one of chlorinated lime. It is a transparent, greenish-yellow liquid, with a faint smell of chlorine, a sharp saline taste, and an alkaline reaction. It has been used *internally*, to fulfil the same indications as chlorinated lime, in doses of thirty drops to a teaspoonful, diluted, several times a day. It is useful, also, in dilution of various strengths, as an *external* application to every form of fetid ulcer, and it is a most valuable and powerful *disinfectant*.

Peroxide of Hydrogen (H_2O_2), has lately been added to our list of alteratives. It may be prepared in numerous ways, the only practically useful ones being based upon the decomposition of peroxide of barium by means of an acid in presence of water. The most satisfactory method is to pass a rapid current of pure carbonic acid through distilled water, peroxide of barium being added in small quantities, care being taken to have the acid always in excess. After filtration, the solution is concentrated under the receiver of an air pump. It is (in the form of a concentrated aqueous solution) a colourless, transparent liquid, less volatile than water, of a bitter taste, having a sp. gr. 1.452, and is incompatible with many substances, as all vegetable tinctures, the citrates and tartrates of the alkalies and of iron, hydrocyanic acid, sulphate, chloride, and nitrate salts, &c.

Peroxide of hydrogen is an active oxidizing agent, and has been found highly efficacious in diabetes, in the dyspnœa of cardiac and pulmonic diseases, in promoting the blood-action of iron, and its use has also been suggested as an anti-syphilitic remedy, in gout, and in epilepsy and other diseases of irritable action of the nerve-centres. The strength of the solution should be such that the peroxide on decomposition should yield a volume of oxygen ten times as great as the volume of the solvent: dose, one to four fluidrachms three times a day.

Locally, it has been applied with advantage to ill-conditioned ulcers, especially chancres. Under the name of *Ozonic Ether*, a solution of peroxide of hydrogen in ether has been used successfully in diabetes, in doses of from ten to thirty minims, up to a drachm. It is also employed in the form of spray, as a disinfectant, and as an application to ulcerated, fetid, or sloughing surfaces; and it has been inhaled with advantage to relieve the cough of phthisis.

ORDER III.—ANTACIDS.

Antacids are medicinal agents, employed to neutralize acids in the blood, primæ viæ, and secretions. The alkalies and alkaline earths, and their carbonates, are the substances included in this division. The alkalies, in the concentrated state, destroy organization and act as corrosive poisons; they are administered internally only in a state of extreme dilution. The alkaline carbonates produce a less intense chemical action on the tissues than the alkalies; and the bicarbonates are less active than the monocarbonates. The alkaline earths, particularly magnesia, are less energetic in their local action than the alkalies proper; and their carbonates manifest little or no chemical influence over the tissues.

When swallowed in a state of dilution, the *alkaline prepara-*

tions combine with the free acids which they encounter in the stomach. The salts which are thus formed, unless carried off by the bowels, are absorbed into the blood, and are thrown out by the secretions, especially by the kidneys. While in the stomach, besides neutralizing acids, the alkalies also promote the digestion and absorption of fatty substances, by forming with them an emulsion. After absorption, they exert a liquefacient action on the blood, and render the urine alkaline. Their long-continued use disorders the functions of digestion and nutrition, produces a chronic deterioration of the blood, and sets up a cachectic condition somewhat analogous to scurvy.

In the *concentrated* form, the alkalies are employed as *escharotics*. The various alkaline preparations are administered *internally*, in the diluted form: 1. as *antacids*, in dyspepsia, accompanied with excess of acid in the primæ viæ, and they are probably also of advantage, in dyspeptic cases, by promoting the digestion of fatty matters. The neutralization of acid, in dyspepsia, by the alkaline preparations, is chiefly *palliative;* although their continued use often diminishes temporarily the tendency to acid secretion. The vegetable tonics and aromatics are frequently combined with antacids, very advantageously, in the treatment of dyspepsia. Contrary to former views, the opinion is now held that alkalies increase the secretion of the gastric juice, and in fact increase the secreting power of all glands with acid secretions; thus, while useful in morbid excess of acid in the stomach, they may be given also to promote digestion, by increasing the quantity of the gastric fluid; for this purpose, they should be given just *before* a meal. 2. As *antidotes*, in cases of poisoning from acids. 3. As *antilithics*, to neutralize lithic acid, when it is separated in undue quantity by the urine; and, also, as *lithontriptics*, or solvents of calculi, especially lithates. They are improper when there is a tendency to the deposition of phosphates; and, in treating cases of uric acid deposit, it is unnecessary to render the urine more than neutral, as, if it be made alkaline, the phosphates formed may be deposited round the uric acid calculi. 4. In the treatment of acute rheumatism and gout, where they act by neutralizing the excess of acid, with which the blood is charged in these diseases. 5. To relieve irritability of the urinary organs—ardor urinæ in gonorrhœa—cutaneous irritation—uterine irritation—pruritus ani, &c.,—when these conditions of irritability are dependent, as is often the case, on excess of acid in the system. 6. As *diuretics* (see p. 271). 7. As *antiplastics* and *resolvents*, in inflammation.

The antacid preparations should be administered in a state of large dilution, with a view to facilitate their absorption, and to prevent an irritant and purgative action on the bowels.

POTASSII PRÆPARATA—PREPARATIONS OF POTASSIUM.

The preparations of potassium, employed as antacids, are the *Solution of Potassa*, *Carbonate of Potassium*, and *Bicarbonate of Potassium*.

The general effects of the potassium preparations are those previously described. They increase both the solid and watery portions of the urine, and in large doses render it alkaline. Under their use, however, the uric acid, either free or combined is greatly diminished; the uric acid, it is asserted, is converted into oxaluric acid, which is metamorphosed into oxalic acid and urea.

LIQUOR POTASSÆ (*Solution of Potassa*), is prepared by the action of lime on a solution of bicarbonate of potassium; the lime abstracts carbonic acid from the carbonate, and precipitates as carbonate of calcium, leaving the free potassa in solution; or it may be made, more directly, by dissolving a troyounce of potassa in a pint of distilled water. Solution of potassa is a limpid, colourless liquid, without smell, of a very acrid, caustic taste, an alkaline reaction, and imparts a soapy feeling to the fingers when rubbed with it; sp. gr. 1.065; it contains five and eight-tenths per cent. of potassium hydrate (KHO).

Effects and Uses.—The antacid, diuretic, antilithic, and

resolvent properties and indications of this preparation have been deseribed above. It is more irritant to the stomach than the carbonates of potassium, and is therefore less eligible for protracted use. In excessive quantity, it may act as an irritant and corrosive poison; oils and vegetable acids should be administered as antidotes. Dose, gtt. x–xx, largely diluted with sweetened water or mucilage. *Externally*, it is used, in a diluted state, as a stimulant lotion.

Potassii Carbonas (*Carbonate of Potassium*). This salt, as usually kept in the shops, is prepared by the purification of the impure carbonate of potassium, known as *Pearlash*, which is obtained from wood-ashes, by lixiviation. Carbonate of potassium (K_2CO_3) occurs in the form of a white, coarse, granular powder, of a nauseous, alkaline taste, and an alkaline reaction,—very soluble in water, but insoluble in alcohol. It is very deliquescent, forming, if long exposed to the air, an oily liquid with the water which it attracts. Acids, acidulous salts, and many other substances are incompatible with it. It is employed as an antacid, antiplastic, diuretic, anthilithic, &c., in the dose of gr. x–xx, in some sweetened aromatic water. It has been found specially useful in torpor of the liver, and in whooping-cough. In large quantities, it acts as a corrosive poison, for which oils and vegetable acids are the antidotes.

As the *purified pearlash* of the shops is always more or less impure, a better salt for internal use is—

Potassii Carbonas Pura (*Pure Carbonate of Potassium*), commonly called *Salt of Tartar*, from its having been formerly obtained from cream of tartar. It is now made by calcining bicarbonate of potassium, which is thus deprived of its water of crystallization and an equivalent of carbonic acid, and is reduced to the state of carbonate. It differs from *purified pearlash* only in containing no impurities.

Potassii Bicarbonas (*Bicarbonate of Potassium*), is made by passing carbonic acid through an aqueous solution of carbonate of potassium, till it is fully saturated. By filtration and evaporation, it is obtained in transparent, colourless crystals, having the shape of irregular eight-sided prisms with two-sided summits ($KHCO_3$). They are inodorous, of a slightly alkaline taste, permanent in the air, soluble in water and insoluble in alcohol. The *effects and uses* of this salt are the same as those of the carbonate, but it is pleasanter in taste and less irritant to the stomach.. It is much used in gout and uric acid lithiasis. Dose, ℈j to ʒj. It is considered the best remedy in acute rheumatism, in which as much as an ounce to an ounce and a half may be given during the day, with opium to relieve pain.

SODII PRÆPARATA—PREPARATIONS OF SODIUM.

The sodium preparations are analogous in effect to those of potassium. Being less irritant and less depressing, they are better anti-dyspeptics, and for the relief of acidity of the primæ viæ. They are inferior in gout and uric acid lithiasis, as they are less powerful solvents of this acid. Their eliminative action as diuretics is also more feeble.

LIQUOR SODÆ (*Solution of Soda*), is prepared by the action of lime on a solution of carbonate of sodium. It is a colourless liquid, having an extremely acrid taste, and a strong alkaline reaction. It has sp. gr. 1.071, and contains five and seven-tenths per cent. of sodium hydrate (NaHo). The dose and administration are the same as those of liquor potassæ.

The preparations of sodium, generally employed as antacids, are the *Carbonates*. There are several sources of carbonated sodium. The native carbonate (called *Natron*), is found in Egypt, Hungary, and other countries. Impure soda, obtained from the ashes of marine plants, is termed *Barilla* or *Kelp*,—barilla, when it is derived from phenogamous plants growing near the sea, and kelp, when procured from cryptogamic plants growing in the sea. Carbonate of sodium is now, however, chiefly made by artificial means, from sulphate of sodium, which is obtained in part from the manufacturers of chlorinated lime, but principally by the action of sulphuric acid on chloride of sodium. The sulphate of sodium is fused with ground limestone and coal, and forms a black mass called

British Barilla, which contains a mixture of carbonate of sodium and sulphide of calcium:—$Na_2SO_4+C_4+CaCO_3=CaS+Na_2CO_3+4CO$. It is afterwards purified by lixiviation, calcination, and other processes. Within a few years past, caustic soda and the carbonates and other salts of sodium have been manufactured near Pittsburgh, in Pennsylvania, from *Cryolite* (a fluoride of sodium and aluminium) ($3NaF,AlF_3$), which is found in an immense deposit in Greenland, and largely imported into Philadelphia. Soda is obtained from cryolite by mixing it with lime and subjecting it to heat; the fluorine combines with the calcium, forming fluoride of calcium, while the remaining metals take the oxygen of the lime and also absorb it from the air, and become alumina and soda, carbonic acid being afterwards passed through the solution, to form carbonate of sodium, the insoluble alumina being deposited. Another new and cheap process of manufacturing soda has lately been introduced, termed the ammonia process, in which sodium chloride is converted directly into sodium carbonate by the use of ammonium carbonate; the ammonium chloride formed is decomposed by calcium hydrate, and the ammonia is again converted into carbonate by the excess of carbonic acid, obtained by heating the sodium carbonate. Recently, too, sodium carbonate has been found in large amount in a lake in Nevada.

SODII CARBONAS (*Carbonate of Sodium*), crystallizes in large, oblique, rhombic prisms (Na_2CO_3), which are transparent, very efflorescent, of an alkaline, disagreeable taste, soluble in water, but insoluble in alcohol. When heated, they undergo the watery fusion, and part with their water of crystallization, which is entirely expelled at a red heat. Perfect crystals have ten equivalents of water of crystallization. It is apt to contain sulphate of sodium and common salt as impurities. Acids, acidulous salts, lime-solution, earthy and metallic salts, &c., are incompatible with carbonate of sodium.

Effects and Uses.—Carbonate of sodium is less irritant, and has a milder and more agreeable taste, than carbonate of potassium. Its effects are otherwise similar, and it is administered in the same cases. In overdoses, it is a corrosive poison, for which oils and acids are the *antidotes*. Dose, gr. x to ʒss, in powder, or dissolved in some bitter infusion. Owing to the variable quantity of water of crystallization which it contains, as kept in the shops, it is best given in the *dried* state.

SODII CARBONAS EXSICCATA (*Dried Carbonate of Sodium*). This salt is deprived of its water of crystallization by heat, and occurs in the form of a white powder. Dose, gr. v–xv, in pill, made with soap and aromatics.

SODII BICARBONAS (*Bicarbonate of Sodium*), is prepared by saturating the carbonate with carbonic acid. In the process followed in this country, the water contained in the carbonate, which is liberated during the process of its saturation, is drained off. Thus obtained, the crystals have the form of the carbonate, retaining only one equivalent of water, but are opaque and porous. They usually occur in granular masses, or in the form of a white, opaque powder, which contains variable amounts of soda, not fully saturated with carbonic acid, and is known as SODII BICARBONAS VENALIS (*Commercial Bicarbonate of Sodium*). This is purified for medicinal use by the percolation of 64 troyounces with 6 pints of distilled water, and the purified salt occurs as a snow-white powder, soluble in 13 parts of water, of a mild, slightly alkaline taste. It is a permanent salt ($NaHCO_3$). By exposure to heat, it gradually parts with its carbonic acid, and at a red heat is converted into the anhydrous carbonate.

The *effects and uses* of this salt are the same as those of the carbonate, but it is less irritant and of a more agreeable taste. It has been used as a liquefacient, in infantile croup, in the dose of gr. j, every five minutes, to promote the expulsion of false membrane. Dose, for an adult, gr. x to ʒss, which may be pleasantly taken in carbonic acid water, or made into *lozenges* with sugar and mucilage of tragacanth. *Soda Powders* (*Pulveres Effervescentes—Effervescing Powders*), consist of tartaric acid (gr. xxv) in one paper, and bicarbonate of sodium (gr. xxx) in another. They are dissolved in separate portions of water, to the amount of half a pint in all, and, when mixed, form a pleasant *effervescing* draught. Bicarbonate of sodium is an ingredient also of *Seidlitz Powders* (see p. 246). *Troches* of bicarbonate of sodium are made by mixing 3 troyounces of bicarbonate of sodium with 9 troyounces of sugar, and 60 grains of nutmeg, and making a mass with mucilage of tragacanth, to be divided into 480 troches, each containing 3 grains of bicarbonate. Equal parts of bicarbonate of sodium and common salt make a good application to the bites of bees, hornets, spiders, &c.

SODII SILICAS (*Silicate of Sodium*), (*Soluble Glass*), is prepared by fusing silica with carbonate of sodium, dissolving in boiling water, and filtering; the solution, on cooling, drops crystals of the salt. Although not officinal, it has been used with advantage, to eliminate uric acid, in gout, &c., in doses of 10 to 15 grains, 2 or 3 times a day, dissolved in water. A solution of 5 grains in 2 fluidounces of water is a good injection in gonorrhœa. In solution of syrupy consistence, it is applied to bandages for the preparation of immovable dressings. *Silicate of Potassium* is also employed for the same therapeutic uses.

LITHII PRÆPARATA—PREPARATIONS OF LITHIUM.

Lithia is found in several minerals, as lepidolite, &c., but in minute amount. It is extracted chiefly by the agency of hydrochloric acid, and from the chloride, the CARBONATE (*Lithii Carbonas*) (L_2CO_3) is prepared by the addition of carbonate of ammonium. It is a white powder, of a mild alkaline taste, soluble in 100 parts of water, more soluble in carbonic acid water, and insoluble in alcohol.

It is a very valuable antacid in gout, from the fact of its low combining number, and the great solubility of the urate of lithium, thus enabling the carbonate to act powerfully in eliminating uric acid from the system. It probably diminishes also the formation of uric acid, and the author has found it highly efficacious in the cure of gout. It is a good diuretic. Dose, 3 to 5 grains, 2 or 3 times daily, largely diluted, and best given in carbonic acid water.

Lithii Citras (*Citrate of Lithium*) ($L_3C_6H_5O_7$), a deliquescent white powder, soluble in 25 parts of water, is made by adding a solution of citric acid to the carbonate of lithium. It is converted into a carbonate in the system, and is, therefore, possessed of the same properties, but is more refrigerant. Strong solutions of lithium salts have been found useful externally in removing gouty enlargements.

AMMONII PRÆPARATA—PREPARATIONS OF AMMONIUM.

The preparations of ammonium (previously noticed under the head of *Stimulants*, p. 188), are administered as *antacids*, in cases in which a *stimulant* action is not objectionable. *Spiritus Ammoniæ Aromaticus* (*Aromatic Spirit of Ammonia*), is the preparation usually employed, and is an excellent antacid carminative in heartburn, attended with flatulence, nausea with syncope, &c. Dose, gtt. xxx–f℥j.

MAGNESII PRÆPARATA—PREPARATIONS OF MAGNESIUM.

Magnesia (p. 241), and its *Carbonate* (p. 242), are employed as antacids in dyspepsia, sick-headache, gravel, &c., particularly where a laxative effect is also desirable. Dose, gr. x–xxx. *Troches of Magnesia* are made by mixing 3 troyounces of magnesia, 60 grains of nutmeg, and 9 troyounces of sugar, and forming with mucilage of tragacanth a mass, to be divided into 480 troches, each containing 3 grains of magnesia.

CALCII PRÆPARATA—PREPARATIONS OF CALCIUM.

The preparations of calcium, employed as antacids, are *Lime-solution*, *Precipitated Carbonate of Calcium*, *Prepared Chalk*, and *Prepared Oyster-shell*. They are very useful in cases of acidity or irritability of the stomach, but their action on the bowels is the reverse of that of magnesia, and hence they can hardly be administered where there is a tendency to constipation. They are also much employed in diarrhœa, and occasionally as alterative resolvents in glandular enlargements, as antispasmodics in nervous disorders, and to relieve irritability of the bladder from calculus.

LIQUOR CALCIS (*Solution of Lime—Lime-water*), is a saturated solution of lime (four troyounces) in distilled, river, or rain water (eight pints). It is a colourless, inodorous liquid, of a disagreeable, alkaline taste, containing about 16 grains of calcium hydrate (Ca2HO) or 12 grains of lime (CaO) in a pint of water. By exposure to the air it gradually absorbs carbonic acid, with the formation of insoluble carbonate of calcium. It should, therefore, be kept in full, well-stoppered bottles, or they should contain some undissolved lime.

Effects and Uses.—Lime-solution combines antacid and astringent properties, and is applicable to all the cases in which antacids are proper, where an astringent effect on the bowels is not objectionable. It is an excellent remedy in gastric irritability, attended with nausea and vomiting, and may be given mixed with an equal part of milk, which disguises its unpleasant taste. A diet of milk and lime-solution is very useful in dyspepsia, accompanied with vomiting of food. Lime-solution is employed also in diarrhœa, after inflammation has been subdued, in diabetes, and as an alterative resolvent in glandular affections. *Externally*, it is used as a wash in tinea capitis, prurigo, scabies, &c., as an application to foul ulcers, and as an injection in leucorrhœa and gleet; atomized inhalations of lime-solution have been found useful in diphtheria and membranous croup. Dose, internally, f℥ss to f℥iij–iv, several times a day; for children, f℥j. *Linimentum Calcis* (*Lime Liniment*), (eight fluidounces of lime-solution, mixed with seven troyounces of flaxseed oil, sometimes called *Carron Oil*), is an invaluable liniment in burns and scalds, and in small-pox.

CALCII CARBONAS PRÆCIPITATA (*Precipitated Carbonate of Calcium*) ($CaCO_3$), is made by mixing boiling solutions of chloride of calcium and carbonate of sodium. It is a fine white powder, insoluble in water, and free from grittiness, but possessing no superiority over *Prepared Chalk*.

CRETA PRÆPARATA (*Prepared Chalk*) ($CaCO_3$), is made from *chalk* or *whiting*, by levigation and elutriation. It occurs in little white conical loaves, which are tasteless, odourless, insoluble in water, but more soluble in carbonic acid water. Its *effects* are those of an absorbent, antacid, and desiccant astringent. It is *used* in dyspepsia and gout, attended with an excess of acid in the system; also in diarrhœa; and, as it forms soluble salts of calcium with the acids of the stomach, its employment has been suggested in rachitis. Dose, gr. x–xxx, in powder, or suspended in water with gum and sugar. *Mistura Cretæ* (*Chalk Mixture*), consists of prepared chalk (half a troyounce), rubbed up with gum Arabic (120 grains), and water (4 fluidounces), and afterwards mixed with glycerin (half a fluidounce), and cinnamon water (4 fluidounces); dose, f℥ss, repeated. Laudanum, and tincture of kino or of catechu, and aromatics, are often added to this mixture, in the treatment of diarrhœa. *Troches of Chalk* are made by mixing 4 troyounces of prepared chalk, a troyounce of gum arabic, 60 grains of nutmeg, and 6 troyounces of sugar, and forming with water a mass, to be divided into 480 troches, each containing 4 grains of prepared chalk.

TESTA PRÆPARATA (*Prepared Oyster-shell*), is the powdered shell of Ostrea edulis, or common oyster, washed with warm water, and afterwards prepared as the last article; it differs from prepared chalk, in containing animal matter united with the carbonate of calcium, and is thought to be more acceptable to a delicate stomach. Dose, gr. x–xxx.

CLASS IV.—TOPICAL MEDICINES.

ORDER I.—IRRITANTS.

Irritants are medicines which are employed to produce irritation or inflammation of the parts to which they are applied. They may be subdivided into RUBEFACIENTS, EPISPASTICS,

SUPPURANTS, and ESCHAROTICS. *Rubefacients* are used merely to produce redness of the skin. *Epispastics*, or *Vesicants*, cause the exhalation of a serous fluid under the cuticle. *Suppurants* produce a crop of pustules. *Escharotics* have a chemical action on the tissues with which they are placed in contact, and decompose or destroy them.

RUBEFACIENTS.

Rubefacients are employed to remove congestion and inflammation, to rouse the capillary system in cases of local torpor, to relieve pain and spasm, and as stimulants to the general system, in coma, syncope, asphyxia, &c. They are adapted to cases in which a sudden and powerful, but transient, action is called for; but they may also be employed where a slight and long-continued action is desired. In removing congestion and inflammation, rubefacients act by stimulating the capillary vessels of inflamed parts and thereby restoring their tone and elasticity. They are chiefly useful in the forming stages or in light grades of inflammation. They are very serviceable local anodynes, when applied to painful parts—acting by a *substitutive* influence. As general stimulants, their efficacy in rousing the system depends partly on their action on the capillary circulation, and partly on the pain which they produce. They are most valuable in the coma or asphyxia, resulting from poisons, drowning, &c., and are inferior to blisters in the cerebral oppression, which occurs in fevers, inflammations of the brain, &c.

Rubefacients are usually applied till pain and redness supervene. If kept too long on the skin, many of them will produce vesication and even gangrene; and, in cases of coma, particular caution is required, as the patient may not feel them till dangerous inflammation has occurred.

SINAPIS—MUSTARD.

MUSTARD-SEEDS are obtained from two varieties of Sinapis, —S. Nigra, or Black Mustard, and S. Alba, or White Mustard (*Nat. Ord.* Brassicaceæ), small annual European plants, cultivated in our gardens. S. Nigra has become naturalized in some parts of the United States. *Black Mustard-seeds* are small, globular, of a deep-brown colour externally, and internally yellow. They are inodorous, except in powder; and, when rubbed with water, exhale a very strong, pungent smell. Their taste is bitterish, hot, and pungent. *White Mustard-seeds* are larger, yellowish externally, and of a less pungent taste, owing to the presence of a mucilaginous substance in their skin. The *powder* of both varieties (commonly called *Flour of Mustard*) is yellow, and is often adulterated with coloured wheaten flour. Both varieties yield their virtues wholly to *water*, and very slightly to alcohol.

Chemical Constituents.—Mustard-seeds yield, upon pressure, a fixed saponifiable oil, which contains oleic acid and a peculiar acid, termed *erucic* ($HC_{22}H_{41}O_2$). From the *black seeds* a very pungent *volatile oil*, containing sulphur, is afterwards obtained by distillation: *it does not pre-exist in the seeds, but is the result of the action of water upon a peculiar principle called Myronate of Potassium.* It is a sulphocyanide of allyl (C_3H_5CyS), is colourless or pale-yellow, rather heavier than water, of a very pungent odour, and an acrid, burning taste, and is the principle to which the black seeds owe their activity. From the *white seeds* no volatile oil is obtained; but, when treated with water, they yield an *acrid fixed principle*, which is analogous in properties to the volatile oil of the black seeds. *It is the result of the reaction of water upon sinalbin* ($C_{30}H_{44}N_2S_2O_{16}$), a peculiar ingredient of the white seeds. The development of the volatile oil in the black seeds, and of the acrid fixed principle in the white seeds, is supposed to depend upon the presence of an albuminous constituent, called *Myrosyne*, which acts the part of a ferment in determining a reaction between water and the peculiar principles of the seeds. Myrosyne is rendered inert by heat, alcohol, and the acids; and water, of the ordinary temperature, is therefore the proper menstruum of mustard.

Effects and Uses—Mustard is an acrid stimulant. In small quantities it is stomachic; in larger doses, it proves emetic; and, in excessive doses, it will produce gastro-enteric inflammation. When applied to the skin, it is a rapid and powerful local excitant, speedily producing redness and pain, and, if long continued, it will develop vesication, ulceration, and even sphacelus. Mustard-seeds, swallowed whole, have been used as a laxative in dyspepsia, in the dose of a tablespoonful once or twice a day, mixed with molasses—the white seeds are preferred; the practice is, however, of doubtful value, as they may become entangled in the appendicula vermiformis. When mustard is employed *internally*, however, it is chiefly as an emetic, in cases of torpor of the stomach, particularly after narcotic poisoning; and, by its stimulant action, mustard often rouses the gastric susceptibility when other emetics fail. Dose, as an emetic, from a large teaspoonful to a tablespoonful of the bruised seeds or powder. Its use in smaller quantity, as a condiment and stimulant of the digestive organs, is well known. In the form of *whey* (half a troyounce boiled in milk Oj), it is given as a diuretic in dropsy. The most general use of mustard is, however, as a cutaneous stimulant, in the form of *cataplasm* (termed a *sinapism*). This is made by mixing flour of mustard with a sufficient quantity of tepid water to give it proper consistence; and it may be diluted with wheat or rye flour, if a weaker effect is desired. Sinapisms are used, when a speedy and powerful rubefacient effect is required: they should be kept on till pain and redness are produced, usually from a quarter of an hour to an hour, and, in cases of insensibility, their effects should be carefully watched. They are applied spread on linen, and covered with gauze, to prevent adhesion to the skin. Mustard is the most active and at the same time the most easily controlled of the rubefacients; a mild but permanent effect may be kept up by the addition of a teaspoonful to a tablespoonful of mustard to a poultice of Indian meal or flaxseed, with a tablespoonful or two of capsicum.

For ready use, there is now kept in the shops *Charta Sinapis* (*Mustard Paper*), which is prepared by mixing 90 grains of black mustard (in powder), with enough solution of gutta-percha to give it a semi-liquid consistence, and then applying the mixture by a brush to a piece of stiff paper, 4 inches square; before being applied to the skin, it should be dipped for about 15 seconds in warm water.

CAPSICUM.

CAPSICUM has been previously noticed as an *aromatic stimulant* (p. 192). It is an efficient rubefacient, useful in rheumatism, low fevers, &c., and is applied in the form of cataplasm, or the tincture or oleoresin may be used.

OLEUM TEREBINTHINÆ—OIL OF TURPENTINE.

The *Oil of Turpentine* (see p. 290), is a speedy and efficacious rubefacient, and sometimes produces a vesicular eruption. It is employed in low forms of disease, attended with coldness of the surface; as a counter-irritant in inflammation; and as a stimulating liniment in rheumatic and paralytic cases. It is often diluted with olive oil.

LINIMENTUM AMMONIÆ—LINIMENT OF AMMONIA.

This preparation, called also *Volatile Liniment*, consists of one fluidounce of *water of ammonia* (see p. 188), and two troyounces of olive oil. It is an excellent application, as a counter-irritant, in affections of the throat and chest, &c.

PIX BURGUNDICA—BURGUNDY PITCH.

This is the prepared RESINOUS EXUDATION from Abies excelsa or Norway Spruce (*Nat. Ord.* Pinaceæ), a lofty evergreen tree of Europe and Northern Asia. Abies picea, or the European Silver Fir, is said to be also a source of the drug. It is obtained by stripping off the bark, and detaching the flakes of resinous matter which form upon the surface of the wound; they are afterwards melted in boiling water and strained. *Burgundy Pitch* is principally collected in Germany and France, and derives its name from Burgundy, in the latter kingdom. After it is imported into the United States, it is generally re-melted and strained, to free it from impurities; and, as found in the shops, it is a hard, brittle, opaque substance, of a yellowish or brownish-yellow colour, and a weak terebinthinate taste and smell; when applied to the body, it softens and becomes adhesive. It contains two resins, and a much smaller proportion of volatile oil than turpentine.

A *spurious Burgundy Pitch* is made by melting together pitch, resin, and turpentine, and agitating the mixture with water.

Effects and Uses.—This is a gentle rubefacient, producing a slight degree of inflammation and serous effusion, without separating the cuticle. It occasionally produces a papillary or vesicular eruption; and, sometimes, though rarely, occasions painful vesication and even ulceration. It is applied in the form of *plaster* to the chest in chronic and sub-acute pulmonary disorders, to the loins in lumbago, to the joints in chronic articular affections, and for the relief of local rheumatic pains in other parts.

Emplastrum Picis Burgundicæ (*Burgundy Pitch Plaster*), consists of twelve parts of Burgundy Pitch, melted with one part of yellow wax, which is used to give consistence to the pitch. *Emplastrum Picis cum Cantharide* (*Plaster of Pitch with Cantharides*), consists of twelve parts of Burgundy Pitch, melted with one part of cerate of cantharides; this is commonly called the *Warming Plaster*, and is a more active rubefacient than Burgundy Pitch, though it does not usually blister. The *Plaster of Antimony*, *Plaster of Iron*, *Compound Galbanum Plaster*, and *Opium Plaster*, all contain Burgundy Pitch.

PIX CANADENSIS—CANADA PITCH.

This is the prepared RESINOUS EXUDATION from Abies Canadensis, or Hemlock Spruce (*Nat. Ord.* Pinaceæ), a very lofty evergreen tree of Canada and the northern parts of the United States. The pitch (sometimes called *Hemlock Gum*), is a spontaneous exudation on the old trees. The portions of bark upon which it hardens are stripped from the tree and boiled, and the melted pitch is skimmed from the surface of the water. It undergoes a further purification in the shops, by melting and straining, and is found in hard, brittle, opaque masses, of a dark yellowish-brown colour, a weak, peculiar odour, and scarcely any taste. It is more readily softened by heat than Burgundy Pitch, and is therefore sometimes a less convenient application. Its constituents are resin, and a minute portion of volatile oil. Its *effects* and *uses* are the same as those of Burgundy Pitch.

Emplastrum Picis Canadensis (*Plaster of Canada Pitch*), sometimes called *Hemlock Pitch Plaster*, consists of twelve parts of Canada Pitch, melted with one part of yellow wax.

Many other acrid substances are occasionally employed as *rubefacients.* GINGER (see p. 197), BLACK PEPPER (see p. 193), and GARLIC (see p. 287), are particularly deserving of mention. A gentle counter-irritant, often used to the epigastric region, to relieve vomiting, is the *Spice Plaster*, which is made by mixing two ounces of powdered ginger with an ounce of powdered cloves and cinnamon, each, and two drachms of capsicum, adding half a fluidounce of tincture of ginger, and honey enough for proper consistence.

EPISPASTICS.

Epispastics, called also *Vesicants* and *Blisters*, are medicines which, when applied to the skin, produce inflammation, accompanied by effusion of serum beneath the cuticle. Many of the rubefacients will blister, if kept on the skin a sufficient length of time; and, on the other hand, the action of vesicants may be made not to extend beyond rubefaction. The inflammation of the skin, caused by vesicants, is erysipelatous in its character, and may result in suppuration and even sloughing or gangrene. In inflammation of the dermoid tissues, as rubeola and scarlatina, in typhus under certain circumstances, and in extreme infancy,—vesicants may produce fatal consequences.

This class of agents is employed: 1. As *local* stimulants, in the cure of internal inflammations; different explanations have been offered of the antiphlogistic influence of blisters, some therapeutists ascribing it to a *derivative* or *revellent* action, by determining vascular and nervous energy to the seat of their operation, but it is more probably due to a stimulant effect, extended to the capillary vessels of the inflamed organ, and experience has shown that, for the relief of internal inflammation, they cannot be applied too near the affected organ. In affections of the head, blisters are pre-eminently useful. 2. To substitute a healthy therapeutic inflammatory action, which subsides spontaneously, for a morbid action existing in the part to which they are applied. In this way vesicants are used for the cure of various cutaneous eruptions. 3. To relieve pain, which they do partly by a stimulant, and partly by a substitutive influence. 4. To break up a train of morbid associations, by the powerful impression which they make on the nervous system, as in the cure of intermittent fever, spasmodic diseases, &c. 5. To stimulate the absorbing or secreting vessels of parts contiguous to the seat of their application; in this way, they are useful in promoting the absorption of dropsical effusions, in the treatment of ununited fracture, &c. 6. As general stimulants, in typhoid conditions of the system, coma, syncope, &c. 7. As local stimulants, in threatened gangrene, paralysis, &c. 8. As evacuants, chiefly for the purpose of local depletion. 9. In retrocedent gout, and in retrocession of the exanthematous eruptions. 10. To prepare a surface for the endermic application of medicines.

CANTHARIS—CANTHARIDES.

Cantharis vesicatoria, termed also Lytta vesicatoria, the Spanish Fly, is a cylindrical insect from six to ten lines in length, by two or three in breadth, with a large cordate head, an oblong body, and elytra or wing-cases, of a beautiful, shining, golden-green colour. It is found most abundantly in Spain, Italy, and the south of France, but occurs in all the temperate parts of Europe, and in Western Asia. The Spanish flies swarm on certain trees and shrubs, and may be detected at a considerable distance by their strong, fetid odour, which resembles that of mice. They make their appearance in May and June, and are collected in these months by persons protected by masks and gauntlets, who beat or shake them from the trees on which they lodge, and receive them, as they fall, upon linen cloths spread underneath. They are plunged into hot vinegar and water, or exposed to the vapour of boiling vinegar, and are afterwards dried in the sun or by drying stoves. When perfectly dry, they are packed in canisters, which are carefully closed so as to exclude atmospheric moisture. They are usually imported into this country from some Mediterranean port. A highly esteemed variety comes from South Russia, through St. Petersburg, which is distinguished by the larger size and copper colour of the flies.

In the *dried* state, cantharides retain their form, colour, odour, &c.; their taste is acrid, burning, and urinous; their powder is of a grayish-brown colour, interspersed with shining green particles. If exposed to moisture, they are soon decomposed, most speedily when powdered. As, moreover, the powder is liable to adulterations, they should always be purchased whole, and should be powdered as they are wanted for use. They are liable to be attacked by mites, which destroy the interior soft parts: the best mode of preserving them is to expose them, in bottles, to the heat of boiling water, which destroys the eggs of the insect. A little camphor or carbonate of ammonium, or a few drops of strong acetic acid or of chloroform, added to the flies, are also recommended as preservatives.

The most important *constituents* of cantharides are a volatile oil, upon which the odour depends, and a white micaceous, crystalline substance, termed *cantharidin*, which is the vesicating principle. Cantharidin is inodorous, tasteless, soluble in ether, chloroform, the oils, acetic acid, and boiling alcohol, and insoluble in water and cold alcohol; but, notwithstanding this *insolubility* of cantharidin, watery and alcoholic solutions of cantharides possess the medicinal properties of the insect,—the cantharidin being rendered soluble by combination with a yellow colouring matter in the insect. *Cantharidin* ($C_5H_6O_2$), by the aid of heat, in the presence of water, may be made to combine with the alkalies, the cantharidin becoming converted into cantharidic acid ($H_2C_5H_6O_2$). The cantharidate of potassium has been employed as a blistering agent.

Physiological Effects.—Cantharides are an acrid stimulant. Taken internally, in small doses, they excite the secretion of the kidneys, and sometimes produce more or less irritation of the genito-urinary passages, evinced by strangury, priapism, pain, and occasionally the discharge of bloody urine. In large doses, they produce violent gastro-enteric and genito-urinary inflammation; and, in excessive doses, prove fatal, with convulsions, tetanus, delirium, and other cerebro-spinal symptoms. Twenty-four grains have occasioned death. In cases of poisoning, after the stomach has been emptied, opiates, demulcents, and stimulants are to be resorted to; but oils are to be avoided. *Applied to the skin*, cantharides produce inflammation, which terminates in the secretion of serum under the cuticle. Even when they are externally applied, their constitutional effects, as strangury, tenesmus, &c., are frequently manifested.

Medicinal Uses.—The indications which cantharides are capable of fulfilling, when administered *internally*, as a diuretic, emmenagogue, &c., have been already noticed (see *tincture*, p. 282). Their chief use is as an *external application*, to produce *blisters;* but they are sometimes also employed externally, as *rubefacients*, for the purpose of local or general stimulation in low forms of disease. Cantharides are preferred to all other substances as *epispastics*, and they are used for all the medicinal purposes, that are within the range of this class of medicines.

The following are the forms under which Spanish flies are used *externally:*

Ceratum Cantharidis (*Cantharides Cerate*), commonly known as *Blistering Cerate*, is made by mixing powdered cantharides (twelve parts) with melted wax and resin (each seven parts), and lard (ten parts). This is the preparation usually employed to raise a blister. It can be applied without the aid of heat, and should be spread on soft leather or linen or adhesive plaster, and covered with gauze or unsized paper. From four to twelve hours is the period for which the cerate should be applied—on the scalp a longer application may be required. For an ordinary impression, and where the cutaneous sensibility is not impaired by disease, it need not be kept on more than four or five hours. In cases of children, less time is required for the application of the cerate, and great caution is necessary in applying it to infants. A poultice of bread and milk or flaxseed meal should be afterwards applied, which usually produces vesication, if the action of the blister has not extended beyond rubefaction. If it be desirable to heal the blistered surface immediately, cotton wadding or cerate may be placed over it, after the serum has been allowed to escape. To maintain the discharge, the cuticle should be removed, and basilicon ointment applied; if the surface require further irritation, the ointments of savine, mezereon, or cantharides may be used. The open or perpetual blister is, however, not required for ordinary antiphlogistic purposes; and, indeed, as a general rule, the blistered surface should be allowed to heal as speedily as possible. In case of excessive pain, a poultice of bread-crumb and lead water, with grain $\frac{1}{4}$ of sulphate of morphia mixed in it, or a starch poultice, or lime liniment is a soothing application. *Goulard's Cerate* is an excellent application to heal obstinate ulcers from blisters. For the relief of *strangury*, diluents and diuretics are proper, as flaxseed tea, with sweet spirit of nitre, decoction of uva ursi, &c., and an opium or morphia suppository, if the symptoms are severe. *Ceratum Extracti Cantharidis* (*Cerate of Extract of Cantharides*), differs chiefly from the common cerate in being made with an alcoholic extract of the flies instead of the flies themselves; it is a new preparation, and is said to be more active than the old. To prepare it, 5 troyounces of cantharides are to be percolated to exhaustion with stronger alcohol, evaporated to the consistence of a soft extract, and mixed with 3 troyounces of resin, 6 troyounces of yellow wax, and 7 troyounces of lard (melted together). *Ethereal*, *alcoholic*, *hydro-alcoholic*, and *watery extracts* of Spanish flies have been suggested as substitutes for the *blistering cerate*, and, mixed with wax and spread on thin cloth or paper, are termed *vesicating taffetas*. *Unguentum Cantharidis* (*Ointment of Cantharides*), is made by mixing 120 grains of cantharides cerate with 360 grains of resin cerate; it is employed as a stimulating dressing to blistered surfaces, or to produce vesication on delicate skins. *Linimentum Cantharidis* (*Liniment of Cantharides*), consists of a troyounce of cantharides dissolved in eight fluidounces of oil of turpentine; it is a prompt stimulating liniment in low fevers, and may be applied to the skin to prepare it for the action of the blistering cerate. *Collodium cum Cantharide* (*Collodion with Cantharides*), or *Cantharidal Collodion*, is made by percolating 8 troyounces of cantharides with stronger ether until 15 fluidounces have passed, then with stronger alcohol until half a pint more of liquid is obtained, evaporating this to a fluidounce, and mixing it with the reserved liquid; to this are to be added with agitation 100 grains of pyroxolon, 320 grains of Canada turpentine, and 160 grains of castor oil, and the solution is to be kept in a well-stopped bottle. It furnishes a very convenient mode of blistering a small irregular surface, and is applied by means of a camel's-hair brush, in successive layers, which should be covered with a piece of oiled silk. *Charta Cantharidis* (*Cantharides Paper*), is made by boiling gently a mixture of 94 troyounces of white wax, a troyounce and a half of spermaceti, 2 troyounces of olive oil, half a troyounce of Canada turpentine and cantharides each, in 5 fluidounces of water, and, after filtration, passing strips of paper over the surface of the mixture, which, when dry, are cut into rectangular strips. The cantharidal preparations are used externally to promote the growth of the hair. *Dupuytren's Pomatum* is a tincture, made with cantharides, ℨi, and alcohol, f℥i, incorporated with nine parts of lard.

CANTHARIS VITTATA—POTATO FLIES.

Several species of Cantharis are found in the United States, and are good substitutes for C. vesicatoria. C. vittata, or the *Potato Fly* is most used. It resembles the Spanish Fly in shape, but is rather smaller, being about six lines in length, with black elytra or wing-cases, and inhabits chiefly the potato plant. It contains *cantharidin.*

AQUA AMMONIÆ—WATER OF AMMONIA.

Stronger *Water of Ammonia* (see p. 188) may be used for the purpose of speedy vesication. Five parts of this, mixed with spirit of camphor, two parts, and spirit of rosemary, one part, has been used as a prompt vesicant, under the name of *Granville's Lotion.* A piece of flannel, saturated with the liniment, is applied to the skin, which it will generally blister in from three to ten minutes. *Gondret's Vesicating Ointment* is made by melting together 2 parts of expressed oil of almond and 32 parts of lard, and adding to this mixture 17 parts of stronger water of ammonia; it will vesicate in ten minutes. Ammonia is applied locally as an antidote to the poison of venomous reptiles and insects.

SUPPURANTS.

OLEUM TIGLII—CROTON OIL.

Croton Oil (see p. 262), when rubbed on the skin, produces rubefaction, accompanied by a pustular eruption. It is an excellent application to the throat and chest, in subacute or chronic laryngeal and bronchial affections, and to rheumatic joints. It may be applied undiluted, or mixed with one, two, or three parts of olive oil or oil of turpentine, according to the susceptibility of the skin.

UNGUENTUM ANTIMONII—ANTIMONIAL OINTMENT.

This ointment consists of one part of tartrate of antimony and potassium mixed with four parts of lard. The peculiar eruptive effects of tartar emetic have been already noticed (p. 211). It may be used in the form of ointment or solution, in the same cases as croton oil, but it is a more painful and permanent application.

ESCHAROTICS.

ESCHAROTICS (from εσχαρα, *an eschar*), called also *Cauterants*, are medicines which destroy the structure and vitality of the parts to which they are applied. The *eschar*, which their application produces, is followed by inflammation and suppuration in the surrounding tissues, by which the slough is separated from the living parts.

They are employed: 1. to effect the destruction of morbid growths, warts, condylomata, polypi, fungous granulations, &c. 2. To decompose the virus of rabid and venomous animals, and of chancres and malignant pustules, and to prevent their absorption. 3. For the cure of violent inflammation, by their *substitutive* action, as when they are applied to the mucous or cutaneous surfaces, in gonorrhœal ophthalmia, erysipelas, poisoned parts, carbuncles, &c. 4. To stimulate indolent sinuses, ulcers, &c., where there influence is also of a *substitutive* character. 5. To open abscesses; though for the opening of abscesses of internal viscera, as of the liver, the recently introduced method of *aspiration* is to be preferred. 6. To form issues. 7. To remove morbid heterologous growths, as lupus, cancer, &c.

ARGENTI NITRAS FUSA—FUSED NITRATE OF SILVER.

Lunar Caustic (described at length, p. 154), is the most commonly employed of the caustics. It has the advantage of not liquefying when applied, and its action is therefore confined to the parts with which it is brought in contact. It is used to remove fungous granulations in wounds and ulcers, to destroy warts, to decompose and prevent the absorption of the syphilitic virus in chancres, to alter the action of indolent ulcers, sinuses, and fistulæ, to subdue the inflammatory action of paronychia, erythema, &c., to arrest the progress of erysipelas and cancrum oris, to cut short variolous pustules, to cure skin diseases by a substitutive action, and in inflammations of mucous membranes. In dilutions of various strengths, it is resorted to in every variety of inflammation of the mucous membranes; when a full impression is desired, a solution of gr. xx–xxx in distilled water f℥j, may be employed; for ordinary purposes, gr. ij to water f℥j.

POTASSA.

Caustic Potassa is prepared by the rapid evaporation of *Solution of Potassa* (see p. 347) with heat. While in the state of fusion, it is received into cylindrical iron moulds, and it occurs in the form of sticks, of a brownish, grayish, or bluish colour, a fibrous fracture, the odour of slaking lime, and a caustic, urinous taste. It dissolves in alcohol, and in less than its weight of water, and attracts both moisture and carbonic acid rapidly from the air. It is more or less impure as found in the shops. By digestion in alcohol, it is freed from impurities insoluble in this menstruum (as the carbonates of potassium), and it may be afterwards obtained quite white and pure by evaporation; it is then termed *Alcoholic Potassa.* The potassa of the shops is a *hydrate*, consisting of one equivalent of water and one of potassa.

Effects and Uses.—It is the most powerful known escharotic, and differs from lunar caustic, in extending its action to a considerable depth beneath the surface to which it is applied. It is used chiefly to open abscesses and form issues, to destroy the virus of chancres, of malignant pustules, and from the bites of venomous reptiles and rabid animals, and sometimes also to arrest the sloughing of carbuncles, and, from its deep-reaching action, it is preferred to lunar caustic in these cases; applied to the cutaneous surface, in cases of phlegmon, threatened carbuncle, &c., it will sometimes avert the progress of inflammation. When it is applied to the skin, this should be covered with linen spread with adhesive plaster, having a hole the size of the spot to be cauterized. A solution (ʒjss to f℥ij of water), is used as a *rubefacient.*

Potassa cum Calce (*Potassa with Lime*), is prepared by rubbing up equal parts of potassa and lime. It is a grayish-white powder, which is sometimes made into a paste with a little alcohol, and is termed *Vienna Paste;* it has also been formed into sticks. The presence of lime renders this a milder, less deliquescent, and more manageable caustic than potassa; it is a favourite application to chancres.

SODA.

Caustic Soda is prepared by the rapid evaporation of *Solution of Soda* (see p. 349) until ebullition ceases, and the soda melts; when it has congealed, it is broken into grayish-white, opaque, brittle fragments, which are very corrosive, very soluble in water, soluble in alcohol, and deliquescent, though, unlike potassa, it does not become permanently liquid, but, after a time, effloresces. It is employed for the same cauterant purposes as potassa, than which it is somewhat milder in action. *London Paste,* made by rubbing up equal parts of soda and lime, has been used with good effect in the removal of enlarged tonsils.

ACIDUM CHROMICUM—CHROMIC ACID.

Chromic Acid (CrO_3) is obtained by the reaction of sulphuric acid upon a solution of bichromate of potassium. It is properly *chromic anhydride*, and occurs in the form of anhydrous deep-red, needleform crystals, of an acid, metallic taste; they are deliquescent, and very soluble in water, with which they form an orange-yellow solution.

Effects and Uses.—This is an *escharotic* of recent introduction into the Materia Medica. It is of unsurpassed power in this particular, decomposing the tissues by its rapid oxidizing action. Used in the form of paste, or solution more or less diluted, it is a most efficacious application to morbid growths and excrescences, as syphilitic condylomata, &c. It gives less pain than other caustics; but it is to be used with caution, especially to delicate parts like the eye, as its action is deeply penetrating. The solution may be made of the strength of from 100 grains up to a troyounce to a fluidounce of water; and is to be applied by means of a pencil or glass rod.

ACIDUM ARSENIOSUM—ARSENIOUS ACID.

This is a powerful escharotic (see p. 331), and is occasionally applied in lupus, onychia maligna, cancerous ulcers, and to change the action of indolent sinuses; but its use is attended with danger. It may be diluted with one or more parts of sulphur.

ZINCI CHLORIDUM—CHLORIDE OF ZINC.

This is also a powerful escharotic (see p. 151); and, in addition to its corrosive properties, it appears to exercise a greater influence over the vital action of neighbouring parts, than some of the other caustics. The separation of its eschar leaves very healthy and vigorous granulations, and it is one of the best applications that can be made to intractable indolent ulcers and sinuses. It will cure lupus.

LIQUOR HYDRARGYRI NITRATIS—SOLUTION OF NITRATE OF MERCURY.

This preparation (see p. 320), termed also the *acid* nitrate of mercury, is a valuable caustic application to malignant ulcers, hospital gangrene, &c.

HYDRARGYRI CHLORIDUM CORROSIVUM—CORROSIVE CHLORIDE OF MERCURY.

Corrosive Sublimate is more frequently used as a stimulant wash than as a caustic. For its properties, uses, and modes of application, see p. 315.

POTASSII BICHROMAS—BICHROMATE OF POTASSIUM.

This salt, already noticed under the head of alteratives (see p. 341), is a good caustic application, in saturated solution, or powder, to syphilitic and other vegetations.

ACIDA MINERALIA—MINERAL ACIDS.

The mineral acids (see p. 156), are powerful escharotics, but are inconvenient for many uses, on account of the extension of their action beyond the point of application. On the other hand, they can be made to reach the bottoms of sinuses and fistulæ, which are inaccessible to the solid caustics. Nitric acid, for such purposes, has no equal in the list of escharotics; it is also used to destroy warts. Properly diluted, the mineral acids are employed in injections, gargles, &c.; and in the form of ointment, in skin diseases.

SULPHATE OF COPPER (see p. 149), and ALUM (see p. 182), are mild escharotics, but are chiefly used to remove fungous granulations in ulcers. The *actual cautery* and *moxa* have been alluded to under the head of HEAT (see p. 22).

ORDER II.—DEMULCENTS.

Demulcents, or *Lenitives*, are medicines which *soften* and relax the tissues, and, when applied to irritated or inflamed surfaces, diminish heat, tension, and pain. They consist chiefly of gum, or mucilage, or of a mixture of these with saccharine and farinaceous substances, and form with water viscid solutions. Their constitutional effects are principally nutritive, though perhaps to some extent they relieve irritation in distant organs, by modifying the acridity of the secretions. Demulcent solutions are administered internally: 1. To sheathe and protect the gastro-enteric surface from the injurious effects of irritating substances—particularly acrid poisons. 2. To relieve irritation and inflammation of the alimentary canal, as in gastritis, enteritis, diarrhœa, and dysentery; and for this purpose they may be administered either by the mouth or rectum. 3. In catarrhal affections, in which they are probably useful, in part by the transmission of their lubricating and soothing effects on the fauces and œsophagus by reflex action to the laryngeal and bronchial membranes, and in part by modifying the acridity of expectorated matters. 4. In affections of the urinary passages, as ardor urinæ, cystitis, &c., and in these cases, they act chiefly by diminishing the acridity of the secretions. 5. As agreeable drinks, to quench thirst and promote the action of the secreting and exhaling organs, in febrile affections. Their effects, in these cases, are owing partly to the water which they contain, to which they are added merely for the sake of flavour, and partly also to the nutrient which they furnish. When administered with the object of increasing the proportion of the fluid parts of the blood, demulcents are termed *Diluents*. 6. As light diet for the sick. 7. For pharmaceutical purposes, to suspend substances insoluble in water, &c.

Externally, mucilaginous solutions are extensively employed, to relieve the heat, swelling, and pain of inflammations, wounds, burns, &c.; to hasten suppuration, where inflammation is too far advanced for resolution; to cleanse foul and scabby ulcers;

to promote suppuration from granulating surfaces, &c., &c. Mucilaginous and amylaceous substances are applied to inflamed and ulcerated parts, mixed with water so as to form soft masses, termed *cataplasms* or *poultices*. These are useful vehicles of heat and moisture to the skin, and are used also as local applications, in rheumatism and gout, and for the relief of internal inflammations, as when applied to the chest and abdomen in pleurisy, bronchitis, peritonitis, dysentery, &c. Applied externally, this class of medicines is termed *Emollients*.

AQUA—WATER.

Water has important medicinal as well as pharmaceutical uses. The Pharmacopœia directs it to be employed in the *purest attainable state*, which is rain or snow water: for pharmaceutical purposes, *distilled water* (*aqua destillata*), should be used. Pure water is a transparent liquid, without colour, taste, or smell; but, owing to its extensive solvent powers, in the natural state it is more or less contaminated with foreign matters. It is now considered to be a compound of 2 atoms of hydrogen and 1 of oxygen (H_2O).

Effects and Uses.—Water is necessary for the solution and digestion of our food; in either insufficient or excessive amount, it may prove injurious. Thus, without a proper supply of water, not only the absorption of soluble matters in the stomach is interfered with, but also the passage of undigested substances into the intestines, and, besides, some articles, as sugar, do not undergo the fermentation necessary for digestion. On the other hand, an excess of water, taken into the stomach, impairs digestion by overdilution of the gastric juice, and will occasion the acetous fermentation of saccharine articles. Water is eliminated from the system by the intestines, skin, and lungs, but chiefly by the kidneys; and it is believed, in large amounts, to increase not only the water but the solid constituents of the urine, hence its use as a diuretic. As it promotes both the metamorphosis and construction of tissue, it may produce a valuable alterative effect in morbid taints of the system and prove a useful adjunct to more active eliminative agents. Water is the basis of all drinks administered to relieve the thirst of fever, and moderate the undue viscidity of the blood which is present in inflammation; it must not be permitted in excess, however, as undue amounts may produce nausea, flatulence, and even vomiting and diarrhœa. The uses of water, as an external agent, have been noticed under the head of *heat* and *cold.*

Aqua Acidi Carbonici (*Carbonic Acid Water*) (H_2CO_3). Water impregnated with a quantity of *carbonic acid*, equal to five times the bulk of the water (which may be obtained from bicarbonate of sodium or from marble, by means of diluted sulphuric acid), often proves useful in allaying nausea and vomiting, and is also a good vehicle for some of the neutral purgative salts, which are of unpleasant taste.

ACACIA—GUM ARABIC.

Gum Arabic is a *gummy exudation* from Acacia vera, Acacia Arabica, and other species of Acacia (*Nat. Ord* Fabaceæ), thorny or prickly trees or shrubs of Africa and Arabia. The gum exudes, either through natural cracks in the bark, or through incisions made to facilitate its exudation, and hardens on exposure. The most abundant yield is in the hot and dry weather, and is obtained from the sickliest trees. Several commercial varieties are known, as Turkey, Barbary, Senegal, India, &c., of which the two most important are Turkey gum, and Senegal gum. 1. *Turkey gum* comes from the Levant or other parts of the Mediterranean, and is the kind usually found in the shops. It consists chiefly of small, irregular fragments, interspersed with larger pieces, of a whitish colour, which is sometimes slightly tinged with yellow or reddish-yellow. It is lighter-coloured, more brittle, more readily soluble, and purer than other varieties, and is generally characterized by innumerable minute fissures pervading its substance. 2. *Senegal gum* comes from the western coast of Africa. It occurs in roundish or oval unbroken pieces, larger, less brittle, and breaking with a more conchoidal fracture than those of Turkey gum, sometimes whitish, but generally yellowish, reddish, or brownish-red. 3. *Barbary gum* comes from Morocco; it is derived, in part at least, from A. gummifera, and consists of two kinds, one resembling the Turkey, the other the Senegal gum. 4. *India gum*, though brought from India, is collected on the north-eastern coast of Africa, and in the ports of the Red Sea. It is in pieces of varying size, colour, and quality, and is often contaminated with Bassora gum, which is insoluble in water. Gum is also imported into England from the Cape of Good Hope, and from Australia. All the varieties are more or less transparent, hard, brittle, and pulverizable, and form a white powder. They are inodorous, with a feeble, slightly sweetish taste, and, when pure, dissolve wholly in the mouth. When kept in a dry place, they undergo no change by time.

Chemical Constituents.—Gum Arabic consists almost wholly of a peculiar proximate principle, usually termed *Gum*, but latterly designated by chemists as *Arabin*. It is soluble in hot or cold water, forming a viscid solution, called *mucilage*, and is insoluble in alcohol, ether, and the oils. Alcohol precipitates gum from its aqueous solution; subacetate of lead (which is a delicate test), nitrate of lead, and solution of chloride of iron also precipitate it from solution. *Arabin* is now considered to consist chiefly of a soluble acid substance termed *Gummic Acid* ($H_2C_{12}H_{18}O_{10},H_2O$), combined with about 3 per cent. of lime, forming a soluble salt, gummate of calcium. Gums of inferior transparency and solubility contain *bassorin*, an inert principle, insoluble in water and alcohol.

Effects and Uses.—Gum Arabic is extensively employed, internally, as a demulcent in gastro-enteric inflammation, diarrhœa, dysentery, cases of acrid poisoning, &c.; as a lubricant to the fauces in catarrhal affections, and also as a vehicle for anodynes and expectorants in cough mixtures; and as a diluent in fevers and inflammatory cases. It is not now considered to be digestible, and can scarcely rank (as formerly supposed) with nutrients. It is usually administered in solution (a troyounce to boiling water Oj, to be given when cool);

in cases of irritation of the fauces, it may be taken in the mouth, and allowed slowly to dissolve. For pharmaceutical purposes, Gum Arabic is much used to suspend insoluble substances in water, and in making pills and lozenges. *Mucilago Acaciæ* (*Mucilage of Gum Arabic*)—(four troyounces to water Oss),—is used in making pills, emulsions, &c.; it becomes sour by keeping. *Syrupus Acaciæ* (*Syrup of Gum Arabic*),—two troyounces to water f℥viij, with sugar fourteen troyounces),—is used for the same purposes. *Mistura Amygdalæ* (*Almond Mixture*),—is made by dissolving a mixture of half a troyounce of *blanched* sweet almonds, 30 grains of gum arabic, and 120 grains of sugar, in half a pint of distilled water; it is a pleasant demulcent and vehicle for other medicines. By dissolving equal parts of sugar and gum arabic in water and evaporating, an agreeable demulcent is obtained, known as *Gum Pectoral*, which is sold as an imitation of *Jujube Paste*.

TRAGACANTHA—TRAGACANTH.

This is a GUMMY EXUDATION from Astragalus verus and other species of Astragalus (*Nat. Ord.* Fabaceæ). They are small shrubs found in Persia, Asia Minor, and countries bordering on the Levant—with numerous branches, covered with imbricated scales and beset with spines. Tragacanth exudes spontaneously in the hot weather, and hardens as it exudes, in forms of various shapes. It occurs in irregular, tortuous flakes or filaments, of a whitish or yellowish-white or occasionally a slightly reddish colour, somewhat translucent, resembling horn in appearance. It is hard and fragile, but very difficult of pulverization, has no smell and very little taste. When heated with water, it swells and forms a paste, and, if agitated with an additional quantity, it forms a uniform mixture, from which it is, however, almost entirely deposited, upon standing a day or two. It contains two constituents, one soluble in water, resembling *arabin*, the other termed *tragacanthin*, which is probably identical with *bassorin* ($C_{12}H_{10}O_{10}$).

Effects and Uses.—Tragacanth is seldom given internally, on account of its difficult solubility. It is useful in suspending heavy insoluble powders, and answers better than gum arabic to impart consistence to lozenges. *Mucilago Tragacanthæ* (*Mucilage of Tragacanth*),—(a troyounce to boiling water Oj), —is used in making pills and troches, and for the suspension of heavy insoluble metallic substances.

LINUM—FLAXSEED.

This is the SEED of Linum usitatissimum, or Common Flax (*Nat. Ord.* Linaceæ), an annual plant, of the height of two feet, originally a native of Eastern countries, but naturalized in Europe, and cultivated in all parts of the world. The SEED and OIL are both officinal. The seeds are about a line in length, oval, smooth, and glossy, of a brown colour externally, and yellowish-white within; a variety of flax is cultivated in Ohio, the seeds of which are greenish-yellow. Flaxseeds are inodorous, and have an oily, mucilaginous taste. They contain 37 or 38 per cent. of *fixed oil*, a large proportion of *mucilaginous matter*, vegetable albumen, and various other ingredients; the mucilaginous matter, which is found chiefly in the husks of the seeds, consists, about one-half, of a principle soluble in cold water, resembling *arabin*, and, about one-third, of a principle insoluble in water. The *Oil* (*Oleum Lini* or *Linseed Oil*), is obtained by expression from the interior part of the seeds; it is laxative in the dose of f℥i–ij, but it is chiefly used, externally, as an ingredient of *Linimentum Calcis* (see p. 354).

Effects and Uses.—The *compound infusion of Flaxseed* (*infusum lini compositum*), half a troyounce to boiling water Oj, with liquorice root ʒij, is an admirable demulcent, extensively employed *internally*, in catarrh, bowel-complaints, nephritic and calculous complaints, strangury, &c.; and also (without the liquorice root), as an enema in dysentery, or an *external* antiphlogistic application, but after a time it is apt to harden on the skin. Decoction is an improper mode of preparing a demulcent solution of flaxseed, as boiling extracts part of the oil; but it answers very well when it is used as a laxative enema. *Flaxseed meal* (*lini farina*) forms a much-used emollient *poultice*, which is prepared by adding the meal to boiling water, constantly stirring, until it makes a thin and smooth dough. The cake, remaining after the expression of the oil, retains the mucilaginous and albuminous constituents of the seeds, and forms a food for cattle, under the name of *oil-cake*. This is used for making poultices, but it is inferior to the meal made from the seeds which have not been deprived of their oil.

ULMUS—SLIPPERY-ELM BARK.

This is the INNER BARK of Ulmus fulva, or Slippery Elm (*Nat. Ord.* Ulmaceæ), a lofty indigenous tree, which is found throughout the United States, north of Carolina, and grows most abundantly west of the Allegheny Mountains. The inner bark is prepared for use by the removal of the epidermis; it is found in the shops in long flat pieces, of a fibrous texture, tawny on the outer surface and reddish on the inner, of a peculiar but not unpleasant smell, and a very mucilaginous taste. It affords a light, grayish, fawn-coloured powder. A large quantity of mucilaginous matter is contained in it, which is readily yielded to water, also some mimo-tannic acid. Much of the bark lately brought into the market is inferior, containing but little mucilage; it is less fibrous and more brittle than the genuine bark.

Effects and Uses.—Slippery-elm bark is a valuable demulcent, extensively and advantageously employed in dysentery, diarrhœa, genito-urinary diseases, catarrhs, &c. It is also highly nutritious. Externally, it is an excellent emollient application, in the form either of infusion, or of poultice made with the powder. It has been also recommended for the dilatation of strictures and fistulæ, and, made into a spongy mass, as a tent to dilate the os uteri. The infusion—*Mucilago Ulmi* (*Mucilage of Slippery-elm Bark*),—(a troyounce to boiling water Oj),—may be used *ad libitum.*

SASSAFRAS MEDULLA—SASSAFRAS PITH.

Sassafras pith is the PITH of the stems of Sassafras officinale (see p. 270). It occurs in light, spongy, whitish, slender, cylindrical pieces, of a mucilaginous taste. It abounds in a gummy matter, which it yields readily to water, forming a limpid, viscid mucilage. This *mucilage* (ʒj to boiling water Oj), is a pleasant demulcent drink in dyspeptic, nephritic, and catarrhal affections, and is much used as a soothing application in ophthalmia.

ALTHÆA—MARSHMALLOW.

The ROOTS of Althæa officinalis (*Nat. Ord.* Malvaceæ), and other Malvaceæ, herbaceous European plants, occasionally found, too, on the borders of salt marshes in our own country, are much used in Europe as demulcents. They are imported in pieces three or four inches in length, of nearly the thickness of the finger, light, easily broken, white externally, of a peculiar faint smell, and a mild, mucilaginous, sweetish taste. The chief constituents of marshmallow are mucilage and starch, the former soluble in cold water, the latter requiring boiling water. It contains also *asparagin* or *malamide* ($C_4H_8N_2O_3,H_2O$), a crystalline principle found in asparagus shoots and other plants.

Uses.—Marshmallow decoction is employed as a demulcent in inflammatory and irritated conditions of the mucous membranes of the respiratory, digestive, and urinary organs, and poultices made of the bruised or powdered root are used externally.

SESAMUM—BENNE.

This is the product of Sesamum Indicum and Sesamum Orientale (*Nat. Ord.* Bignoniæ), annual plants, growing to the height of four or five feet, with ovate-lanceolate, lobed leaves, reddish-white axillary flowers, and an oblong capsule containing small, oval, yellowish seeds. They are natives of India, but are now raised in Asia, Egypt, Italy, and also in South Carolina, and in the neighbourhood of Philadelphia. The seeds contain a FIXED OIL, and the LEAVES yield to cold water a large quantity of mucilage, resembling that of sassafras pith. This is a highly esteemed demulcent drink, used in cholera infantum and infantile bowel-complaints. The seeds are eaten as food by the negroes in Carolina, in broths, puddings, &c. The OIL (*oleum sesami*), which is inodorous, of a bland, sweetish taste, and keeps well, may be used internally or externally as a substitute for olive oil.

CYDONIUM—QUINCE SEED.

This is the SEED of Cydonia vulgaris (*Nat. Ord.* Pomaceæ), a native of Europe, but cultivated in the United States for the fruit. The seeds are ovate, angular, reddish-brown externally, white within, inodorous, insipid, and abound in mucilage. They are used externally, in solution, two drachms to a pint of boiling water.

GLYCYRRHIZA—LIQUORICE ROOT.

This is the ROOT of Glycyrrhiza glabra (*Nat. Ord.* Fabaceæ), a small, herbaceous, perenial plant, of the countries around the Mediterranean. It is imported from Sicily and Spain; and a portion of the Sicilian root is said to be the product of G. echinata. As found in the shops, liquorice root is in long wrinkled pieces, often worm-eaten, varying from a few lines to more than an inch in thickness, externally grayish-brown, internally yellowish, without smell, and of a sweet, mucilaginous, sometimes slightly acrid taste. The best pieces are of the brightest yellow internally. The powder is grayish-yellow, or, if it is powdered with the epidermis removed, pale sulphur-yellow. The constituents of liquorice root are, a peculiar, transparent, yellow, uncyrstallizable sugar, termed *glycyrrhizin* (which is scarcely soluble in cold water, but soluble in boiling water and alcohol, and is insusceptible of the vinous fermentation), starch, albumen, an acrid resin, &c.

Effects and Uses.—A decoction of liquorice root (a troyounce boiled for a few minutes in water Oj), is a useful demulcent in dysenteric, catarrhal, and nephritic affections; it is also added to decoctions of acrid substances, to cover their taste and acridity. It should be made of the root, *deprived of its cortical part*, which is acrid and without demulcent virtues; by long boiling, the acrid resin is extracted. The powder is used in making pills (see p. 31). A *fluid extract* is officinal.

EXTRACTUM GLYCYRRHIZÆ (*Liquorice*), is made by the evaporation of a decoction of the half-dried root. It comes to this country chiefly from Leghorn and Messina, and in part, also, from Spain; good liquorice is prepared, too, in New York and in England. *Crude Liquorice*, when good, occurs in black, flattened, cylindrical rolls, about an inch in diameter, which are dry, brittle, with a shining fracture, of a very sweet, peculiar, slightly acrid taste, and are quite soluble in water. It is, however, much sophisticated, and for internal use is, generally, *refined*, by dissolving the impure extract in water, without ebullition, straining the solution, and evaporating: sugar is often mixed with it, and sometimes mucilage or glue. *Refined Liquorice* is in small cylindrical pieces, not thicker than a pipestem. Liquorice is a pleasant demulcent, much used as an addition to cough mixtures and lozenges, and to acrid infusions and decoctions. *Mistura Glycyrrhizæ Composita* (*Compound Mixture of Liquorice*), commonly called *Brown Mixture*, consists of liquorice, gum arabic, sugar, each half a troyounce; paregoric, f℥ij; antimonial wine, f℥j; sweet spirit of nitre, f℥ss; water, f℥xij; dose, f℥ss. Liquorice enters into the composition of several *troches* already noticed.

CETRARIA—ICELAND MOSS.

Cetraria Islandica, or Iceland Moss (*Nat. Ord.* Lichenaceæ), is a foliaceous, erect lichen, from two to four inches high, found in the northern latitudes and mountainous districts of the new and old continents. It is principally obtained from Norway and Iceland, but is said to be abundant also in New England; as found in the shops, it consists of irregularly lobed and channeled coriaceous leaves, fringed at their edges with rigid hairs, of a brownish or grayish-white colour, darker on the upper surface, and sometimes marked with blood-red spots. It is almost odourless, and has a bitter, mucilaginous taste; its powder is whitish-gray. It gives up its virtues to boiling water, and consists chiefly of a kind of amylaceous matter (which is coloured blue by iodine, and is termed *Lichenin*), and a bitter principle, termed *Cetrarin* or *Cetraric Acid* ($H_2C_{34}H_{30}O_{16}$); it contains, besides, other principles.

Effects and Uses.—Iceland Moss is a demulcent tonic, and is also highly nutritious. It is adapted to cases requiring a light aliment combined with a mild and acceptable tonic; and, from its demulcent properties, has a soothing influence in inflammations of the various mucous membranes. It is chiefly used in chronic affections of the pulmonary and digestive organs, in the form of *decoction* (*decoctum cetrariæ*), (half a troyounce boiled in water enough to make a pint), which may be taken *ad libitum*. By maceration in water or a weak alkaline solution, Iceland Moss may be deprived of its bitter principle; and it is then used as a mild nutritive demulcent.

CHONDRUS—IRISH MOSS.

Chondrus crispus, Carrageen or Irish Moss (*Nat. Ord.* Algaceæ), is a marine alga, found chiefly on the west coast of Ireland, and also on the coast of New England; it is prepared for use by washing, bleaching, and drying. As found in the shops, it consists of fronds, from two to three or four inches long, mostly yellowish or dirty-white, but intermixed with purplish-red portions, nearly inodorous, and of a mucilaginous taste. It swells up in warm water, and is almost entirely dissolved when boiled. Its chief constituent is a peculiar mucilaginous principle, for which the term *Carrageenin* has been proposed; and it contains also some mucus, resins, &c.

Effects and Uses.—It is a very agreeable nutritive demulcent, useful in bowel-complaints and pectoral affections. It may be given in the form of *decoction* (half a troyounce to water, Ojss, boiled to Oj) flavoured with lemon-juice and sugar; or it may be made with milk or cream into *blanc-mange*, which forms an excellent light diet for the sick.

AMYLUM—STARCH.

This term is applied by the Pharmacopœia to the FECULA of the SEED of Triticum vulgare, the well-known wheat (*Nat. Ord.* Graminaceæ). It is a proximate principle, however, which pervades the vegetable kingdom, being found in various parts of plants, especially in seeds, tubers, and bulbous roots. It is obtained by bringing the substances in which it exists to a state of minute division, agitating or washing them with cold water, straining or pouring off the liquid, and allowing it to stand until the fecula which it holds in suspension has subsided. It occurs as a white, opaque, odourless, tasteless powder, or in columnar masses, of a crystalline aspect, and produces a peculiar sound when compressed between the fingers. It is insoluble in alcohol, ether, and cold water. Examined under the microscope, starch is seen to consist of minute cells or granules, varying in size and shape in the different varieties of amylaceous substances. The *envelope* of these granules is insoluble in *cold* water, but is ruptured by heat, so that the interior portion is exposed and becomes dissolved; hence starch is said to be insoluble in cold, but soluble in boiling water. Starch is $C_6H_{10}O_5$. By the action of heat, or by long boiling with diluted sulphuric, hydrochloric, or muriatic acid, it is converted into *dextrin*, an isomeric soluble principle, and by the same process this may be converted into grape sugar. The same change takes place in grains, after germination, through the agency of a nitrogenous principle, termed *diastase*. The test for starch is iodine, which forms with starch-solution a rich blue iodide; with bromine, starch strikes an orange precipitate; nitric acid converts it into oxalic acid.

Effects and Uses.—The starchy or farinaceous articles form an important group of nutrients. Their assimilation is effected by the albuminous principles of the digestive tube (salivin, pepsin, &c.), which change starch into grape sugar. This is converted in part into fatty tissue, and is partly fermented into lactic acid, which acts as a calefacient. Starch is used externally as a dusting powder to excoriated surfaces, as an emollient poultice, and in solution as a vehicle for laudanum as an enema. It is the antidote for iodine.

MARANTA—ARROW-ROOT.

Arrow-root is a FECULA, obtained from the RHIZOME of Maranta arundinacea (*Nat. Ord.* Marantaceæ), a perennial herbaceous plant, of the height of two or three feet, originally found in the West Indies, and now cultivated in both the West and East Indies, Georgia, Florida, Ceylon, and Sierra Leone. Other plants also furnish some of the arrow-root of commerce. The ROOT of M. arundinacea is a white, fleshy, scaly, articulated, cylindrical tuber, from six inches to a foot or more in length, furnished with long fibres, and giving origin to several tuberous stoles, similar to itself. It consists principally of fecula or starch, which is extracted from the roots, when they are about a year old: they are washed and beaten into a pulp, which is stirred in water, and the fibrous part wrung out by the hands; the milky liquor is strained and suffered to settle, and the subsiding mass is dried in the sun. It occurs in the form of a light, opaque, white powder, or small pulverulent masses, without odour or taste; and is brought to our market chiefly from the West Indies, and to some amount, also, from Georgia and Florida. The preferred kind is that which comes from Bermuda.

Arrow-root is a pure starch, insoluble in cold water. Its peculiar characteristic is the structure and appearance of its granules, *when viewed under a microscope;* and this affords the best means of distinguishing it from other feculæ, which are mixed with or sold for it. The granules of the genuine arrow-root are ovate-oblong, irregularly convex, from the $\frac{1}{2000}$ to the $\frac{1}{750}$ of an inch long, with fine rings, a hilum or central cavity, and often short processes or spines.

Effects and Uses.—Arrow-root is a valuable nutritive demulcent, forming a very pleasant light diet in bowel-complaints and pulmonary and urinary affections. It is also much used as an article of food for infants. It is prepared by mixing a tablespoonful with a little cold water until it is reduced to a paste, and then gradually adding a pint of boiling water or milk, or due proportions of each, stirring the mixture at the same time. Lemon-juice and sugar, or wine and spices may be added, according to the indication. It is generally made with milk, when used as a diet for infants.

CANNA.

Canna (known also by the French name of *Tous Les Mois*), is a fecula prepared from the RHIZOME of an undetermined species of canna, generally believed, however, to be C. edulis. It comes from the West Indies and Central America, and occurs in the form of a light, very white powder, of a shining appearance. Its granules are longer than those of any other variety of starch, are ovate or oblong, with numerous regular, unequally distant rings, and have a glistening or satiny appearance. It is used and prepared like arrow-root.

TAPIOCA.

This is the FECULA of the ROOT of Janipha Manihot (*Nat. Ord.* Euphorbiaceæ), a South American shrub, some six or eight feet in height, cultivated also in the West Indies, where it is termed the *Cassava* plant. The ROOT is a very large, white, fleshy tuber, and is found under two varieties, the *sweet* and *bitter;* the latter contains an acrid, poisonous juice (in which prussic acid is present), which is, however, volatile, and dissipated by heat. Tapioca is obtained from the expressed juice of both varieties, from which it is deposited as a *starchy pow-*

der; it is afterwards dried by heat, which partially ruptures the starch-grains and causes them to swell and agglomerate into small masses or lumps. It occurs in the form of irregular, hard, white, rough grains, of little taste, and partially soluble in cold water. In boiling water it swells up, and forms a transparent jelly-like mass, which constitutes an admirable *demulcent artiçle of diet*, applicable to the same cases as arrow-root. This is prepared by soaking two tablespoonfuls (previously washed) in half a pint of cold water for 3 or 4 hours; then adding a pint of milk or water; simmering till it becomes soft; stirring well, as it cools; and flavouring with sugar, lemon-juice, wine, and nutmeg.

SAGO.

Sago is the prepared FECULA of the PITH of Sagus Rumphii, or the Sago Palm, and of other species of Sagus (*Nat. Ord.* Palmaceæ), small trees of the Moluccas and other East India Islands. The immature stems contain a great mass of spongy medullary matter, which is extracted in the state of a coarse powder; this is mingled with water, and the mixture, upon standing, deposits the insoluble farina, which, when dried, constitutes sago. The sago of commerce is prepared by forming the meal into a paste with water, and rubbing it into grains. It is *refined* at Malacca and Singapore, so as to give the grains a fine pearly lustre, and in this state is called *Pearl Sago*. *Pearl Sago* is the preferred variety, and is that which is now in general use. It is in small grains, about the size of a pin's head, hard, whitish, of a light-brown colour, inodorous, and nearly tasteless. *Common Sago* is in larger, duller, browner grains, often mixed with a dirty-looking powder.

Sago is, chemically, a starch. Common Sago is insoluble in cold water; but Pearl Sago is partly dissolved by it, owing to the heat which it has undergone. The only use of sago is as a bland, unirritating article of diet. It is prepared by mixing and allowing to stand for half an hour, two tablespoonfuls of sago and a pint of water, with the juice and rind of a lemon, and a proper amount of sugar ; this mixture is boiled till the particles are dissolved, with constant stirring; and afterwards wine and nutmeg may be added.

HORDEUM—BARLEY.

Barley, as prepared for medicinal use, consists of the decorticated SEED of Hordeum distichon, and other species of Hordeum (*Nat. Ord.* Graminaceæ); well-known grains, supposed to be derived from Tartary, and now in cultivation in most parts of the world. The SEEDS are oval, oblong, marked with a longitudinal furrow, of a yellowish colour externally, white within, a faint odour, and a mild, sweetish taste. They contain starch (about 32 per cent.), gluten, gum, sugar, and a peculiar principle termed *Hordein*, analogous to lignin.

When made to germinate by warmth and moisture, and afterwards baked to deprive them of vitality, barley-seeds are termed *Malt;* this process increases the nutritious properties of the grain, by increasing the proportions of sugar, starch, and gum, at the expense of the hordein. Deprived of its husk, the grain is termed *Hulled Barley,* and hulled barley, when ground, is *Barley Meal.* PEARL BARLEY is the grain with all the investments removed, and afterwards rounded and polished in a mill; it is thus freed from its fibrous matter, and is the only fit form for medicinal use. It consists of small white, oval grains, with a dark longitudinal furrow on one side, and yields its virtues to boiling water. In the form of *decoction*, and suitably flavoured, it makes an exceedingly bland, demulcent, nutritive drink, in fevers and inflammatory cases; (two troyounces, previously washed with cold water, are mixed with water Oss, and boiled for a short time; this water should be thrown away, and Oiv boiling hot are poured upon the barley, and boiled to Oij). A decoction of *Malt* is more nutritious; mixed with hops, it is termed *Wort.*

AVENÆ FARINA (*Oatmeal*),—the meal prepared from the seed of Avena Sativa (*Nat. Ord.* Graminaceæ),—furnishes a pleasant diet for the sick, more nutritious than the pure starches, as it contains 16 per cent. of albuminoid constituent, with 65 per cent. of starch. It has a slight laxative influence on the bowels, and is often administered to assist the action of cathartics. *Oatmeal gruel* is prepared by boiling from one to two troyounces of the meal in three pints of water to a quart, straining the decoction, allowing it to stand till it cools, and then pouring off the clear liquor from the sediment. It may be flavored with sugar, and lemon-juice or raisins.

ORYZA (*Rice*),—the FRUIT of Oryza Sativa (*Nat. Ord.* Graminaceæ), containing about 85 per cent. of starch, and nearly 4 per cent. of gluten, is an excellent demulcent diet for the sick, in affections of the bowels. *Rice-Water*, made by boiling a troyounce in a pint of water for an hour, may be used as a drink.

ZEA MAYS—the FRUIT of our well-known Indian Corn or Maize, is highly nutritive, containing nearly 9 per cent. of vegetable albumen and 55 per cent. of starch. The *meal* is used externally as a poultice (the *mush* poultice), which is a very good application for the maintenance of heat.

SALEP—the prepared BULBS of Orchis mascula (*Nat. Ord.* Orchidaceæ), consists of small, oval, hard, heavy, semi-transparent masses, of a yellowish colour, a feeble odour, and a mild mucilaginous taste. It contains, like tragacanth, two gums (one insoluble, the other soluble), and also starch. It is demulcent and nutritive, and is used in the same way as tapioca sago, &c. The *Castillon Powders*, consisting of salep, sago, and tragacanth (in powder), each a drachm, prepared oyster-shell a scruple, and cochineal enough to give colour to the mixture, constitute an excellent article of diet in bowel complaints. A drachm may be taken boiled in a pint of milk.

GELATINA (*Gelatin*), a solid, transparent, corneous substance, obtained from the bones and other tissues of animals (soluble in boiling water, and forming, on cooling, a transparent jelly), may be noticed with demulcents. When dried, it is found in the form of whitish or yellowish, semi-transparent, hard and tough, tasteless, inodorous strips. It is used to make soups and jellies for the sick, but it is not of easy digestion, and it does not nourish the nitrogenous tissues. In solution, it has been used as an enema in dysentery and hemorrhoids. And in pharmacy, it is employed to make capsules for the administration of disagreeable liquid medicines, and as a coating for pills.

ICHTHYOCOLLA (*Isinglass*), prepared from the swimming bladder of Acipenser huso (the sturgeon), and of other fishes, is the purest form of gelatin. *Court Plaster* is made by coating oiled silk with a solution of isinglass.

For *external use*, the ANIMAL FATS are employed as *emollients*.

ADEPS (*Lard*), is the PREPARED FAT of sus scrofa (the hog); the internal fat of the abdomen is preferred, which is washed, melted, and strained. Below the temperature of 90°, it occurs as a soft, white solid, which, for medicinal use, should be free from saline matter. It consists of olein and stearin. It is used in pharmacy as an addition to poultices, and as an inunction in the exanthemata, particularly scarlatina. *Cerate* (*Ceratum*) (formerly termed *Simple Cerate*), is made by melting together two parts of lard and one part of white wax. *Unguentum* (*Ointment*), is made by melting together four parts of lard and one part of yellow wax. *Lard Oil* (the olein of lard), is a good vehicle for anodyne enemata.

SEVUM (*Suet*), is the PREPARED FAT of ovis aries (the sheep). It is composed almost exclusively of stearin.

CETACEUM (*Spermaceti*), is a peculiar CONCRETE SUBSTANCE, obtained from Physeter macrocephalus (the spermaceti whale). It is the *Palmitate of Cetyl* ($C_{16}H_{33}C_{16}H_{31}O_2$), or *Cetine*. *Spermaceti Cerate* (*Ceratum Cetacei*), is made by melting together one part of spermaceti and three parts of white wax, and then adding five parts of olive oil, previously heated. Ointment of rose water (see p. 173) contains spermaceti.

CERA FLAVA (*Yellow Wax*), is a peculiar CONCRETE SUBSTANCE, prepared by Apis mellifica (the honey bee).

CERA ALBA (*White Wax*), is yellow wax bleached. They are chiefly used in making cerates, ointments, and plasters.

OLEUM THEOBROMÆ—OIL OF THEOBROMA.

This oil, commonly known as *Butter of Cacao*, is the CONCRETE OIL of the KERNELS of the FRUIT of Theobroma Cacao (*Nat. Ord.* Sterculiaceæ), a handsome tree, from twelve to twenty feet in height, growing in Mexico, the West Indies, Central America, and South America. The fruit is an ovate-oblong capsule or berry, half a foot in length, with a thick, coriaceous, ligneous rind, inclosing a whitish pulp, in which numerous ovate seeds are imbedded, about the size of an almond. Separated from the matter in which they are enveloped, these constitute the *Chocolate-nuts* of commerce (see p. 106). They contain FIXED OIL (*Cacao Butter*), *Theobromia*, and other matters. *Thebromia* is a nitrogenous alkaloid, analogous to caffeina. *Cacao Butter* is obtained by expression, decoction, or the action of a solvent. It occurs in whitish or yellowish, oblong cakes, of the consistence of tallow, and of an agreeable odour and taste. It contains a large proportion of stearin, also palmitin and olein. It is used in pharmacy for coating pills, and also largely in preparing suppositories, for which it is well adapted from its consistence and blandness.

GLYCERINA—GLYCERIN.

This is a substance which exists in oils in combination with the fatty acids (stearic, margaric, oleic, &c.), and is liberated from them, when they unite with bases in the process of saponification. It is usually obtained in the process for making lead plaster, by mixing litharge (oxide of lead) with olive oil and boiling water, by which the fatty acid unites with the lead and is precipitated, and the glycerin remains in solution. It is freed from any lead it may contain by means of a stream of sulphuretted hydrogen gas, and is afterwards filtered through animal charcoal; or it may be made more directly by blowing steam through fat, which causes a separation of the glycerin and fatty acids. Glycerin (C_3H_53HO), or Glyceric Alcohol, is the hydrate of *Glyceryl*, *Glycyl*, or *Propenyl*. It is a thick, syrupy liquid, colourless or straw-coloured, unctuous to the touch, inodorous, and of a sharp, sweet taste. When pure, its sp. gr. is 1.26, when it contains 98 per cent. of anhydrous glycerin; the Pharmacopœia directs its sp. gr. to be 1.25. It is soluble in oils, alcohol, and water, but is insoluble in ether and chloroform, and does not evaporate when exposed to the air, but absorbs one half its weight of water. It has remarkable solvent properties, dissolving iodine, bromine, the alkalies, tannic and other vegetable acids, a large number of neutral salts, and many organic principles. Officinal solutions of medicinal substances in glycrin are termed *Glycerites* (*glycerita*).

Effects and Uses.—Glycerin is a bland and unirritating substance. It has the capacity of diffusing itself freely over and through organic matter, incorporating itself between organic molecules, by which it is absorbed and appropriated. It has been used *internally* as a nutrient and demulcent, and has been deemed of value in cachectic, strumous, and asthenic conditions in *children*, but the weight of opinion is against its efficacy as an alterative. It is as a *topical* application that it is chiefly employed. As an enema in dysentery, to soften hardened mucus in the air-passages, in various cutaneous affections, in diphtheria, in deafness attended with dryness of the meatus, and as a vehicle or solvent for active medicines, glycerin is a valuable article. The name *Plasma* is applied to a compound of glycerin (f℥i) and starch (grs. 70), mixed at 240° F.; this is used as a substitute for ointments, and is a good excipient for pills.

PYROXYLON.

Pyroxylon, or Soluble Gun Cotton, is made by adding half a troyounce of cotton, freed from impurities, to a mixture of 3½ troyounces of nitric acid gradually added to 4 troyounces of sulphuric acid, and allowing it to macerate for 15 hours; it is to be washed first with cold water, and then with boiling water, and, after being drained on filtering paper, it is dried by means of a water-bath. Pyroxylon has the appearance of ordinary cotton, but is harsh to the touch. It is insoluble in water, nearly so in alcohol, but, when *freshly* prepared, it dissolves in ether, forming collodion; it is liable to *decomposition* if kept for some time.

COLLODIUM—COLLODION.

This is a solution of pyroxylon (200 grains), in stronger ether (12½ fluidounces), and stronger alcohol (3½ fluidounces). Collodion is a slightly opalescent, syrupy liquid, with a strong ethereal smell. By long standing, it deposits a layer of fibrous matter, and becomes more transparent; this layer should be reincorporated by agitation, before the collodion is used. When applied to the skin, the solvent evaporates and it forms a colourless, transparent, flexible, and strongly contractile film. In this way it proves antiphlogistic, by driving the blood away from a part, limiting effusion, and promoting absorption, and at the same time, acts as an admirable emollient by protecting an inflamed surface from the action of the air. It is a useful application to ulcers, fissures, and skin diseases, and erysipelatous parts. It is used also in surgery as a substitute for adhesive plaster, and in pharmacy as a vehicle for other medicines. *Iodized Collodion* (a very good solution of iodine for external application), contains from ten to twenty grains of iodine in a fluidounce of collodion. Collodion containing tannic acid (gr. xx–f℥i), is a good styptic application.

Collodium Flexile (*Flexible Collodion*) is made by mixing

a pint of collodion, 320 grains of Canada turpentine, and 160 grains of castor oil. This is a softer, more pliable, and more elastic preparation, useful in cases where the strongly contractile power of ordinary collodion is objectionable. Collodion, in all forms, is to be kept in well-stoppered bottles.

LIQUOR GUTTA-PERCHÆ—SOLUTION OF GUTTA-PERCHA.

This is a solution of a troyounce and a half of gutta-percha in 17 troyounces of purified chloroform. In preparing it, carbonate of lead is employed to free it from colouring matter. It is a clear, colourless, or nearly colourless solution, and should be kept in well-stoppered glass vials. By the evaporation of the chloroform, this proves an admirable application to inflamed or abraded parts, in skin affections, chaps, &c.; also an excellent protective coating to parts threatened with bed-sores or liable to excoriation.

FERMENTUM—YEAST.

This well-known product of fermentation is a flocculent, frothy, somewhat viscid substance, of a dirty-yellowish colour, a sour, vinous odour, and a bitter taste. It is insoluble in alcohol or water. Its most important characteristic is its power of exciting the vinous fermentation in saccharine and starchy liquids, which it owes to the presence of a cryptogamic plant, *Torula Cerevisiæ*. It is occasionally used in low fevers, attended with irritability of the stomach, in the dose of f℥ss–ij, every two or three hours, which sometimes proves laxative. *Externally*, it is added to farinaceous poultices, applied to sloughing ulcers.

SACCHARUM—SUGAR.

Sugar is a principle diffused through the vegetable world, under many forms, distinguished all by a sweet taste. They are divided into two chief groups—*Cane Sugar* and *Grape Sugar*. Cane sugar is the product of Saccharum officinarum (*Nat. Ord.* Graminaceæ), a native of tropical countries, cultivated most successfully in the West Indies, and to some extent in Louisiana. It has a general resemblance to Indian corn. (Cane sugar is made also in France from the beet-root.) The juice of the sugar-cane is extracted by crushing and expressing the stalks; it is then boiled with quicklime, strained, and reduced by evaporation to a thick syrup, which is cooled and granulated in shallow vessels. *Raw* sugar is *refined* by the agency of animal charcoal. When pure, cane sugar is white, crystallized in translucent double oblique prisms, very sweet, soluble in one third its weight of water, in alcohol, but not in ether. At a heat of 320° F., it melts and cools into a glassy, amorphous mass, known as *Barley-sugar;* from a strong solution, it can be made to crystallize slowly upon a string as *Rock-candy*.

The uncrystallizable portion, which is drawn off in the granulation of sugar, is MOLASSES (SYRUPUS FUSCUS), or *Treacle*, a dark, brownish-black, syrupy liquid.

Grape sugar is the sugar of grapes and other acid fruits; it is also found in the liver and blood of mammalia, and in the urine of diabetes mellitus. It may be procured artificially by acting on starch with diluted sulphuric acid. It occurs as whitish or grayish-white, non-crystalline masses, or as a dense transparent syrup.

Cane sugar ($C_{12}H_{22}O_{11}$) combines with alkalies to form saccharates. Grape sugar ($C_6H_{12}O_6,H_2O$), when boiled with an alkali, is transformed into the acid of molasses, melassic acid; mixed with solution of potassa and a weak solution of cupric sulphate, it attracts oxygen and causes the precipitation of a reddish cuprous oxide (Cu_2O).

Effects and Uses.—Sugar, especially in the form of barley-sugar, is an excellent demulcent to relieve catarrhal irritation; much of the cough-relieving action of cough syrups is due to the sugar they contain. It abates thirst, and is used to flavour refrigerant drinks. For pharmaceutical purposes, sugar is much employed, for its agreeable taste, and also as a preservative of vegetable substances, and to protect mineral medicines from oxidation. Molasses is slightly laxative as well as demulcent.

MEL—HONEY.

This *saccharine* liquid, the familiar product of the bee (*Apis Mellifica*), best used in the form of *Mel Despumatum* (*Clarified Honey*), is a slightly laxative article of food, and is used in pharmacy, and as an agreeable demulcent ingredient in gargles.

SACCHARUM LACTIS (*Sugar of Milk*) ($C_{12}H_{22}O_{11},H_2O$), the saccharine principle of milk, obtained from whey, is used as a bland non-nitrogenous article of diet. By fermentation, sugar of milk gives rise to *Lactic Acid* (*Acidum Lacticum*), a limpid, syrupy liquid, of a pale-wine colour, which has been used in certain forms of dyspepsia, and for the removal of phosphatic deposits in the urine, in the dose of ʒi–iij during the day.

CARBO LIGNI—CHARCOAL.

Although not strictly ranking with demulcents, the medicinal uses of charcoal may, perhaps, be appropriately noticed under this head. Charcoal is prepared by the exposure of wood to a red heat without access of air. For medicinal purposes, the charcoal prepared from young willow-shoots, for the manufacture of gunpowder, is preferred. It is a black, shining, brittle, porous substance, without odour or taste, and insoluble in water.

Effects and Uses.—It is employed internally as an absorbent of acrid secretions in dyspepsia (in which it is often very useful), in gastric irritation, diarrhœa, and dysentery; dose, from one to four teaspoonfuls. Externally, it is used with effect to absorb the offensive gases given off by foul sores, in the form of poultice, mixed with flaxseed meal, or with bread-crumb, which is better, from its porosity; dry charcoal is sprinkled with advantage over sloughing ulcers, and appears to promote the separation of the sloughs.

ORDER III.—COLOURING AGENTS.

These are employed exclusively for pharmaceutical purposes. The following articles enter into officinal preparations, to which they are intended to communicate their peculiar colour.

CROCUS—SAFFRON.

This is the STIGMAS of Crocus Sativus (*Nat. Ord.* Iridaceæ), a small perennial plant, the native country of which is Greece and Asia Minor, but now cultivated all over Europe and in our own country. In Lancaster county, Pennsylvania, it has been raised to considerable extent. The stigmas are an inch or more in length, of a rich deep-orange colour, a peculiar aromatic odour, and a warm, pungent, bitter taste; they contain a principle termed *Saffranin* or *Polychroite.*

Saffron is now admitted to possess little, if any, medicinal activity, and is used only to impart colour and flavour to officinal preparations.

SANTALUM—RED SAUNDERS.

This is the WOOD of Pterocarpus Santalinus, a large tree of India and Ceylon (*Nat. Ord.* Fabaceæ). It comes in roundish or angular billets, internally of a blood-red colour, externally brown, of little smell or taste; in the shops, it is found in the form of chips, raspings, or coarse powder; it contains a resinoid matter, *Santalin* ($C_{16}H_{16}O_3$). It is employed solely to give colour to spirits and tinctures.

COCCUS—COCHINEAL.

This is an insect, termed Coccus Cacti, of Mexico and Central America, naturalized in Teneriffe and other places. The *female* insect, *dried,* constitutes the article of the shops. It occurs in the form of roundish or somewhat angular grains, about an eighth of an inch in diameter, convex on one side, concave or flat on the other, and wrinkled. Two varieties are distinguished, one reddish-gray, the other nearly black, known as *silver* grains and *black* grains. It has a faint, heavy odour, and a bitter, slightly acidulous taste; its colouring principle is *Carminic Acid* ($C_{14}H_{14}O_8$).

Cochineal has had antispasmodic virtues attributed to it, and has been used in whooping-cough, especially in combination with carbonate of potassium; dose, to infants, a third of a grain three times a day. It is chiefly employed, however, to colour tinctures and ointments.

ORDER IV.—ANTHELMINTICS.

Anthelmintics are medicines which promote the destruction and expulsion of worms from the alimentary canal. They act in different ways; some weaken or destroy the worms by a direct poisonous influence, others by mechanical means; the drastic cathartics have an anthelmintic effect, from the increased secretion and exhalation which they induce from the alimentary canal.

SPIGELIA.

Spigelia, called also Pinkroot, is the ROOT of Spigelia Marilandica, or Carolina Pink (*Nat. Ord.* Spigeliaceæ), an herbaceous, indigenous plant, found chiefly in our Southern and Southwestern States. The root is perennial, and consists of a number of slender fibres; the stems are numerous, from a foot to a foot and a half high, of a purplish colour, furnished with sessile, opposite, ovate-lanceolate leaves, and terminate in spikes, bearing carmine-coloured, funnel-shaped flowers, which appear from May to July. The ROOT, as found in the shops, consists of numerous slender, wrinkled, branching, brownish fibres, attached to a dark-brown caudex, and has a faint peculiar smell, and a sweetish, slightly bitter taste; its activity is diminished by time. Boiling water extracts its virtues, which are thought to depend upon a *bitter principle;* it contains also volatile oil, resin, a little tannic acid, and other matters.

Effects and Uses.—In ordinary doses, Spigelia often proves anthelmintic without any sensible effect on the system. In

Fig. 28.

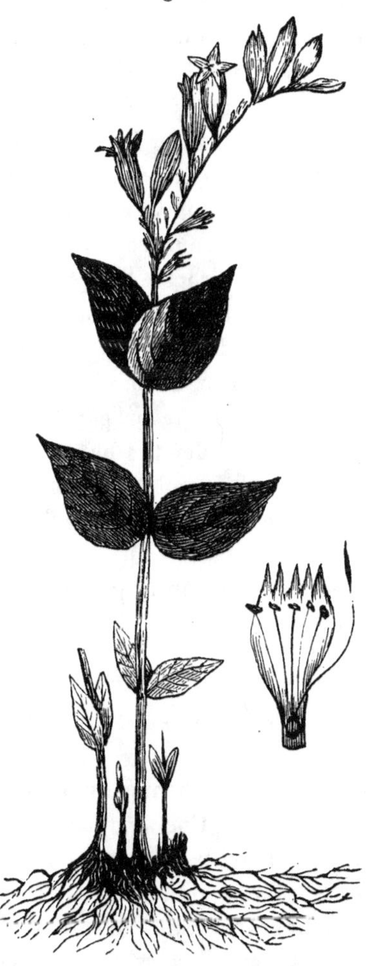

larger doses, it purges and sometimes vomits; and, in excessive doses, it operates as a narcotic poison, producing vertigo, dilated pupils, convulsions, and death. It is less apt to occasion narcotic effects when it acts on the bowels, and hence it is usually combined with or followed by cathartics. As an anthelmintic against lumbrici (or round worms), it is considered the most reliable article we possess.

Administration.—Dose of the *powdered root*, ʒi–ij, for an adult; for a child three or four years old, gr. x–xx, to be repeated night and morning, for three or four days, and followed by a brisk cathartic; calomel is sometimes combined with it. The *infusion* is the usual form of administration (half a troyounce to boiling water Oj, with frequently senna half a troyounce); dose f℥ss–j for a child two or three years old, f℥iv–viij for an adult, night and morning. The *fluid extract* contains in a fluidounce a troyounce of spigelia—dose, for a child two years old, ten drops. The *Fluid Extract of Spigelia and Senna* (made by mixing 10 fluidounces of fluid extract of spigelia with 6 fluidounces of fluid extract of senna, and dissolving, in the mixture, 20 minims of the oils of anise and caraway, each), is a pleasant preparation; dose, f℥ss for an adult, fʒj for a child. Under the name of *Worm Tea*, preparations containing spigelia and cathartics are kept in the shops, as in the following formula: Spigelia, ℥ss, manna, ℥i, senna and fennel each, ʒij, savine, ℈ij—to be infused in a pint of boiling water, and a tablespoonful given to a child two years old, three times a day.

CHENOPODIUM—WORMSEED.

Wormseed is the FRUIT of Chenopodium anthelminticum, or Jerusalem Oak (*Nat. Ord.* Chenopodiaceæ), an indigenous, herbaceous, perennial plant, from two to five feet high, with alternate, oblong-lanceolate, sinuated and toothed, yellowish-green leaves, with numerous small flowers of the same colour, arranged in long terminal panicles. Wormseed, as found in the shops, is in small spherical grains, not larger than a pin's head, of a dull, greenish-yellow or brownish colour, a peculiar offensive smell, and a rather aromatic, pungent taste. Their sensible and medicinal properties are owing to a VOLATILE OIL (OLEUM CHENOPODII), obtained by distillation.

Effects and Uses.—Wormseed is a very efficient anthelmin-

Fig. 29.

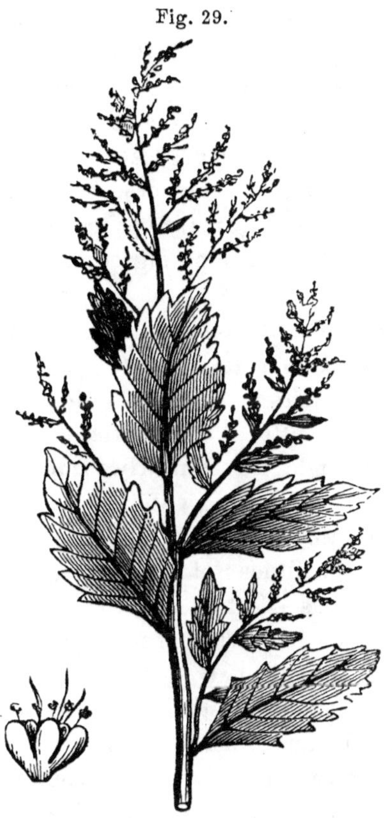

tic, particularly adapted to the expulsion of lumbrici from children. Dose, ℈i–ij for a child two or three years old, in molasses, night and morning, for three or four days, to be followed by a brisk cathartic. The *oil* is more used than the fruit; dose, gtt. v–x for a child, in emulsion with sugar. The expressed juice of the leaves, and a decoction made with milk, are also used.

SANTONICA.

The unexpanded FLOWERS of Artemisia Cina, a native of Persia, and of other species of Artemisia, are used in Europe as an anthelmintic (in the dose of 10 to 30 grains), under the name of *Levant Wormseed.* They resemble small seeds in appearance, are about a line in length, oval, obtuse at both ends, of a greenish-brown colour, a strong, somewhat terebinthinate odour, and a bitter, camphoraceous taste. They contain volatile oil, resin, and a peculiar principle, termed *Santonin*—*Santoninum*, which is made by digesting santonica and lime in diluted alcohol, adding acetic acid, crystallizing, boiling with alcohol, digesting the tincture with animal charcoal, filtering, and crystallizing. It is a weak acid ($C_{15}H_{18}O_3$), and occurs in colourless, shining, flattened prisms, without smell, nearly tasteless at first, but after a time bitter; it becomes yellow on exposure to the light. It is nearly insoluble in cold water, soluble in 250 parts of boiling water, in 43 parts of cold and 3 parts of boiling alcohol, and in 75 parts of ether. This is the anthelmintic constituent of Santonica, and is much employed for a poisonous effect on lumbrici; but, in large doses, it is capable of producing serious if not fatal poisoning in man. The symptoms are (occasionally but not invariably) vomiting, giddiness, stupor, coldness of the skin with clammy perspiration, dilated pupils, and, finally, tetanic convulsions. A remarkable effect of santonin, even in moderate amounts, is a change in the field of vision, so that objects are seen as if through a *yellow* medium. It is eliminated through the kidneys, producing a yellow discoloration of the urine. Dose, 2 or 3 grains, two or three times a day, in the form of syrup. *Troches of Santonin* (*Trochisci Santonini*), are made by rubbing together half a troyounce of santonin and tragacanth each, and eighteen troyounces of sugar, and then, with orange-flower water forming a mass, to be divided into 480 troches, each troche containing half a grain of santonin. The use of santonin has been suggested also in amaurosis.

AZEDARACH.

This is the BARK of the ROOT of Melia Azedarach, or Pride of China (*Nat. Ord.* Meliaceæ), an Asiatic tree, cultivated extensively as an ornamental tree in our Southern States. It has a bitter, nauseous taste, and yields its virtues to boiling water; but, as it is used only in the recent state, it is not found in our shops. Its effects are said to resemble those of Spigelia. The *decoction* is the preferred form of administration (four troyounces to water Oij, boiled to Oj); dose for a child f℥ss, every two or three hours, till it affects the stomach and bowels; or night and morning for several days.

MUCUNA—COWHAGE.

The HAIRS of the PODS of Mucuna pruriens (*Nat. Ord.* Fabaceæ), a West India perennial climbing plant, act as an anthelmintic, by a mechanical penetration of the worms. The PODS are about four inches long, shaped like the Italic letter *ſ*, and are covered with brown BRISTLY HAIRS, which, when handled, stick in the fingers, and produce an intense itching. For *administration*, the pods are dipped into syrup or molasses, and the hairs scraped off with the liquid, which should have the consistence of thick honey. Dose, a tablespoonful for an adult, a teaspoonful for a child, night and morning, for several days, and followed by a cathartic.

FILIX MAS—MALE FERN.

Aspidium Filix Mas, or Male Fern (*Nat. Ord.* Filicales), is an indigenous plant, common to all parts of the world, with a perennial, horizontal root, from which spring numerous annual, oval, lanceolate, acute, bright-green pinnate fronds or leaves, from a foot to four feet in height; the leaflets are deeply lobate, oval, crenate at their edges, and gradually diminish from the base of the pinna to the apex. The RHIZOME is the portion used. It is a long, cylindrical caudex, *covered with portions of the stipes*, and, as found in the shops, it is generally broken into fragments, of a brown colour externally, internally yellowish-white or greenish, with a peculiar feeble odour, and a sweetish, bitter, astringent, nauseous taste. It deteriorates by keeping. It contains volatile oil, fixed oil, resin, tannic and gallic acids, &c., &c.; and ether is the best solvent to extract its virtues.

Effects and Uses.—Male fern possesses tonic and astringent properties; but its chief use is to cause the expulsion of tænia, which it destroys by a specific action. Its efficacy in this respect has been long and well attested, but it is most used to destroy the Swiss variety of tænia, (borthriocephalus latus). Dose, of the *powder*, ʒi–iij, in electuary or emulsion, night and morning, for one or two days. The *oleoresin* (*oleoresina filicis*) is the best preparation; it is a dark, thick liquid, of a bitterish, nauseous, slightly acrid taste—dose fʒss to fʒi, night and morning, for a day or two, to be followed by a cathartic. The administration of the tæniacide agents should be always preceded by a twenty-four hours' fast.

GRANATI RADICIS CORTEX—BARK OF POMEGRANATE ROOT.

The BARK of the ROOT of Punica granatum (see p. 172), is used for the expulsion of tænia. It is a powerful styptic, and may act in this way. It is given in *decoction* (two troyounces to water Oij, boiled to Oj), dose, f℥ij, or more.

OLEUM TEREBINTHINÆ (*Oil of Turpentine*), (see p. 288), is used as a remedy for tænia and other worms. Dose, f℥j, combined with or followed by castor oil.

CALOMEL (see p. 313), is a valuable anthelmintic, given in cathartic doses.

BRAYERA (*Koosso*). The FLOWERS and UNRIPE FRUIT of Brayera anthelmintica (*Nat. Ord.* Rosaceæ), a native of Abyssinia, have been introduced into European practice, as a remedy for tænia, under the name of *Koosso*. The dried flowers occur in unbroken, compressed clusters, of a greenish-yellow colour, a fragrant balsamic odour, and a faint taste, which after a time becomes acrid and disagreeable. They are said to impart their virtues best to hot water, and to yield gum, resin, fatty matter, tannic acid, &c. They are best given upon an empty stomach, after a previous evacuation of the bowels, in the dose of half a troyounce of the *powder*, mixed with half a pint of warm water.

ROTTLERA—KAMEELA.

This is the *glandular* POWDER and HAIRS, obtained from the capsules of Rottlera tinctoria (*Nat. Ord.* Euphorbiaceæ), a small tree of Hindostan and the East India islands. It is an orange-red, granular, inflammable powder, with little smell or taste, insoluble in cold, and nearly so in boiling water; soluble in boiling alcohol and ether. It consists chiefly of resinous substances, to one of which, soluble in ether, and considered the active constituent, the name of *Rottlerin* has been given.

Uses.—Kameela, or *Kamala*, is a highly esteemed tæniacide in India, and has lately been introduced into Europe and our own country. Dose of the *powder*, ʒi–ij, suspended in syrup. A tincture (six troyounces to alcohol Oj), is given in the dose of fʒi–iv. Castor Oil should be taken after the medicine.

PEPO—PUMPKIN SEED.

The SEED of Cucurbita pepo, or common Pumpkin, is probably the most efficacious remedy known in the expulsion of tapeworm. These seeds are oval, flattish, grooved, 9 lines long by 5 or 6 in breadth, of a light brownish-white colour, a sweetish, oily taste, and aromatic smell. They owe their activity to a principle, soluble in ether, chloroform, and especially alcohol. One or two troyounces of the *fresh seeds*, deprived of their outer envelope, beaten to a paste with finely powdered sugar, and diluted with water or milk, should be taken after a twenty-four hours' fast, and followed in two or three hours, by a dose of castor oil. A fluid extract, made with alcohol and glycerin, is probably the best preparation; dose fʒss–i.

APPENDIX.

SIGNS AND ABBREVIATIONS USED IN PRESCRIPTIONS.

℞, *Recipe*, take.
āā, *Ana*, (ανα), of each.
℔, *Libra*, *libræ*, a pound, pounds.
℥, *Uncia*, *unciæ*, an ounce, ounces.
ʒ, *Drachma*, *drachmæ*, a drachm, drachms.
℈, *Scrupulus*, *scrupuli*, a scruple, scruples.
O, *Octarius*, *octarii*, a pint, pints.
f℥, *Fluiduncia*, *fluidunciæ*, a fluidounce, fluidounces.
fʒ, *Fluidrachma*, *Fluidrachmæ*, a fluidrachm, fluidrachms.
♏, *Minimum*, *minima*, a minim, minims.

Ad 2 Vic., *Ad duas vices*, at two takings.
Ad Lib., *Ad libitum.*
Add., *Adde*, *addantur*, add, let be added.
Altern. Horis, *Alternis horis*, every other hour.
Aq. Destil., *Aqua destillata*, distilled water.
Aq. Ferv., *Aqua fervens*, hot water.
Aq. Fluvial., *Aqua fluvialis*, river water.
Aq. Font., *Aqua fontana*, spring water.
Aq. Pluv., *Aqua pluvialis*, rain water.
Bis Ind., *Bis indies*, twice a day.
Bull., *Bulliat*, *bulliant*, let it or them boil.
Cap., *Capiat*, *capiendum*, let the patient take it, it must be taken.
Chart., *Chartula*, *chartulæ*, a small paper, or papers.
Cochleat., *Cochleatim*, by spoonfuls.
Coch. Mag., *Cochleare magnum*, a tablespoonful.
Coch. Med., *Cochleare medium*, a dessertspoonful.
Coch. Parv., *Cochleare parvum*, a teaspoonful.
Col., *Cola*, *coletur*, strain, let it be strained.
Collyr., *Collyrium*, an eye-water.
Comp., *Compositus*, compounded.
Cong., *Congius*, *congii*, a gallon, gallons.
C. M. S., *Cras mane sumendus*, to be taken to-morrow morning.
C. N., *Cras nocte*, to-morrow night.
Decoc., *Decoctum*, a decoction.
De D. in D., *De die in diem*, from day to day.

DIEB. ALTER., *Diebus Alternis*, every other day.
DIL., *Dilue, dilutus*, dilute, diluted.
DIM., *Dimidius*, one-half.
DIV., *Divide*, divide.
D., *Doses*, a dose.
ELEC., *Electuarium*, an electuary.
ENEM., *Enema, enemata*, a clyster, clysters.
EXHIB., *Exhibeatur*, let it be administered.
F. H., *Fiat haustus*, let a draught be made.
FIL., *Filtra*, filter.
FT., *Fiat, fiant*, let there be made.
GARG., *Gargarysma*, a gargle.
GR., *Granum, grana*, a grain, grains.
GTT., *Gutta, guttæ*, a drop, drops.
GUTTAT., *Guttatim*, by drops.
HAUST., *Haustus*, a draught.
IND., *Indies*, daily.
INF., *Infunde*, pour in.
INFUS., *Infusum*, an infusion.
INJ., *Injiciatur*, let it be injected.
JUL., *Julepus, julepum*, a julep.
M., *Misce*, mix.
MANE, in the morning.
MIST., *Mistura*, a mixture.
MIC. PAN., *Mica panis*, crumb of bread.
NO., *Numero*, in number.
OMN. HOR., *Omni horâ*, every hour.
OMN. BID., *Omni biduo*, every two days.
OMN. BIH., *Omni bihorâ*, every two hours.
OMN. MAN., *Omni mane*, every morning.
OMN. NOCTE, *Omni nocte*, every night.
OMN. QUADR. HOR., *Omni quadrante horæ*, every quarter of an hour.
PH., Pharmacopœia.
POCUL., *Poculum*, a cup.
P. R. N., *Pro re natâ*, as the symptoms may call for.
PULV., *Pulvis*, a powder.
Q. P., *Quantum placeat*, as much as you please.
Q. S., *Quantum sufficiat*, enough.
QUOR., *Quorum*, of which.
REDIG. IN PULV., *Redigatur in pulverem*, let it be reduced to powder.
REPET., *Repetatur, repetantur*, let it or them be repeated.
S., *Signa*, write.
S. A., *Secundum artem*, according to art.
SEMIH., *Semihorâ*, half an hour.
SIGN., *Signatura*, a label.
SS., *Semis*, a half.
SUM., *Sume, sumendus*, take, let it be taken.
TABEL., *Tabella*, a lozenge.
TROCH., *Trochiscus*, a lozenge.
TRIT., *Tritura*, triturate.

TABLE OF ANTIDOTES.

NEUROTIC POISONS.

Poisons.	*Antidotes.*
Opium, Chloral, Calabar Bean,	Stomach pump; emetics; cold affusions; counter-irritation; strong decoction of coffee; hypodermic injection of atropia; electro-magnetism; artificial respiration.
Belladonna, Stramonium, Hyoscyamus, Dulcamara,	Stomach pump; emetics; cathartics; cold affusions; hypodermic injection of a morphia-salt; electro-magnetism.
Tobacco, Lobelia, Aconite, Digitalis, Conium, Veratrum Viride,	After emptying the stomach, the diffusible stimuli, especially alcohol.
Alcohol,	The same as for opium; except that ammonia is the physiological antidote.
Hydrocyanic Acid and Cyanides,	Ammonia; chlorine; cold affusions.
Strychnia, Veratria,	Tannic acid; opium; conium; extr. hemp; camphor; chloral; calabar bean; bromide of potassium; atropia; inhalations of ether or chloroform.

CORROSIVE POISONS.

Acids, Mineral and Vegetable,	Magnesia; chalk; the alkaline solutions; the fixed oils; emetics are not to be used.
Salt of Sorrel,	Calcium salts.
Cream of Tartar,	Sodium carbonates in solution.
Alkalies,	Vinegar; lemon-juice; citric acid; oils.
Alum,	Ammonium or sodium carbonate.
Baryta and its soluble salts,	Magnesium, sodium, or potassium sulphates.
Arsenious acid,	Hydrated oxide of iron; hydrated magnesia.
Soluble arsenites,	Ferric subacetate.
Corrosive sublimate and soluble mercuric salts, Soluble cupric salts,	White of egg; blood; milk; flour; for cupric salts, also ferrocyanide of potassium.
Soluble zinc salts,	Albumen; sodium carbonates; magnesia.

Poisons.	*Antidotes.*
Soluble lead salts,	The alkaline or soluble earthy sulphates.
Tartar Emetic,	Tannic acid.
Nitrate of Silver,	Chloride of Sodium.
Sulphates and Chloride of Iron,	Alkaline carbonates.
Bichromate of Potassium,	Magnesia; soap; alkaline carbonates.

IRRITANT POISONS.

Cantharides,	Emetics; opiates and demulcents; oils are objectionable.
Drastic Cathartics,	Opiates; demulcents; stimulants.
Phosphorus,	Magnesia; oil of turpentine.
Iodine,	Starch.
Bromine,	Ammonia.
Chlorine Gas,	The cautious inhalation of ammonia.
Creasote, Carbolic Acid,	Albuminous substances.
Asphyxiating Gases,	Cold affusions; electro-magnetism; artificial respiration.

INDEX.

LINDSAY & BLAKISTON'S

PHYSICIAN'S VISITING LIST.

Published Annually. Now Ready for 1875.

FOR VARIOUS STYLES AND PRICES, SEE PAGE 25 OF THIS CATALOGUE.

No. 25 South Sixth Street,

PHILADELPHIA,
April, 1875.

CATALOGUE

OF

LINDSAY & BLAKISTON'S

MEDICAL,

DENTAL AND PHARMACEUTICAL

PUBLICATIONS.

MESSRS. LINDSAY & BLAKISTON ask the attention of the Medical Profession to the extensive list and varied character of their publications and to the Classified Index of them annexed.

ALL THEIR PUBLICATIONS can be had from or through BOOKSELLERS in any of the large cities of the United States or Canada. When, for any reason, it is inconvenient thus to procure them, they will be furnished direct by mail or express upon receipt of a Post-office order, draft or check for the amount ordered.

IN ADDITION to their own publications, they keep on hand a full and complete assortment of all Medical Books published in the United States; and, by special arrangement with Messrs. J. & A. CHURCHILL and other Medical Publishers of London, they can supply many important English Medical Works at greatly reduced prices; such as are not on hand they can import promptly to order.

AS SPECIAL AGENTS OF THE SYDENHAM SOCIETY in the United States, they are prepared to receive Subscribers at Ten Dollars per Annum, and supply any of the back years. Complete lists of works published will be furnished upon application.

DEALERS IN MEDICAL BOOKS will be supplied on the most favorable terms, and will be furnished with copies of this Catalogue, without charge, for distribution among their customers if desired.

CLASSIFIED INDEX

TO

LINDSAY & BLAKISTON'S PUBLICATIONS.

ANATOMY.

BRAIN AND NERVOUS SYSTEM.

CHEST, HEART, THROAT, ETC.

CHILDREN (DISEASES OF).

CANCER.

CHEMISTRY, BOTANY, ETC.

DEFORMITIES.

DENTAL SCIENCE.

DICTIONARIES.

EYE AND EAR.

ELECTRICITY.

FEMALES (DISEASES OF).

FEVERS.

FORENSIC MEDICINE & TOXICOLOGY.

GENERATIVE & URINARY ORGANS, SYPHILIS, ETC.

HYGIENE AND POPULAR MEDICINE.

KIDNEYS AND THE LIVER.

MATERIA MEDICA AND THERAPEUTICS.

MICROSCOPICAL.

MANUALS, ETC., FOR STUDENTS.

MISCELLANEOUS.

OBSTETRICS.

PRACTICE OF MEDICINE.

PATHOLOGY.

PHYSIOLOGY.

PHARMACEUTICAL.

RHEUMATISM, GOUT, ETC.

SURGERY.

STIMULANTS AND NARCOTICS.

SCIENTIFIC.

STOMACH, DIGESTION, ETC.

SKIN AND HAIR.

ATTHILL (LOMBE), M. D.,

Fellow and Examiner in Midwifery, King and Queen's College of Physicians, Dublin.

CLINICAL LECTURES ON DISEASES PECULIAR TO WOMEN. Second Edition, Revised and Enlarged, with Six Lithographic Plates and other Illustrations on Wood. Price $2.25

The value and popularity of this book is proved by the rapid sale of the first edition, which was exhausted in less than a year from the time of its publication. It appears to possess three great merits: First, It treats of the diseases very common to females. Second, It treats of them in a thoroughly clinical and practical manner. Third, It is concise, original, and illustrated by numerous cases from the author's own experience. His style is clear and the volume is the result of the author's large and accurate clinical observation recorded in a remarkable, perspicuous, and terse manner, and is conspicuous for the best qualities of a practical guide to the student and practitioner. — *British Medical Journal.*

ADAMS (WILLIAM), F. R. C. S.,

Surgeon to the Royal Orthopedic and Great Northern Hospitals.

CLUB-FOOT: ITS CAUSES, PATHOLOGY, AND TREATMENT. Being the Jacksonian Prize Essay of the Royal College of Surgeons. A New Revised and Enlarged Edition, with 106 Illustrations engraved on Wood, and Six Lithographic Plates. A large Octavo Volume. Price $6.00

ADAMS (ROBERT), M. D.,

Regius Professor of Surgery in the University of Dublin, &c., &c.

RHEUMATIC GOUT, OR CHRONIC RHEUMATIC ARTHRITIS OF ALL THE JOINTS. The Second Edition. Illustrated by numerous Woodcuts, and a quarto Atlas of Plates. 2 Volumes. Price $8.50

ALTHAUS (JULIUS), M.D.,

Physician to the Infirmary of Epilepsy and Paralysis.

A TREATISE ON MEDICAL ELECTRICITY, Theoretical and Practical, and its Use in the Treatment of Paralysis, Neuralgia, and other Diseases. Third Edition, Enlarged and Revised, with One Hundred and Forty-six Illustrations. In one volume octavo. Price . $6.00

In this work both the scientific and practical aspects of the subject are ably, concisely, and thoroughly treated. It is much the best work treating of the remedial effects of electricity in the English language. — *New York Medical Record.*

ARNOTT (HENRY), F.R.C.S.

CANCER: its Varieties, their Histology and Diagnosis. With Five Lithographic Plates and Twenty-two Wood Engravings. Price $2.25

AGNEW (D. HAYES), M.D.,

Professor of Surgery in the University of Pennsylvania.

THE LACERATIONS OF THE FEMALE PERINEUM, AND VESICO-VAGINAL FISTULA, their History and Treatment, with numerous Illustrations. Octavo. Price $2.00

Prof. Agnew has been a most indefatigable laborer in this department, and his work stands deservedly high in the estimation of the profession. It is well illustrated, and full descriptions of the operations and instruments employed are given. — *Canada Lancet.*

ACTON (WILLIAM), M.R.C.S., ETC.

THE FUNCTIONS AND DISORDERS OF THE REPRODUCTIVE ORGANS. In Childhood, Youth, Adult Age, and Advanced Life, considered in their Physiological, Social, and Moral Relations. Third American from the Fifth London Edition. Carefully revised by the Author, with additions. $3.00

Mr. Acton has done good service to society by grappling manfully with sexual vice, and we trust that others, whose position as men of science and teachers enable them to speak with authority, will assist in combating and arresting the evils which it entails. The spirit which pervades his book is one which does credit equally to the head and to the heart of the author. — *British and Foreign Medico-Chirurgical Review.*

SAME AUTHOR.

PROSTITUTION: Considered in its Moral, Social, and Sanitary Aspects. Second Edition, Enlarged. Price $5.00

ANSTIE (FRANCIS E.), M.D.,

Lecturer on Materia Medica and Therapeutics, etc.

STIMULANTS AND NARCOTICS. Their Mutual Relations, with Special Researches on the Action of Alcohol, Ether, and Chloroform on the Vital Organism. Octavo. $3.00

ANDERSON (M'CALL), M.D.,

Professor of Clinical Medicine in the University of Glasgow, &c.

ECZEMA. The Pathology and Treatment of the various Eczematous Affections or Eruptions of the Skin. The Third Revised and Enlarged Edition. Octavo. Price $2.75

BUZZARD (THOMAS), M. D.,

Physician to the National Hospital for Paralysis and Epilepsy.

CLINICAL ASPECTS OF SYPHILITIC NERVOUS AFFECTIONS. 12mo. Cloth. Price $1.75

BASHAM (W. R.), M.D., F.R.C.P.,

Senior Physician to the Westminster Hospital, &c.

AIDS TO THE DIAGNOSIS OF DISEASES OF THE KIDNEYS. With Ten large Plates. Sixty Illustrations. Price . $2.00

SAME AUTHOR.

ON DROPSY, AND ITS CONNECTION WITH DISEASES OF THE KIDNEYS, HEART, LUNGS AND LIVER. With Sixteen Plates. Third Edition. Octavo. $5.00

M. BARTH AND M. HENRI ROGER.

A MANUAL OF AUSCULTATION AND PERCUSSION. A new Translation, from the Sixth French Edition. $1.25

S. M. BRADLEY, F. R. C. S.

Senior Assistant Surgeon Manchester Royal Infirmary.

A MANUAL OF COMPARATIVE ANATOMY AND PHYSIOLOGY. With 60 Illustrations. Third Edition. Price . $2.50

BEALE (LIONEL S.), M.D.

DISEASE GERMS: AND ON THE TREATMENT OF DISEASES CAUSED BY THEM.

PART I.—SUPPOSED NATURE OF DISEASE GERMS.
PART II.—REAL NATURE OF DISEASE GERMS.
PART III.—THE DESTRUCTION OF DISEASE GERMS.

Second Edition, much enlarged, with Twenty-eight full-page Plates, containing 117 Illustrations, many of them colored. Demy Octavo. Price $5.00

This new edition, besides including the contents revised and enlarged of the two former editions published by Dr. Beale on Disease Germs, has an entirely new part added on "The Destruction of Disease Germs."

SAME AUTHOR.

BIOPLASM. A Contribution to the Physiology of Life, or an Introduction to the Study of Physiology and Medicine, for Students. With Numerous Illustrations. Price $3.00

This volume is intended as a TEXT-BOOK for Students of Physiology, explaining the nature of some of the most important changes which are characteristic of and peculiar to living beings.

PROTOPLASM, OR MATTER AND LIFE. Third Edition, very much Enlarged. Nearly 350 pages. Sixteen Colored Plates. One volume. Price $4.50

PART I. DISSENTIENT. PART II. DEMONSTRATIVE. PART III. SUGGESTIVE.

HOW TO WORK WITH THE MICROSCOPE. Fourth Edition, containing 400 Illustrations, many of them colored. Octavo. Price $7.50

This work is a complete manual of microscopical manipulation, and contains a full description of many new processes of investigation, with directions for examining objects under the highest powers, and for taking photographs of microscopic objects.

ON KIDNEY DISEASES, URINARY DEPOSITS, AND CALCULOUS DISORDERS. Including the Symptoms, Diagnosis, and Treatment of Urinary Diseases. With full Directions for the Chemical and Microscopical Analysis of the Urine in Health and Disease. The Third Edition. Seventy Plates, 415 figures, copied from Nature. Octavo. Price $10.00

THE USE OF THE MICROSCOPE IN PRACTICAL MEDICINE. For Students and Practitioners, with full directions for examining the various secretions, &c., in the Microscope. Fourth Edition. 500 Illustrations. Octavo. Preparing.

BLOXAM (C. L.),

Professor of Chemistry in King's College, London.

CHEMISTRY, INORGANIC AND ORGANIC. With Experiments and a Comparison of Equivalent and Molecular Formulæ. With 276 Engravings on Wood. Second Edition, carefully revised. Octavo. Price, in cloth, $4.50; leather, ... $5.50

SAME AUTHOR.

LABORATORY TEACHING; OR PROGRESSIVE EXERCISES IN PRACTICAL CHEMISTRY. Third Edition. With Eighty-nine Engravings. Crown Octavo. Price $2.00

BRODHURST (B. E.), F.R.C.S.,

Surgeon to the Orthopedic Department of St. George's Hospital, &c.

THE DEFORMITIES OF THE HUMAN BODY. A System of Orthopœdic Surgery. With numerous Illustrations. Octavo. Price $3.00

BIRCH (S. B.), M.D.,

Member of the Royal College of Physicians, &c.

CONSTIPATED BOWELS; the Various Causes and the Different Means of Cure. Third Edition. Price $1.00

BUCKNILL (JOHN CHARLES), M.D., & TUKE (DANIEL H.), M.D.

A MANUAL OF PSYCHOLOGICAL MEDICINE: containing the Lunacy Laws, the Nosology, Œtiology, Statistics, Description, Diagnosis, Pathology (including Morbid Histology), and Treatment of Insanity. Third Edition, much enlarged, with Ten Lithographic Plates, and numerous other Illustrations. Octavo. Price $8.00

This edition contains upwards of 200 pages of additional matter, and, in consequence of recent advances in Psychological Medicine, several chapters have been rewritten, bringing the Classification, Pathology, and Treatment of Insanity up to the present time.

There are ten lithographic plates representing the handwriting of the insane and the morbid cerebral changes revealed by the microscope, assisted by wood-engravings indicating the classification of the convolutions of the brain.

Thirty tracings of the pulse in various forms of insanity, made by the Sphygmograph, have also been added.

BIDDLE (JOHN B.), M. D.,

Professor of Materia Medica and Therapeutics in the Jefferson Medical College, Philadelphia, &c.

MATERIA MEDICA, FOR THE USE OF STUDENTS. With Illustrations. Sixth Edition, Revised and Enlarged. Price $4.00

This new and thoroughly revised edition of Professor Biddle's work has incorporated in it all the improvements as adopted by the New United States Pharmacopœia just issued. It is designed to present the leading facts and principles usually comprised under this head as set forth by the standard authorities, and to fill a vacuum which seems to exist in the want of an elementary work on the subject. The larger works usually recommended as text-books in our Medical schools are too voluminous for convenient use. This will be found to contain, in a condensed form, all that is most valuable, and will supply students with a reliable guide to the course of lectures on Materia Medica as delivered at the various Medical schools in the United States.

BYFORD (W. H.), A.M., M.D.,

Professor of Obstetrics and Diseases of Women and Children in the Chicago Medical College, &c.

PRACTICE OF MEDICINE AND SURGERY. Applied to the Diseases and Accidents incident to Women. Second Edition, Revised and Enlarged. Octavo. Price, cloth, $5.00; sheep . . $6.00

This work treats well-nigh all the diseases incident to women, diseases and accidents of the vulva and perineum, stone in the bladder, inflammation of the vagina, menstruation and its disorders, the uterus and its ailments, ovarian tumors, diseases of the mammæ, puerperal convulsions, phlegmasia alba dolens, puerperal fever, &c. Its scope is thus of the most extended character, yet the observations are concise, but convey much practical information. —*London Lancet.*

SAME AUTHOR.

ON THE CHRONIC INFLAMMATION AND DISPLACEMENT OF THE UNIMPREGNATED UTERUS. A New, Enlarged, and Thoroughly Revised Edition, with Numerous Illustrations. Octavo. $3

Dr. Byford writes the exact present state of medical knowledge on the subjects presented; and does this so clearly, so concisely, so truthfully, and so completely, that his book on the uterus will always meet the approval of the profession, and be everywhere regarded as a popular standard work. —*Buffalo Medical and Surgical Journal.*

BLACK (D. CAMPBELL), M. D.,

L. R. C. S. Edinburgh, Member of the General Council of the University of Glasgow, &c., &c.

THE FUNCTIONAL DISEASES OF THE RENAL, URINARY, and Reproductive Organs, with a General View of Urinary Pathology. Price $2.50

CONTENTS.

Chap. 1. On the Conditions that affect the Secretion of the Urine, with special reference to Suppression.
" 2. Retention of Urine; its Varieties, Causes, and Treatment.
" 3. Irritable Bladder, Strangury.
Chap. 4. On the Pathology and Treatment of Nocturnal Enuresis, and Spermatic Incontinence.
" 5. Sterility in the Male.
" 6. Male Impotence.
" 7. Anomalous Urethral Discharges.

The style of the author is clear, easy, and agreeable, . . . his work is a valuable contribution to medical science, and being penned in that disposition of unprejudiced philosophical inquiry which should always guide a true physician, admirably embodies the spirit of its opening quotation from Professor Huxley. — *Philada. Med. Times.*

BEASLEY (HENRY).

THE BOOK OF PRESCRIPTIONS. Containing over 3000 Prescriptions, collected from the Practice of the most Eminent Physicians and Surgeons—English, French, and American; comprising also a Compendious History of the Materia Medica, Lists of the Doses of all Officinal and Established Preparations, and an Index of Diseases and their Remedies. Fourth Edition, Revised and Enlarged. Price, $2.50

This NEW edition of Dr. Beasley's Prescription Book, although presented in a much more compact form and at a greatly reduced price, has been thoroughly revised, and an account of all the new medicines lately introduced, with the formulas of the new Pharmacopœias added. Carefully selecting from the mass of materials at his disposal, the author has aimed to compile a volume sufficiently comprehensive, in which both physician and druggist, prescriber and compounder, may find under the head of each remedy the manner in which that remedy may be most effectively administered, or combined with other medicines in the treatment of disease. The alphabetical arrangement of the book renders this easy. A short description of each medicine is also given, and a list of the doses in which its several preparations may be prescribed.

BY SAME AUTHOR.

THE POCKET FORMULARY: A Synopsis of the British and Foreign Pharmacopœias. Ninth Revised Edition. Price . $2.50

THE DRUGGIST'S GENERAL RECEIPT BOOK AND VETERINARY FORMULARY. Seventh Edition. Price. . . $3.50

BRUNTON (T. LAUDER), M.D., D.Sc.,

Lecturer on Materia Medica in the Medical College of St. Bartholomew's Hospital.

EXPERIMENTAL INVESTIGATION OF THE ACTION OF MEDICINES: A Hand-Book of Practical Pharmacology, with Engravings. Preparing.

BRANSTON (THOMAS F.).

HAND-BOOK OF PRACTICAL RECEIPTS. For the Chemist, Druggist, &c.; with a Glossary of Medical and Chemical Terms. $1.50

BEETON (MRS.).

BOOK OF HOUSEHOLD MANAGEMENT. Colored and other Illustrations. 1100 pages. $3.25

COHEN (I. SOLIS), M. D.

Lecturer on Laryngoscopy and Diseases of the Throat and Chest in Jefferson Medical College.

ON INHALATION. ITS THERAPEUTICS AND PRACTICE. Including a Description of the Apparatus employed, &c. With Cases and Illustrations. Price $2.50

SAME AUTHOR.

CROUP. In its Relations to Tracheotomy. Price . . $1.00

CARSON (JOSEPH), M.D.,

Professor of Materia Medica and Pharmacy in the University.

A HISTORY OF THE MEDICAL DEPARTMENT OF THE UNIVERSITY OF PENNSYLVANIA, from its Foundation in 1765: with Sketches of Deceased Professors, &c. $2.00

The history of the University of Pennsylvania has a national as well as a local interest, from the early date of its origination, and the connection with it of men of illustrious public reputation, such as Drs. Franklin, Rush, Physick, Gibson, Dewees, Chapman, Wood, &c., &c. For the labor and love which he has spent in preparing this most interesting and valuable work, Prof. Carson has earned the gratitude of the alumni of the University, and of all others interested in medical education in this country. — *American Journal of Medical Science.*

CARPENTER (W. B.), M.D., F.R.S.

THE MICROSCOPE AND ITS REVELATIONS. The Fifth London Edition, Revised and Enlarged, with more than 500 Illustrations. $5.50

SAME AUTHOR.

PRINCIPLES OF HUMAN PHYSIOLOGY. The Seventh Revised and Enlarged Edition. With nearly 300 Illustrations on Steel and Wood. Edited by Mr. HENRY POWER. Octavo. . . $11.25

CHAVASSE (P. HENRY), F.R.C.S.,

Author of Advice to a Wife, Advice to a Mother, &c.

APHORISMS ON THE MENTAL CULTURE AND TRAINING OF A CHILD, and on various other subjects relating to Health and Happiness. Addressed to Parents. Price $1.50

Dr. Chavasse's works have been very favorably received and had a large circulation, the value of his advice to WIVES and MOTHERS having thus been very generally recognized. This book is a sequel or companion to them, and it will be found both valuable and important to all who have the care of families, and who want to bring up their children to become useful men and women. It is full of fresh thoughts and graceful illustrations.

CLARKE (W. FAIRLIE), M.D.,

Assistant Surgeon to Charing Cross Hospital.

CLARKE'S TREATISE ON DISEASES OF THE TONGUE. With Lithographic and Wood-cut Illustrations. Octavo. Price $5.00

It contains The Anatomy and Physiology of the Tongue, Importance of its Minute Examination, Its Congenital Defects, Atrophy, Hypertrophy, Parasitic Diseases, Inflammation, Syphilis and its effects, Various Tumors to which it is subject, Accidents, Injuries, &c., &c.

COOPER (S.).

A DICTIONARY OF PRACTICAL SURGERY AND ENCYCLOPÆDIA OF SURGICAL SCIENCE. New Edition, brought down to the present time. By SAMUEL A. LANE, F.R.C.S., assisted by other eminent Surgeons. In two vols., of over 1000 pages each. $15.00

CLAY (CHARLES), M. D.

Fellow of the London Obstetrical Society, &c.

THE COMPLETE HAND-BOOK OF OBSTETRIC SURGERY, or, Short Rules of Practice in Every Emergency, from the Simplest to the most Formidable Operations in the Practice of Surgery. First American from the Third London Edition. With numerous Illustrations. In one volume. $2.25

CHAMBERS (THOMAS K.), M. D.,

LECTURES, CHIEFLY CLINICAL. Illustrative of a Restorative System of Medicine.

CHEW (SAMUEL), M.D.,

Late Professor of the Practice of Medicine in the University of Maryland.

MEDICAL EDUCATION. A Course of Lectures on the Proper Method of Studying Medicine. $1.00

This is a most excellent manual for the student, as well as a refreshing and suggestive one to the practitioner. —*Lancet and Observer.*

COBBOLD (T. SPENCER), M.D., F.R.S.

WORMS: a Series of Lectures delivered at the Middlesex Hospital on Practical Helminthology. Post Octavo. $2.00

CLEAVELAND (C. H.), M.D.,

Member of the American Medical Association, &c.

A PRONOUNCING MEDICAL LEXICON. Containing the Correct Pronunciation and Definition of Terms used in Medicine and the Collateral Sciences. Improved Edition, Cloth, $1.25; Tucks, $1.50

This work is not only a Lexicon of all the words in common use in Medicine, but it is also a Pronouncing Dictionary, a feature of great value to Medical Students. To the Dispenser it will prove an excellent aid, and also to the Pharmaceutical Student. It has received strong commendation both from the Medical Press and from the profession.

COLES (OAKLEY), D.D.S.

Dental Surgeon to the Hospital for Diseases of the Throat, &c.

A MANUAL OF DENTAL MECHANICS. Containing much information of a Practical Nature for Practitioners and Students.

INCLUDING

The Preparation of the Mouth for Artificial Teeth, on Taking Impressions, Various Modes of Applying Heat in the Laboratory, Casting in Plaster of Paris and Metal, Precious Metals used in Dentistry, Making Gold Plates, Various Forms of Porcelain used in Mechanical Dentistry, Pivot Teeth, Choosing and Adjusting Mineral Teeth, the Vulcanite Base, the Celluloid Base, Treatment of Deformities of the Mouth, Receipts for Making Gold Plate and Solder, etc., etc.

With 140 Illustrations. Price $2.50

SAME AUTHOR.

ON DEFORMITIES OF THE MOUTH, CONGENITAL AND ACQUIRED, with their Mechanical Treatment. By JAMES OAKLEY COLES, D.D.S., Member of the Odontological Society, etc., etc. Second Edition, Revised and Enlarged. With Eight Colored Engravings and Fifty-one Illustrations on Wood. Price . . $2.50

The second edition of this work shows that the author has continued to devote himself with zeal to the investigation and treatment of a very interesting class of cases. He has especially studied the congenital cleft palate, and has, with the mirror, detected in several cases growths in the naso-pharyngeal tonsil. We recommend the work to the study of both surgeons and dentists. —*London Lancet.*

CLARK (F. LE GROS), F. R. S.,

Senior Surgeon to St. Thomas's Hospital.

OUTLINES OF SURGERY AND SURGICAL PATHOLOGY, including the Diagnosis and Treatment of Obscure and Urgent Cases, and the Surgical Anatomy of some Important Structures and Regions. Assisted by W. W. WAGSTAFFE, F. R. C. S., Resident Assistant-Surgeon of, and Joint Lecturer on Anatomy at, St. Thomas's Hospital. Second Edition, Revised and Enlarged. Price $3.00

This edition brings the work up to the highest level of our present knowledge, incorporating all that is sound and recent in Physiology so far as it relates to subjects requiring its aid. It is not alone an admirable exposition of the principles of Surgery, but a trusty guide to the emergencies of Practice. We cannot too highly estimate the ability to condense and the results of a ripened experience furnished to us here in a readable and practical form.—*Med. Times and Gazette.*

COOLEY (A. J.).

CYCLOPÆDIA OF PRACTICAL RECEIPTS. Containing Processes and Collateral Information in the Arts, Manufactures, Professions, and Trades, including Medicine, Pharmacy, and Domestic Economy; designed as a General Book of Reference for the Manufacturer, Tradesman, Amateur, and Heads of Families. The Fifth Edition, Revised and partly Rewritten by RICHARD V. TUSON, F.C.S., &c. Over 1000 royal-octavo pages, double columns. With Illustrations. Price $10.00

Every part of this edition has been subjected to a thorough and complete revision by the editor, assisted by other scientific gentlemen. In the chemical portion of the book, every subject of practical importance has been retained, corrected, and added to; to the name of every substance of established composition a formula has been attached; while to the Pharmaceutist its value has been greatly increased by the additions which have been made from the British, Indian, and United States Pharmacopœias.

CAZEAUX (P.), M. D.,

Adjunct Professor of the Faculty of Medicine, Paris, etc.

A THEORETICAL AND PRACTICAL TREATISE ON MIDWIFERY, including the Diseases of Pregnancy and Parturition. Translated from the Seventh French Edition, Revised, Greatly Enlarged, and Improved, by S. TARNIER, Clinical Chief of the Lying-In Hospital, Paris, etc., with numerous Lithographic and other Illustrations. Price, in Cloth, $6.50; in Leather, $7.50.

M. Cazeaux's Great Work on Obstetrics has become classical in its character, and almost an Encyclopædia in its fulness. Written expressly for the use of students of medicine, its teachings are plain and explicit, presenting a condensed summary of the leading principles established by the masters of the obstetric art, and such clear, practical directions for the management of the pregnant, parturient, and puerperal states, as have been sanctioned by the most authoritative practitioners, and confirmed by the author's own experience.

DOBELL (HORACE), M. D.,

Senior Physician to the Hospital.

WINTER COUGH (CATARRH, BRONCHITIS, EMPHYSEMA, ASTHMA). Lectures Delivered at the Royal Hospital for Diseases of the Chest. The Third Enlarged Edition, with Colored Plates. Octavo. Price $3.50

This work has been thoroughly revised. Two new Lectures have been added—viz., Lecture IV., "On the Natural Course of Neglected Winter Cough, and on the Interdependence of Winter Cough with other Diseases;" Lecture IX., "On Change of Climate in Winter Cough." Also additional matter on Post-nasal Catarrh, Ear-Cough, Artificial Respiration as a means of Treatment, Laryngoscopy, New Methods and Instruments in Treating of Emphysema, a good Index, and Colored Plates, with appended Diagnostic Physical signs.

DIXON (JAMES), F.R.C.S.,

Surgeon to the Royal London Ophthalmic Hospital, &c.

A GUIDE TO THE PRACTICAL STUDY OF DISEASES OF THE EYE, with an Outline of their Medical and Operative Treatment, with Test Types and Illustrations. Third Edition, thoroughly Revised, and a great portion Rewritten. Price $2.50

Mr. Dixon's book is essentially a practical one, written by an observant author, who brings to his special subject a sound knowledge of general Medicine and Surgery.—*Dublin Quarterly*.

DILLNBERGER (DR. EMIL).

A HANDY-BOOK OF THE TREATMENT OF WOMEN AND CHILDREN'S DISEASES, according to the Vienna Medical School. Part I. The Diseases of Women. Part II. The Diseases of Children. Translated from the Second German Edition, by P. NICOL, M.D. Price $1.75

Many practitioners will be glad to possess this little manual, which gives a large mass of practical hints on the treatment of diseases which probably make up the larger half of every-day practice. The translation is well made, and explanations of reference to German medicinal preparations are given with proper fulness. — *The Practitioner*.

DARLINGTON (WILLIAM), M.D.

FLORA CESTRICA; OR, HERBORIZING COMPANION. Containing all the Plants of the Middle States, their Linnæan Arrangement, a Glossary of Botanical Terms, a complete Index, &c. Third Edition. 12mo. $2.25

DUCHENNE (DR. G. B.).

LOCALIZED ELECTRIZATION AND ITS APPLICATION TO PATHOLOGY AND THERAPEUTICS. Translated by HERBERT TIBBITS, M.D. With Ninety-two Illustrations. Price . $3.00

Duchenne's great work is not only a well-nigh exhaustive treatise on the medical uses of Electricity, but it is also an elaborate exposition of the different diseases in which Electricity has proved to be of value as a therapeutic and diagnostic agent.

PART II., illustrated by chromo-lithographs and numerous wood-cuts, is preparing.

DURKEE (SILAS), M.D.,

Fellow of the Massachusetts Medical Society, &c.

GONORRHŒA AND SYPHILIS. The Fifth Edition, Revised and Enlarged, with Portraits and Eight Colored Illustrations. Octavo. Price $5.00

Dr. Durkee's work impresses the reader in favor of the author by its general tone, the thorough honesty everywhere evinced, the skill with which the book is arranged, the manner in which the facts are cited, the clever way in which the author's experience is brought in, the lucidity of the reasoning, and the care with which the therapeutics of venereal complaints are treated. — *Lancet*.

DRUITT (ROBERT), F.R.C.S.

THE SURGEON'S VADE-MECUM. A Manual of Modern Surgery. The Tenth Revised and Enlarged Edition, with 350 Illustrations. $5.00

DALBY (W. B.), F. R. C. S.,

Aural Surgeon to St. George's Hospital.

LECTURES ON THE DISEASES AND INJURIES OF THE EAR. Delivered at St. George's Hospital. With Illustrations. Price $1.50

This admirable little volume by Mr. Dalby, the accomplished aural surgeon to St. George's Hospital, consists of eleven lectures delivered by him at that institution. With a modest aim, this work, the latest issued by the English press on Aural Surgery, is happy in conception and pleasantly written; further, it shows that its author is thoroughly *au fait* in his specialty. The subject of which the volume treats is handled in a terse style, and this, if we mistake not, will make it acceptable to the student and practitioner who have a just horror of unnecessary details. In conclusion, we hope that we have succeeded in interesting our readers in the volume. We cordially recommend it as a trustworthy guide in the treatment of the affections of the ear. The book is moderate in price, beautifully illustrated by wood-cuts, and got up in the best style. — *Glasgow Medical Journal.*

DUNGLISON (ROBLEY), M. D.,

Late Professor of Institutes of Medicine, &c., in the Jefferson Medical College.

A HISTORY OF MEDICINE, from the Earliest Ages to the Commencement of the Nineteenth Century. Edited by his son, RICHARD J. DUNGLISON, M.D. $2.50

ELLIS (EDWARD), M. D.

Physician to the Victoria Hospital for Sick Children, &c.

A PRACTICAL MANUAL OF THE DISEASES OF CHILDREN, with a Formulary. Second Edition, Revised and Improved. One volume. $2.75

The AUTHOR, in issuing this new edition of his book, says: "I have very carefully revised each chapter, adding several new sections, and making considerable additions where the subjects seemed to require fuller treatment, without, however, sacrificing conciseness or unduly increasing the bulk of the volume."

ELAM (CHARLES), M.D., F.R.C.P.

ON CEREBRIA AND OTHER DISEASES OF THE BRAIN. Octavo. $2.50

FOTHERGILL (J. MILNER), M. D.

THE HEART AND ITS DISEASES, AND THEIR TREATMENT. With Illustrations. Octavo. Price $5.00

This work gives to the reader a concise view of Cardiac Diseases, uniting the most recent information as to the cause of heart-disease, with German Pathology and the latest advances in Therapeutics. It is designed to fill the gap between our standard works and the present position of our knowledge in diseases of the heart.

BY SAME AUTHOR.

DIGITALIS. Its Mode of Action and its Use, illustrating the Effect of Remedial Agents over Diseased Conditions of the Heart. Price $1.25

FAGGE (C. HILTON), M. D., F.R.C.P.,

Senior Assistant Physician and Demonstrator of Morbid Anatomy at Guy's Hospital.

THE PRINCIPLES AND PRACTICE OF MEDICINE. In preparation.

FOX (JOSEPH), D.D.S.,

Lecturer on the Structure and Diseases of the Teeth at Guy's Hospital.

THE NATURAL HISTORY, DISEASES AND STRUCTURE OF THE HUMAN TEETH, with 250 Illustrations. Price . $4.00

FOSTER (BALTHAZAR), M.D.,

Professor of Medicine in Queen's College.

LECTURES AND ESSAYS ON CLINICAL MEDICINE. Revised and Enlarged by the Author. With Engravings. Octavo. Price $3.50

FRANKLAND (E.), M. D., F. R. S., &c.

HOW TO TEACH CHEMISTRY, being the substance of Six Lectures to Science Teachers. Reported, with the Author's sanction, by G. George Chaloner, F. C. S., &c. Nearly ready.

FENWICK (SAMUEL), M.D., F.R.C.P.

THE MORBID STATES OF THE STOMACH AND DUODENUM, AND THEIR RELATIONS TO THE DISEASES OF OTHER ORGANS. With Ten Plates. $5.00

FLINT (AUSTIN), M.D.,

Professor of the Principles and Practice of Medicine, &c., Bellevue Hospital College, New York.

CLINICAL REPORTS ON CONTINUED FEVER. Based on an Analysis of One Hundred and Sixty-four Cases, with Remarks on the Management of Continued Fever; the Identity of Typhus and Typhoid Fever; Diagnosis, &c., &c. Octavo. Price . . $2.00

GANT (FREDERICK J.), F. R. C. S.,

Surgeon to the Royal Free Hospital, &c.

THE IRRITABLE BLADDER. Its Causes and Curative Treatment; including a Practical View of Urinary Pathology, Deposits, and Calculi. Third Edition, Revised and Enlarged. With New Illustrations. Price $2.50

The fact that a third edition of this book has been required seems to be sufficient proof of its value. The author has carefully revised and added such additional matter as to make it more complete and practically useful.

GODFREY (BENJAMIN), M.D., F.R.A.S.

THE DISEASES OF HAIR: a Popular Treatise upon the Affections of the Hair System. $1.50

GROSS (SAMUEL D.), M.D.,

Professor of Surgery in the Jefferson Medical College, Philadelphia, &c.

AMERICAN MEDICAL BIOGRAPHY OF THE NINETEENTH CENTURY. With a Portrait of BENJAMIN RUSH, M.D. Octavo. $3.50

GREENHOW (E. HEADLAM), M.D.,

Fellow of the Royal College of Physicians, &c.

ON CHRONIC BRONCHITIS, Especially as Connected with Gout, Emphysema, and Diseases of the Heart. Price . . . $2.00

Of all works yet written on Chronic Bronchitis, this is undoubtedly the best. The style is clear and to the point, and the principles of pathology and treatment eminently correct and practical. It is a positive addition to our medical literature.—*Journal Psychological Medicine.*

HARLEY (GEORGE), M. D., F. R. C. P.,

Physician to University College Hospital.

THE URINE AND ITS DERANGEMENTS: With the Application of Physiological Chemistry to the Diagnosis and Treatment of Constitutional as well as Local Diseases; being a Course of Lectures delivered at University College. With Engravings. Price $2.75

CONTENTS.

1. What is Urine?
2. Changes in the Composition of the Urine, induced by Food, Drink, Medicine, and Disease.
3. Urea, Ammonæmia, Uræmia.
4. Uric Acid.
5. Hippuric Acid, Chloride of Sodium.
6. Urohæmatin, Abnormal Pigments in Urine.
7. Phosphoric Acid, Phosphatic Gravel and Calculi.
8. Oxalic Acid, Oxaluria, Mulberry Calculi.
9. Inosite in Urine, Creatin and Creatinine, Cholesterin, Cystin, Xanthin, Leucin, Tyrosin.
10. Diabetes Mellitus.
11. Albuminuria.

On the whole, we have here a valuable addition to the library of the practising physician; not only for the information which it contains, but also for the suggestive way in which many of the subjects are treated, as well as for the fact that it contains the ideas of one who thoroughly believes in the future capabilities of Therapeutics based on Physiological facts, and in the important service to be rendered by Chemistry to Physiological investigation.
American Journal of the Medical Science.

HABERSHON (S. O.), M. D.,

Physician to Guy's Hospital, &c.

ON THE DISEASES OF THE LIVER. Their Pathology and Treatment. Being the Lettsonian Lectures, delivered at the Medical Society of London, 1872. Price $1.50

These Lectures contain within a brief compass a large amount of information and many practical suggestions that cannot fail to be of great value to every practitioner.
Dublin Medical Journal.

HEWITT (GRAILY), M. D.,

Physician to the British Lying-in Hospital, and Lecturer on Diseases of Women and Children, &c.

THE DIAGNOSIS, PATHOLOGY, AND TREATMENT OF DISEASES OF WOMEN, including the Diagnosis of Pregnancy. Founded on a Course of Lectures delivered at St. Mary's Hospital Medical School. The Third Edition, Revised and Enlarged, with new Illustrations. Octavo. Price in Cloth . . . $5.00
" Leather . . . 6.00

This new edition of Dr. Hewitt's book has been so much modified, that it may be considered substantially a new book; very much of the matter has been entirely rewritten, and the whole work has been rearranged in such a manner as to present a most decided improvement over previous editions. Dr. Hewitt is the leading clinical teacher on Diseases of Women in London, and the characteristic attention paid to Diagnosis by him has given his work great popularity there. It may unquestionably be considered the most valuable guide to correct Diagnosis to be found in the English language.

HILLIER (THOMAS), M.D.,

Physician to the Hospital for Sick Children, &c.

A CLINICAL TREATISE ON THE DISEASES OF CHILDREN. Octavo. Price $3.00

We have said enough to indicate and illustrate the excellence of Dr. Hillier's volume. It is eminently the kind of book needed by all medical men who wish to cultivate clinical accuracy and sound practice.—*London Lancet.*

HOLDEN (LUTHER), F.R.C.S.

HUMAN OSTEOLOGY, comprising a Description of the Bones with Delineations of the Attachments of the Muscles, &c. With numerous Illustrations. Fifth Edition, carefully Revised. Price, $6.00

HOLDEN'S MANUAL OF DISSECTIONS. Price . $5.00

HARRIS (CHAPIN A.), M. D., D. D. S.

Late President of and Professor of the Principles and Practice of Dental Surgery in the Baltimore College, &c.

THE PRINCIPLES AND PRACTICE OF DENTISTRY. Tenth Revised Edition. In great part rewritten, rearranged, and with many new and important Illustrations. Including—1. Dental Anatomy and Physiology. 2. Dental Pathology and Therapeutics. 3. Dental Surgery. 4. Dental Mechanics. Edited by P. H. AUSTEN, M.D., Professor of Dental Science and Mechanism in the Baltimore College of Dental Surgery. With nearly 400 Illustrations, including many new ones made especially for this edition. Royal octavo. Price, in cloth, $6.50; in leather $7.50

This new edition of Dr. Harris's work has been thoroughly revised in all its parts—more so than any previous edition. So great have been the advances in many branches of dentistry, that it was found necessary to rewrite the articles or subjects, and this has been done in the most efficient manner by Professor Austen, for many years an associate and friend of Dr. Harris, assisted by Professor Gorgas and Thomas S. Latimer, M.D. The publishers feel assured that it will now be found the most complete text-book for the student and guide for the practitioner in the English language.

SAME AUTHOR.

A DICTIONARY OF MEDICAL TERMINOLOGY, DENTAL SURGERY, AND THE COLLATERAL SCIENCES. Third Edition, Carefully Revised and Enlarged, by FERDINAND J. S. GORGAS, M. D., D.D.S., Professor of Dental Surgery in the Baltimore College, &c., &c. Royal octavo. Price, in cloth, $6.50; in leather . . . $7.50

The many advances in Dental Science rendered it necessary that this edition should be thoroughly revised, which has been done in the most satisfactory manner by Professor Gorgas, Dr. Harris's successor in the Baltimore Dental College, he having added nearly three thousand new words, besides making many additions and corrections. The doses of the more prominent medicinal agents have also been added, and in every way the book has been greatly improved, and its value enhanced as a work of reference.

HANDY (WASHINGTON R.), M.D.

Late Professor of Anatomy, &c., in the Baltimore College.

A TEXT-BOOK OF ANATOMY, AND GUIDE TO DISSECTIONS. For the Use of Students of Medicine and Dental Surgery. With 312 Illustrations. Octavo. Price $4.00

Dr. Handy's work was prepared with special reference to the wants of the Student and Practitioner of Dental Surgery. Directing particular attention to the Mouth, it shows step by step the important Anatomical and Physiological relations which it has with each and all the organs and functions of the general system.

HARDWICH AND DAWSON.

HARDWICH'S MANUAL OF PHOTOGRAPHIC CHEMISTRY. With Engravings. Eighth Edition. Edited and Rearranged by G. DAWSON, Lecturer on Photography, &c., &c. 12mo. . . $2.00

The object of the Editor has been to give practical instruction in this fascinating art, and to lead the novice from first principles to the higher branches, impressing him with the value of care and exactness in every operation.

HEADLAND (F. W.), M. D.,

Fellow of the Royal College of Physicians, &c., &c.

ON THE ACTION OF MEDICINES IN THE SYSTEM. Sixth American from the Fourth London Edition. Revised and Enlarged. Octavo. Price $3.00

Dr. Headland's work gives the only scientific and satisfactory view of the action of medicine; and this not in the way of idle speculation, but by demonstration and experiments, and inferences almost as indisputable as demonstrations. It is truly a great scientific work in a small compass, and deserves to be the hand-book of every lover of the Profession. It has received the approbation of the *Medical Press*, both in this country and in Europe, and is pronounced by them to be the most *original* and practically useful work that has been issued for many years.

HILLES (M. W.),

Formerly Lecturer on Anatomy, &c., at Westminster Hospital.

THE POCKET ANATOMIST. Being a Complete Description of the Anatomy of the Human Body; for the Use of Students. Price, in cloth, $1.00; in Pocket-book form $1.25

HEATH (CHRISTOPHER), F.R.C.S.,

Surgeon to University College Hospital, &c.

INJURIES AND DISEASES OF THE JAWS. The Jacksonian Prize Essay of the Royal College of Surgeons of England, 1867. Second Edition, Revised, with over 150 Illustrations. Octavo. Price, $5.00

SAME AUTHOR.

A MANUAL OF MINOR SURGERY AND BANDAGING, for the Use of House Surgeons, Dressers, and Junior Practitioners. With a Formulæ and Numerous Illustrations. 16mo. Price . $2.25

HOLMES (T. M. A.),

Surgeon and Lecturer on Surgery to St. George's Hospital, &c.

THE SURGICAL TREATMENT OF THE DISEASES OF INFANCY AND CHILDHOOD. Second Edition, Revised and Enlarged, containing Seven large Colored Plates and over One Hundred other Illustrations. Price $5.00

HUFELAND (C. W.), M. D.

THE ART OF PROLONGING LIFE. Edited by ERASMUS WILSON, M. D., F. R. S., &c. 12mo. Cloth. $1.25

The highly practical character of Dr. Hufeland's book, the sound advice which it contains, and its elevated moral tone, recommend it for extensive circulation both among professional and non-professional readers.

HEWSON (ADDINELL,) M. D.

Attending Surgeon Pennsylvania Hospital, &c.

EARTH AS A TOPICAL APPLICATION IN SURGERY. Being a full Exposition of its use in all the Cases requiring Topical Applications admitted in the Surgical Wards of the Pennsylvania Hospital during a period of Six Months. With Four full-page Illustrations.

CONTENTS.

Preface; Introduction; Histories of Cases; Comments as to the Effects of the Contact of the Earth; Its Effects on Pain; Its Power as a Deodorizer; Its Influence over Inflammation; Its Influence over Putrefaction; Its Influence over the Healing Processes; Modus Operandi of the Earth; As a Deodorizer and other Putrefaction; In its Effects on Living Parts.

Price, ... $2.50

It presents the results of researches by the author into the action of Earth as a surgical dressing, and embraces the histories of over ninety cases which occurred in the wards of the Pennsylvania Hospital some three years since, but whose publication has been delayed, for the double purpose of weighing them by subsequent experience, and of interpreting their meaning by a careful study of the various subjects which they involve.

HODGE (HUGH L.), M. D.

Emeritus Professor in the University of Pennsylvania.

HODGE ON FŒTICIDE, OR CRIMINAL ABORTION. Fourth Edition. Price, in paper covers, ... $0.30
" flexible cloth, ... 0.50

This little book is intended to place in the hands of professional men and others the means of answering satisfactorily and intelligently any inquiries that may be made of them in connection with this important subject.

HOLDEN (EDGAR), A. M., M. D.,

Of Newark, New Jersey.

CONTAINING THREE HUNDRED ILLUSTRATIONS.

THE SPHYGMOGRAPH. Its Physiological and Pathological Indications. The Essay to which was awarded the Stevens Triennial Prize in the College of Physicians and Surgeons in New York, April, 1873. Illustrated by Three Hundred Engravings on Wood. One volume octavo. Price. $3.00

HOOD (P.), M.D.

A TREATISE ON GOUT, RHEUMATISM, AND THE ALLIED AFFECTIONS. Crown octavo. $4.25

HANCOCK (HENRY), F.R.C.S.

ON THE OPERATIVE SURGERY OF THE FOOT AND ANKLE. Numerous Illustrations. Octavo. . . . $6.00

JONES (T. WHARTON), F.R.S.

DEFECTS OF SIGHT AND HEARING. Their Nature, Causes, Prevention, &c. Second Edition. Price $1.25

JONES, SIEVEKING, AND PAYNE.

A MANUAL OF PATHOLOGICAL ANATOMY. By C. HANDFIELD JONES, M. D., F. R. S., Physician to St. Mary's Hospital; and EDWARD H. SIEVEKING, M.D., F.R.C.P., Physician to St. Mary's Hospital. A New and Enlarged Edition. Edited by J. F. PAYNE, M.B., F.R.C.P., Assistant Physician and Lecturer on Morbid Anatomy at St. Thomas's Hospital. With Numerous Illustrations. . . $6.00

LAWSON (GEORGE), F.R.C.S.,

Surgeon to the Royal London Ophthalmic Hospital.

DISEASES AND INJURIES OF THE EYE, THEIR MEDICAL AND SURGICAL TREATMENT. Containing a Formulary, Test Types, and Numerous Illustrations. Price $2.50

This Manual is admirably clear and eminently practical. The reader feels that he is in the hands of a teacher who has a right to speak with authority, and who, if he may be said to be positive, is so from the fulness of knowledge and experience, and who, while well acquainted with the writings and labors of other authorities on the matters he treats of, has himself practically worked out what he teaches. — *London Medical Times and Gazette.*

LEBER & ROTTENSTEIN (DRS.).

DENTAL CARIES AND ITS CAUSES. An Investigation into the Influence of Fungi in the destruction of the Teeth, translated by THOMAS H. CHANDLER, D.M.D., Professor of Mechanical Dentistry in the Dental School of Harvard University. With Illustrations. Octavo. Price $1.50

This work is now considered the best and most elaborate work on Dental Caries. It is everywhere quoted and relied upon as authority by the profession, who have seen it in the original, and by authors writing on the subject.

LEGG (J. WICKHAM), M. D.

Member of the Royal College of Physicians, &c.

A GUIDE TO THE EXAMINATION OF THE URINE. For the Practitioner and Student. Third Edition. 16mo. Cloth. Price, $0.75

Dr. Legg's little manual has met with remarkable success; the speedy exhaustion of two editions has enabled the author to make certain emendations which add greatly to its value. It can confidently be commended to the student as a safe and reliable guide.

LEARED (ARTHUR), M.D., F.R.C.P.

IMPERFECT DIGESTION: ITS CAUSES AND TREATMENT. The Fifth Edition, Revised and Enlarged. $1.75

LESCHER (F. HARWOOD).

THE ELEMENTS OF PHARMACY. For Students. The Fourth Edition, Revised and Enlarged. Octavo. $3.00

LIEBREICH (DR.).

ATLAS OF OPHTHALMOSCOPY: Representing the Normal and Pathological Conditions of the Fundus Oculi as seen with the Ophthalmoscope. Composed of Twelve Chromo-lithographic Plates (containing Fifty-nine Figures), accompanied by an Explanatory Text, translated into English. Second Edition, Enlarged and Revised. 4to. $15.00

LIVEING (EDWARD), M.D.

ON MEGRIM, SICK-HEADACHE, AND SOME ALLIED DISORDERS. With Colored Plate. Octavo. $6.00

LEWIN (DR. GEORGE).

Professor at the Fr.-Wilh. University, and Surgeon-in-Chief of the Syphilitic Wards and Skin Diseases of the Charity Hospital, Berlin.

THE TREATMENT OF SYPHILIS by Subcutaneous Sublimate Injections. With a Lithographic Plate illustrating the Mode and Proper Place of administering the Injections, and of the Syringe used for the purpose. Translated by CARL PRŒGLER, M.D., late Surgeon in the Prussian Service, and E. H. GALE, M.D., late Surgeon in the United States Army. Price $2.25

The great number of cases treated, some fourteen hundred, within a period of four years, in the wards of the Charity Hospital, Berlin, only twenty of which were returned on account of Syphilitic relapses, certainly entitles the method of treatment advocated by this distinguished syphilographer to the attention of all physicians under whose notice syphilitic cases come.

LIZARS (JOHN), M. D.

Late Professor of Surgery in the Royal College of Surgeons, Edinburgh.

THE USE AND ABUSE OF TOBACCO. From the Eighth Edinburgh Edition. 12mo. Price, in flexible cloth, . $0.60

This little work contains a History of the introduction of Tobacco, its general characteristics; practical observations upon its effects on the system; the opinion of celebrated professional men in regard to it, together with cases illustrating its deleterious influence, &c., &c.

MACNAMARA (C.).

Surgeon to the Ophthalmic Hospital, and Professor of Ophthalmic Medicine in the Medical College, Calcutta.

MANUAL OF THE DISEASES OF THE EYE. The Second Edition, carefully Revised; with Additions, and numerous Colored Plates, Diagrams of the Eye, many Illustrations on Wood, Snellen's Test Types, &c., &c. Price $5.00

"This work when first published took its place in medical literature as the most complete, condensed, and well-arranged manual on ophthalmic surgery in the English language. Arranged especially for medical students, it became, however, the work of reference for the busy practitioner, who could obtain nearly all that was best worth knowing on this subject, tersely stated, and easily found by the aid of the excellent marginal notes on the contents of the paragraphs." —*Philadelphia Medical Times.*

MACKENZIE (MORELL), M. D.

Physician to the Hospital for Diseases of the Throat, London, &c.

GROWTHS IN THE LARYNX. Their History, Causes, Symptoms, Diagnosis, Pathology, Prognosis, and Treatment. With Reports and Analysis of One Hundred Consecutive Cases treated by the Author; and a Tabular Statement of every published case treated since the invention of the Laryngoscope. With numerous Colored and other Illustrations. Octavo. Price $3.00

Dr. Mackenzie's position has given him great advantages and a large experience in the treatment of Diseases of the Throat, and for many years he has been regarded as a leading authority in this department of Surgery. The Illustrations have been prepared with great care and expense.

OTHER WORKS BY SAME AUTHOR.

THE LARYNGOSCOPE IN DISEASES OF THE THROAT. With an Appendix on Rhinoscopy, and an Essay on Hoarseness and Loss of Voice. With Additions by J. SOLIS COHEN, and Numerous Illustrations on Wood and Stone. Price $3.00

PHARMACOPŒIA OF THE HOSPITAL for Diseases of the Throat; with One Hundred and Fifty Formulæ for Gargles, &c., &c. Price $1.25

MEIGS AND PEPPER.

A PRACTICAL TREATISE ON THE DISEASES OF CHILDREN. By J. FORSYTH MEIGS, M.D., Fellow of the College of Physicians of Philadelphia, &c., &c., and WILLIAM PEPPER, M.D., Physician to the Philadelphia Hospital, &c. Fifth Edition, thoroughly Revised and greatly Enlarged, forming a Royal Octavo Volume of over 1000 pages. Price, bound in cloth, $6.00; leather $7.00

It is the most complete work on the subject in our language. It contains at once the results of personal, and the experience of others. Its quotations from the most recent authorities, at home and abroad, are ample, and we think the authors deserve congratulations for having produced a book unequalled for the use of the student and indispensable as a work of reference for the practitioner. — *American Medical Journal.*

MURPHY (JOHN G.), M.D.

A REVIEW OF CHEMISTRY FOR STUDENTS. Adapted to the Courses as Taught in the Principal Medical Schools in the United States. $1.25

MENDENHALL (GEORGE), M.D.,

Professor of Obstetrics in the Medical College of Ohio, &c.

MEDICAL STUDENT'S VADE MECUM. A Compendium of Anatomy, Physiology, Chemistry, the Practice of Medicine, Surgery, Obstetrics, Diseases of the Skin, Materia Medica, Pharmacy, Poisons, &c., &c. Eleventh Edition, Revised and Enlarged, with 224 Illustrations. $2.50

MAXSON (EDWIN R.), M.D.,

Formerly Lecturer on the Practice of Medicine in the Geneva Medical College, &c.

THE PRACTICE OF MEDICINE. $4.00

MARSHALL (JOHN), F.R.S.,

Professor of Surgery, University College, London.

PHYSIOLOGICAL DIAGRAMS. Life-size, and Beautifully Colored. An Entirely New Edition, Revised and Improved, illustrating the whole Human Body, each Map printed on a single sheet of paper, seven feet long and three feet nine inches broad.

No. 1. The Skeleton and Ligaments.
No. 2. The Muscles, Joints, and Animal Mechanics.
No. 3. The Viscera in Position. — The Structure of the Lungs.
No. 4. The Organs of Circulation.
No. 5. The Lymphatics or Absorbents.
No. 6. The Digestive Organs.
No. 7. The Brain and Nerves.
No. 8. The Organs of the Senses and Organs of the Voice. Plate 1.
No. 9. The Organs of the Senses. Plate 2.
No. 10. The Microscopic Structure of the Textures. Plate 1.
No. 11. The Microscopic Structure of the Textures. Plate 2.

Price of the Set, Eleven Maps, in Sheets, ... $50.00
" " " " handsomely Mounted on Canvas, with Rollers, and varnished, ... $80.00
An Explanatory Key to the Diagram. Price 50

SAME AUTHOR.

DESCRIPTION OF THE HUMAN BODY. Its Structure and Functions. Illustrated by Physiological Diagrams, Designed for the Use of Teachers in Schools, Students of Medicine, &c. New Edition. A Quarto Volume of Text and a Folio Volume containing 193 Colored Illustrations. Price $10.00

MAUNDER (C. F.), F. R. C. S.

Surgeon to the London Hospital; formerly Demonstrator of Anatomy at Guy's Hospital.

OPERATIVE SURGERY. Second Edition, with One Hundred and Sixty-four Engravings on Wood. Price . . . $2.50

MAYNE (R. G.), M. D., AND MAYNE (J.), M. D.

MEDICAL VOCABULARY: An Explanation of all Names, Synonyms, Terms, and Phrases used in Medicine and the Relative Branches of Medical Science, giving their correct Derivation, Meaning, Application, and Pronunciation. Intended especially as a book of reference for Physicians and Students. Fourth Edition, Revised and Enlarged. Post 8vo. 450 pages. Price $3.50

MARTIN (JOHN H.).

Author of Microscopic Objects, &c.

A MANUAL OF MICROSCOPIC MOUNTING. With Notes on the Collection and Examination of Objects, and upwards of One Hundred Illustrations on Stone and Wood, drawn by the Author. Price $3.00

"This book is more than its title indicates. It gives a description of the apparatus necessary for microscopical research, as well as the methods of preparation and preserving the various objects. It is a complete and well-illustrated work on its subject, which is daily becoming more valuable to the scientist and more cultivated as an elegant and interesting study." — *Scientific American.*

MEADOWS (ALFRED), M. D.

Physician to the Hospital for Women, and to the General Lying-in Hospital, &c.

MANUAL OF MIDWIFERY. A New Text-Book. Including the Signs and Symptoms of Pregnancy, Obstetric Operations, Diseases of the Puerperal State, &c., &c. First American from the Second London Edition. With numerous Illustrations. Price $3.00

This book is especially valuable to the Student as containing in a condensed form a large amount of valuable information on the subject which it treats. It is also clear and methodical in its arrangement, and therefore useful as a work of reference for the practitioner. The Illustrations are numerous and well executed.

MILLER (JAMES), F. R. C. S.

Professor of Surgery University of Edinburgh.

ALCOHOL, ITS PLACE AND POWER. From the Nineteenth Glasgow Edition. 12mo. Cloth flexible. Price $0.75

This work was prepared by Professor Miller at the special request of the Scottish Temperance League, who were anxious to have a work of high authority, presenting the medical view of the subject that could be freely disseminated among all classes.

MILLER AND LIZARS.

ALCOHOL: Its Place and Power. By JAMES MILLER, F.R.S.E., late Professor of Surgery in the University of Edinburgh, &c.—THE USE AND ABUSE OF TOBACCO. By JOHN LIZARS, late Professor to the Royal College of Surgeons, &c. The Two Essays in One Volume. 12mo. $1.00

MARSDEN (ALEXANDER), M.D.

A NEW AND SUCCESSFUL MODE OF TREATING CERTAIN FORMS OF CANCER. Second Edition, Colored Plates. $3.50

NORRIS (GEORGE W.), M.D.

Late Surgeon to the Pennsylvania Hospital, &c.

CONTRIBUTIONS TO PRACTICAL SURGERY, including numerous Clinical Histories, Drawn from a Hospital Service of Thirty Years. In one volume, Octavo. Price $4.00

OTT (ADOLPH),

Practical and Analytical Chemist.

ON SOAPS AND CANDLES. Including the Most Recent Discoveries in the Manufacture of all kinds of Ordinary Hard, Soft, and Toilet Soaps, and Tallow and Composite Candles. With Illustrations. Price $2.50

OVERMAN (FREDERICK),

Mining Engineer, &c.

PRACTICAL MINERALOGY, ASSAYING AND MINING. With a Description of the Useful Minerals, and Instructions for Assaying, according to the Simplest Methods. $1.25

PHYSICIAN'S VISITING LIST, PUBLISHED ANNUALLY.

SIZES AND PRICES.

For 25 Patients weekly.	Tucks, pockets, and pencil,	$1.00
50 " "	" " "	1.25
75 " "	" " "	1.50
100 " "	" " "	2.00
50 " " 2 vols.	{ Jan. to June / July to Dec. } "	2.50
100 " " 2 vols.	{ Jan. to June / July to Dec. } "	3.00

INTERLEAVED EDITION.

For 25 Patients weekly,	interleaved, tucks, pockets, &c.,	1.50
50 " "	" " " "	1.75
50 " " 2 vols.	{ Jan. to June / July to Dec. } " "	3.00

This Visiting List has now been published *Twenty-four Years*, and has met with such uniform and hearty approval from the Profession, that the demand for it has steadily increased from year to year.

POWER, HOLMES, ANSTIE, AND BARNES.

REPORTS ON THE PROGRESS OF MEDICINE AND SURGERY, PHYSIOLOGY, OPHTHALMIC MEDICINE, MIDWIFERY, DISEASES OF WOMEN AND CHILDREN, MATERIA MEDICA, &c. Edited for the Sydenham Society of London. Octavo. Price $2.00

PARKES (EDWARD A.), M. D.,

Professor of Military Hygiene in the Army Medical School, &c.

A MANUAL OF PRACTICAL HYGIENE. The Fourth Revised and Enlarged Edition, for Medical Officers of the Army, Civil Medical Officers, Boards of Health, &c., &c. With many Illustrations. One volume Octavo. Price $6.00

This work, previously unrivalled as a text-book for medical officers of the army, is now equally unrivalled as a text-book for civil medical officers. The first book treats in successive chapters of water, air, ventilation, examination of air, food, quality, choice, and cooking of food, beverages, and condiments; soil, habitations, removal of excreta, warming of houses, exercise, clothing, climate, meteorology, individual hygienic management, disposal of the dead, the prevention of some common diseases, disinfection, and statistics. The second book is devoted to the service of the soldier, but is hardly less instructive to the civil officer of health. It is, in short, a comprehensive and trustworthy text-book of hygiene for the scientific or general reader. —*London Lancet.*

POWER (HENRY), M.B., F.R.C.S.,

Senior Ophthalmic Surgeon to St. Bartholomew's Hospital.

THE STUDENT'S GUIDE TO THE DISEASES OF THE EYE. With Engravings. Preparing.

PENNSYLVANIA HOSPITAL REPORTS.

EDITED BY A COMMITTEE OF THE HOSPITAL STAFF. J. M. DA COSTA, M.D., and WILLIAM HUNT, M.D. Vols. 1 and 2; each volume containing upwards of Twenty Original Articles, by former and present Members of the Staff, now eminent in the Profession, with Lithographic and other Illustrations. Price per volume . $4.00

The first Reports were so favorably received, on both sides of the Atlantic, that it is hardly necessary to speak for them the universal welcome of which they are deserving. The papers are all valuable contributions to the literature of medicine, reflecting great credit upon their authors. The work is one of which the Pennsylvania Hospital may well be proud. It will do much towards elevating the profession of this country. —*American Journal of Obstetrics.*

PAGET (JAMES), F.R.S.,

Surgeon to St. Bartholomew's Hospital, &c.

SURGICAL PATHOLOGY. Lectures delivered at the Royal College of Surgeons of England. Third London Edition, Edited and Revised by WILLIAM TURNER, M. D. With Numerous Illustrations. Price, in cloth, $7.50; in leather $8.50

A new and revised edition of Mr. Paget's Classical Lectures needs no introduction to our readers. Commendation would be as superfluous as criticism out of place. Every page bears evidence that this edition has been "carefully revised."—*American Medical Journal.*

PEREIRA (JONATHAN), M.D., F.R.S., &c.

PHYSICIAN'S PRESCRIPTION BOOK. Containing Lists of Terms, Phrases, Contractions, and Abbreviations used in Prescriptions, with Explanatory Notes, the Grammatical Constructions of Prescriptions, Rules for the Pronunciation of Pharmaceutical Terms, a Prosodiacal Vocabulary of the Names of Drugs, &c., and a Series of Abbreviated Prescriptions illustrating the use of the preceding terms, &c.; to which is added a Key, containing the Prescriptions in an unabbreviated Form, with a Literal Translation, intended for the use of Medical and Pharmaceutical Students. From the Fifteenth London Edition. Price, in cloth, $1.25; in leather, with Tucks and Pocket, . $1.50

PROCTOR (BARNARD S.).

PRACTICAL PHARMACY. A Course of Lectures comprising Descriptions of General Processes, Lessons in Dispensing, Pharmacopœial Testing, Qualitative and Quantitative, &c. With Illustrations. Octavo. Price $5.00

PARKER (LANGSTON), F.R.C.S.L.

THE MODERN TREATMENT OF SYPHILITIC DISEASES. Containing the Treatment of Constitutional and Confirmed Syphilis, with numerous Cases, Formulæ, &c., &c. Fifth Edition, Enlarged. $4.25

PRINCE (DAVID), M.D.

PLASTIC AND ORTHOPEDIC SURGERY. Containing 1. A Report on the Condition of, and Advances made in, Plastic and Orthopedic Surgery up to the Year 1871. 2. A New Classification and Brief Exposition of Plastic Surgery. With numerous Illustrations. 3. Orthopedics: A Systematic Work upon the Prevention and Cure of Deformities. With numerous Illustrations. Octavo. Price . . . $4.50

This is a good book upon an important practical subject; carefully written, and abundantly illustrated. It goes over the whole ground of deformities — from cleft-palate and club-foot to spinal curvatures and ununited fractures. It appears, moreover, to be an original book. —*Medical and Surgical Reporter.*

SAME AUTHOR.

GALVANO-THERAPEUTICS. A Revised reprint of A Report made to the Illinois State Medical Society. With Illustrations. Price, $1.25

PIESSE (G. W. SEPTIMUS),

Analytical Chemist.

WHOLE ART OF PERFUMERY. And the Methods of Obtaining the Odors of Plants; the Manufacture of Perfumes for the Handkerchief, Scented Powders, Odorous Vinegars, Dentifrices, Pomatums, Cosmetics, Perfumed Soaps, &c.; the Preparation of Artificial Fruit Essences, &c. Second American from the Third London Edition. With Illustrations. $3.00

PIGGOTT (A. SNOWDEN), M.D.,

Practical Chemist.

COPPER MINING AND COPPER ORE. Containing a full Description of some of the Principal Copper Mines of the United States, the Art of Mining, the Mode of Preparing the Ore for Market, &c., &c. $1.50

PAVY (F. W.), M. D., F. R. S.

DIABETES. Researches on its Nature and Treatment. Third Revised Edition. Octavo . . . .

PHYSICIAN'S PRESCRIPTION BLANKS, with a Margin for Duplicates, Notes, Cases, &c., &c. Price, per package, .
Price, per dozen . .

RINDFLEISCH (DR. EDWARD).

Professor of Pathological Anatomy, University of Bonn.

TEXT-BOOK OF PATHOLOGICAL HISTOLOGY. An Introduction to the Study of Pathological Anatomy. Translated from the German, by WM. C. KLOMAN, M.D., assisted by F. T. MILES, M.D., Professor of Anatomy, University of Maryland, &c., &c. Containing Two Hundred and Eight elaborately executed Microscopical Illustrations. Octavo. Price, bound in Cloth, ... $6.00
" " Leather, ... 7.00

This is now confessedly the leading book, and the only complete one on the subject in the English language. The *London Lancet* says of it: "Rindfleisch's work forms a mine which no pathological writer or student can afford to neglect, who desires to interpret aright pathological structural changes, and his book is consequently well known to readers of German medical literature. What makes it especially valuable is the fact that it was originated, as its author himself tells us, more at the microscope than at the writing-table. Altogether the book is the result of honest hard labor. It is admirably as well as profusely illustrated, furnished with a capital Index, and got up in a way that is worthy of what must continue to be the standard book of the kind."

ROBERTS (FREDERICK T.)., M. D., B. Sc.

Assistant Physician and Teacher of Clinical Medicine in the University College Hospital; Assistant Physician Brompton Consumption Hospital, &c.

A HAND-BOOK OF THE THEORY AND PRACTICE OF MEDICINE. One volume medium octavo, containing over 1000 pages. Price . . . . $5.00.

This work has been prepared mainly for the use of Students, and its object is to present in as condensed a form as the present extent of Medical Literature will permit, and in one volume, such information with regard to the Principles and Practice of Medicine, as shall be sufficient not only to enable them to prepare for the various examinations which they may have to undergo, but also to guide them in acquiring that Clinical Knowledge which can alone properly fit them for assuming the active duties of their profession. The work is also adapted to the wants of very many members of the profession who are already busily engaged in general Practice, and consequently have but little leisure and few opportunities for the perusal of the larger works on Practice or of the various special monographs.

REYNOLDS (J. RUSSELL), M. D., F. R. S.,

Lecturer on the Principles and Practice of Medicine, University College, London.

LECTURES ON THE CLINICAL USES OF ELECTRICITY. Delivered at University College Hospital. Second Edition, Revised and Enlarged. Price $1.25

RYAN (MICHAEL), M. D.

Member of the Royal College of Physicians.

PHILOSOPHY OF MARRIAGE, in its Social, Moral, and Physical Relations; with an Account of the Diseases of the Genito-Urinary Organs, &c. Price $1.00

This is a philosophical discussion of the whole subject of Marriage, its influences and results in all their varied aspects, together with a medical history of the reproductive functions of the vegetable and animal kingdoms, and of the abuses and disorders resulting from it in the latter. It is intended both for the professional and general reader.

RADCLIFFE (CHARLES BLAND), M.D.,

Fellow of the Royal College of Physicians of London, &c.

LECTURES ON EPILEPSY, PAIN, PARALYSIS, and other Disorders of the Nervous System. With Illustrations. . . $2.00

The reputation which Dr. Radcliffe possesses as a very able authority on nervous affections will commend his work to every medical practitioner. We recommend it as a work that will throw much light upon the Physiology and Pathology of the Nervous System. — *Canada Medical Journal.*

ROBERTSON (A.), M.D., D.D.S.

A MANUAL ON EXTRACTING TEETH. Founded on the Anatomy of the Parts involved in the Operation, the kinds and proper construction of the instruments to be used, the accidents likely to occur from the operation, and the proper remedies to retrieve such accidents. A New Revised Edition. $1.50

The author is well known as a contributor to the literature of the profession, and as a clear, terse, and practical writer. The subject is one to which he has devoted considerable attention, and is treated with his usual care and ability. The work is valuable not only to the dental student and practitioner, but also to the medical student and surgeon. — *Dental Cosmos.*

REESE (JOHN J.), M.D.,

Professor of Medical Jurisprudence and Toxicology in the University of Pennsylvania.

AN ANALYSIS OF PHYSIOLOGY. Being a Condensed View of the most important Facts and Doctrines, designed especially for the Use of Students. Second Edition, Enlarged. . . . $1.50

SAME AUTHOR.

THE AMERICAN MEDICAL FORMULARY. Price . $1.50

A SYLLABUS OF MEDICAL CHEMISTRY. Price . $1.00

RICHARDSON (JOSEPH), D.D.S.

Late Professor of Mechanical Dentistry, &c., &c.

A PRACTICAL TREATISE ON MECHANICAL DENTISTRY. Second Edition, much Enlarged. With over 150 beautifully executed Illustrations. Octavo. Price, in leather $4.50

This work does infinite credit to its author. Its comprehensive style has in no way interfered with most elaborate details where this is necessary; and the numerous and beautifully executed wood-cuts with which it is illustrated make the volume as attractive as its instructions are easily understood. —*Edinburgh Med. Journal.*

ROBERTS (LLOYD D.), M.D.,

Vice-President of the Obstetrical Society of London, Physician to St. Mary's Hospital, Manchester.

THE STUDENT'S GUIDE TO THE PRACTICE OF MIDWIFERY. With Engravings. In Preparation.

REEVES (H. A.), F. R. C. S.

THE STUDENT'S GUIDE TO PRACTICAL HISTOLOGY, Histo-Chemistry, and Embryology. With Engravings on Wood. 12mo. Preparing.

RIGBY AND MEADOWS.

DR. RIGBY'S OBSTETRIC MEMORANDA. Fourth Edition, Revised and Enlarged, by ALFRED MEADOWS, M.D., Author of "A Manual of Midwifery," &c. Price 50

RIHL AND O'CONNOR.

THE PHYSICIAN'S DIARY. Monthly, Semi-Annual, and Annual Journal and Cash-Book Combined. The Fourth Revised Edition. A large folio volume, with printed Heads, Index, &c., &c. Bound in full leather. Price $7.50

RUPPANER (ANTOINE), M.D.

THE PRINCIPLES AND PRACTICE OF LARYNGOSCOPY AND RHINOSCOPY IN DISEASES OF THE THROAT, &c. Fifty-nine Illustrations. Price $1.50

SANDERSON, KLEIN, FOSTER, AND BRUNTON.

A HAND-BOOK FOR THE PHYSIOLOGICAL LABORATORY. Being Practical Exercises for Students in Physiology and Histology, by E. KLEIN, M. D., Assistant Professor in the Pathological Laboratory of the Brown Institution, London; J. BURDON-SANDERSON, M. D., F. R. S., Professor of Practical Theology in University College, London; MICHAEL FOSTER, M.D., F.R.S., Fellow of and Prælector of Physiology in Trinity College, Cambridge; and T. LAUDER BRUNTON, M.D., D.Sc., Lecturer on Materia Medica in the Medical College of St. Bartholomew's Hospital. Edited by J. BURDON-SANDERSON. The Illustrations consist of One Hundred and Twenty-three octavo pages, including over Three Hundred and Fifty Figures, with appropriate letter-press explanations attached and references to the text, and bound in a separate volume. Price of the two volumes, text and plates, $8.00

We feel that we cannot recommend this work too highly. To those engaged in physiological work as students or teachers, it is almost indispensable; and to those who are not, a perusal of it will by no means be unprofitable. The execution of the plates leaves nothing to be desired. They are mostly original, and their arrangement in a separate volume has great and obvious advantages. — *Dublin Journal of Medical Sciences.*

SIEVEKING (E. H.), M.D., F.R.C.S.

THE MEDICAL ADVISER IN LIFE ASSURANCE. Price $2.25

This book supplies, in a concise and available form, such facts and figures as are required by the Physician or Examiner to assist him in arriving at a correct estimate of the many contingencies upon which life insurance rests.

SWAIN (WILLIAM PAUL), F.R.C.S.,

Surgeon to the Royal Albert Hospital, Devonport.

SURGICAL EMERGENCIES: A MANUAL CONTAINING CONCISE DESCRIPTIONS OF VARIOUS ACCIDENTS AND EMERGENCIES, WITH DIRECTIONS FOR THEIR IMMEDIATE TREATMENT. With numerous Wood Engravings. In one volume, 12mo. Cloth. Price $2.00

STILLE (ALFRED), M.D.,

Professor of the Theory and Practice of Medicine in the University of Pennsylvania, &c.

EPIDEMIC MENINGITIS; or, Cerebro-Spinal Meningitis. In one volume, Octavo. $2.00

This monograph is a timely publication, comprehensive in its scope, and presenting within a small compass a fair digest of our existing knowledge of the disease, particularly acceptable at the present time. It is just such a one as is needed, and may be taken as a model for similar works. — *American Journal Medical Sciences.*

SAME AUTHOR.

ELEMENTS OF GENERAL PATHOLOGY. A Practical Treatise on the Causes, Forms, Symptoms, and Results of Disease. Second Edition preparing.

SCHULTZE (DR. B. S.),

Professor of Midwifery at the University of Jena.

LECTURE DIAGRAMS FOR INSTRUCTION IN PREGNANCY AND MIDWIFERY. Twenty Plates of the largest Imperial size, printed in colors. Drawn and Edited with Explanatory Notes, and a 4to volume of letter-press. Prices, in sheets, $15.00. Handsomely mounted on rollers for hanging up. . . . $30.00

SANSOM (ARTHUR ERNEST), M.B.,

Physician to King's College Hospital, &c.

CHLOROFORM. Its Action and Administration. Price $2.00

This work may be characterized as most excellent. Written not alone from a theoretical point of view, but showing very considerable experimental study, and an intimate clinical acquaintance with the administration of these remedies, — passing concisely over the whole ground, giving the latest information upon every point. It is just the work for the student and practitioner. — *American Medical Journal.*

SCANZONI (F. W. VON),

Professor in the University of Wurzburg.

A PRACTICAL TREATISE ON THE DISEASES OF THE SEXUAL ORGANS OF WOMEN. Translated from the French. By A. K. GARDNER, M.D. With Illustrations. Octavo. . $5.00

STOKES (WILLIAM),

Regius Professor of Physic in the University of Dublin.

THE DISEASES OF THE HEART AND THE AORTA. Octavo. $3.00

SYDENHAM SOCIETY'S PUBLICATIONS. New Series, 1859 to 1873 inclusive, 15 years, 56 vols. Subscriptions received, and back years furnished at $10.00 per year. Full prospectus, with the Reports of the Society and a list of the Books published, furnished free upon application.

SANKEY (W. H. O.), M.D., F.R.C.P.

LECTURES ON MENTAL DISEASES. Octavo. . . $3.25

SWERINGEN (HIRAM V.).

Member American Pharmaceutical Association, &c.

PHARMACEUTICAL LEXICON. A Dictionary of Pharmaceutical Science. Containing a concise explanation of the various subjects and terms of Pharmacy, with appropriate selections from the collateral sciences. Formulæ for officinal, empirical, and dietetic preparations; selections from the prescriptions of the most eminent physicians of Europe and America; an alphabetical list of diseases and their definitions; an account of the various modes in use for the preservation of dead bodies for interment or dissection; tables of signs and abbreviations, weights and measures, doses, antidotes to poisons, &c., &c. Designed as a guide for the Pharmaceutist, Druggist, Physician, &c. Royal Octavo. Price in cloth $5.00
" leather 6.00

"We have received from publishers so many English reprints ill adapted to the needs of this country, that it is with pleasure we welcome a thorough American book, written for the uses of the American pharmaceutist. Besides, the work is well written, creditably arranged, and neatly printed. It will be found very useful to the druggist as well as to the physician. Being in the form of a dictionary, its aim is to give *immediate* information in a concise manner, and not a complete treatise on each subject. So far as we have been able to see, the PHARMACEUTICAL LEXICON is remarkably correct." —*Druggist's Circular.*

SHEPPARD (EDGAR), M. D.

Professor of Psychological Medicine in King's College, London.

MADNESS, IN ITS MEDICAL, SOCIAL, AND LEGAL ASPECTS. A series of Lectures delivered at King's College, London. Octavo. Price $2.50

SAVAGE (HENRY), M. D., F. R. C. S.

Consulting Physician to the Samaritan Free Hospital, London.

THE SURGERY, SURGICAL PATHOLOGY, and Surgical Anatomy of the Female Pelvic Organs, in a Series of Colored Plates taken from Nature: with Commentaries, Notes, and Cases. Third Edition, greatly enlarged. A quarto volume. Price . .

SAME AUTHOR.

AN EXPOSITION OF THE NATURE OF THE SURGICAL DISEASES OF THE FEMALE PELVIC ORGANS. With a View to their Rational Treatment. Preparing.

SUTTON (FRANCIS), F. C. S.

A SYSTEMATIC HAND-BOOK OF VOLUMETRIC ANALYSIS, or the Quantitative Estimation of Chemical Substances by Measure, Applied to Liquids, Solids, and Gases. Third Edition, enlarged. With numerous Illustrations.

SMITH (EUSTACE), M.D.

Physician to the East London Hospital for Diseases of Children, &c.

CLINICAL STUDIES OF DISEASES IN CHILDREN.

Preparing.

TANNER (THOMAS HAWKES), M. D., F.R.C.P., &c.

THE PRACTICE OF MEDICINE. Sixth American from the last London Edition. Revised, much Enlarged, and thoroughly brought up to the present time. With a complete Section on the Diseases Peculiar to Women, an extensive Appendix of Formulæ for Medicines, Baths, &c., &c. Royal Octavo, over 1100 pages. Price, in cloth, $6.00; leather $7.00

There is a common character about the writings of Dr. Tanner—a characteristic which constitutes one of their chief values: they are all essentially and thoroughly practical. Dr. Tanner never, for one moment, allows this utilitarian end to escape his mental view. He aims at teaching how to recognize and how to cure disease, and in this he is thoroughly successful. . . . It is, indeed, a wonderful mine of knowledge.—*Medical Times.*

SAME AUTHOR.

A PRACTICAL TREATISE ON THE DISEASES OF INFANCY AND CHILDHOOD. Third American from the last London Edition, Revised and Enlarged. By ALFRED MEADOWS, M.D., London, M.R.C.P., Physician to the Hospital for Women and to the General Lying-in Hospital, &c., &c. Price $3.50

This book of Dr. Tanner's has been much enlarged and the plan altered by Dr. Meadows. As it now stands, it is probably one of the most complete in our language. It no longer deals with children's diseases only, but includes the peculiar conditions of childhood, both normal and abnormal, as well as the therapeutics specially applicable to that class of patients. The articles on Skin Diseases have been revised by Dr. Tilbury Fox, and those on Diseases of the Eye by Dr. Brudenell Carter, both gentlemen distinguished in these specialties.—*Medical Times and Gazette.*

A MEMORANDA OF POISONS. A New and much Enlarged Edition. Price 75

AN INDEX OF DISEASES AND THEIR TREATMENT. The last London Edition. 12mo. Price $3.00

TYSON (JAMES), M.D.,

Lecturer on Microscopy in the University of Pennsylvania, &c.

THE CELL DOCTRINE. Its History and Present State, with a Copious Bibliography of the Subject, for the use of Students of Medicine and Dentistry. With Colored Plate, and numerous Illustrations on Wood. Price $2.00

BY SAME AUTHOR.

A PRACTICAL GUIDE TO THE EXAMINATION OF URINE. For the use of Physicians and Students. With a Colored Plate and numerous Illustrations Engraved on Wood. A 12mo Volume. Price, $1.50

TAFT (JONATHAN), D. D. S.,

Professor of Operative Dentistry in the Ohio College, &c.

A PRACTICAL TREATISE ON OPERATIVE DENTISTRY. Second Edition, thoroughly Revised, with Additions, and fully brought up to the Present State of the Science. Containing over 100 Illustrations. Octavo. Price, in leather, ... $4.50

Professor Taft has done good service in thus embodying, in a separate volume, a comprehensive view of operative dentistry. This gentleman's position as a teacher must have rendered him familiar with the most recent views which are entertained in America on this matter, while his extensive experience and well-earned reputation in practice must have rendered him a competent judge of their merits. We willingly commend Professor Taft's able and useful work to the profession.—*London Dental Review.*

TROUSSEAU (A.),

Professor of Clinical Medicine to the Faculty of Medicine, Paris, &c.

LECTURES ON CLINICAL MEDICINE. Delivered at the Hôtel Dieu, Paris. Translated from the Third Revised and Enlarged Edition by P. VICTOR BAZIRE, M.D., London and Paris; and JOHN ROSE CORMACK, M.D., Edinburgh, F.R.S., &c. With a full Index, Table of Contents, &c. Complete in Two volumes, royal octavo, bound in cloth. Price $10.00; in leather $12.00

Trousseau's Lectures have attained a reputation both in England and this country far greater than any work of a similar character heretofore written; and, notwithstanding but few medical men could afford to purchase the expensive edition issued by the Sydenham Society, it has had an extensive sale. In order, however, to bring the work within the reach of all the profession, the publishers now issue this edition, containing all the lectures as contained in the five-volume edition, at one-half the price. The *London Lancet*, in speaking of the work, says: "It treats of diseases of daily occurrence and of the most vital interest to the practitioner. And we should think any medical library absurdly incomplete now which did not have alongside of Watson, Graves, and Tanner, the 'Clinical Medicine' of Trousseau."

The Sydenham Society's Edition of Trousseau can also be furnished in sets, or in separate volumes, as follows: Volumes I., II., and III., $5.00 each. Volumes IV. and V., $4.00 each.

TILT (EDWARD JOHN), M.D.

THE CHANGE OF LIFE IN HEALTH AND DISEASE. A Practical Treatise on the Nervous and other Affections incidental to Women at the Decline of Life. From the Third London Edition. Price $3.00

The work is rich in personal experience and observation, as well as in ready and sensible reflection on the experience and observation of others. The book is one that no practitioner should be without, as the best we have on a class of diseases that makes a constant demand upon our care, and requires very judicious management on the part of the practitioner.—*London Lancet.*

TOYNBEE (J.), F.R.S.

ON DISEASES OF THE EAR. Their Nature, Diagnosis, and Treatment. A new London Edition, with a Supplement. By JAMES HINTON, Aural Surgeon to Guy's Hospital, &c. And numerous Illustrations. Octavo. $5.00

THOMPSON (SIR HENRY), F.R.C.S., &c.

ON THE PREVENTIVE TREATMENT OF CALCULOUS DISEASE, and the Use of Solvent Remedies. Price . . $1.00

SAME AUTHOR.

CLINICAL LECTURES IN DISEASES OF THE URINARY ORGANS. Third London Edition, with additional Lectures and Illustrations. $2.50

PRACTICAL LITHOTOMY AND LITHOTRITY. Second Edition, with Illustrations. $4.00

THOROWGOOD (JOHN C.), M.D.,

Lecturer on Materia Medica at the Middlesex Hospital.

THE STUDENT'S GUIDE TO MATERIA MEDICA. With Engravings on Wood. $2.50

TYLER SMITH (W.), M.D.,

Physician, Accoucheur, and Lecturer on Midwifery, &c.

ON OBSTETRICS. A Course of Lectures. Edited by A. K. GARDNER, M.D. With Illustrations. Octavo. $5.00

THOROWGOOD (J. C.), M. D.

Physician to the City of London Hospital for Diseases of the Chest, and to the West London Hospital, &c.

NOTES ON ASTHMA. Its various Forms, their Nature and Treatment, including Hay Asthma, with an Appendix of Formulæ, &c. Second Edition. Price $1.75

TOMES (JOHN), F. R. S.

Late Dental Surgeon to the Middlesex and Dental Hospitals, &c.

A SYSTEM OF DENTAL SURGERY. The Second Revised and Enlarged Edition, by CHARLES S. TOMES, M.A., Lecturer on Dental Anatomy and Physiology, and Assistant Dental Surgeon to the Dental Hospital of London. With 263 Illustrations. Price . . $5.00

This book has been for some time out of print in this country. The material progress made in the science of Dental Surgery since its first publication has rendered large additions and many revisions necessary to the New Edition: in order to bring it fully up to the time; this has been done without increasing the size of the book more than possible. Many improvements, however, will be found added to the Text, and some Sixty new illustrations are incorporated in the volume.

TOMES (C. S.), B. A.

Lecturer on Anatomy and Physiology, and Assistant Surgeon to the Dental Hospital of London.

A MANUAL OF DENTAL ANATOMY AND PHYSIOLOGY with Numerous Illustrations. Preparing.

TROUSSEAU (A.), M. D.

Professor of Clinical Medicine to the Faculty of Medicine, Paris; Physician to the Hotel Dieu, &c., &c.

LECTURES ON CLINICAL MEDICINE. Delivered at the Hotel Dieu, Paris. Sydenham Society's Edition.

Price of Vols. 1, 2, and 3, each, ... $5.00
" " 4 and 5 " 4 00

TUKE (DANIEL H.), M. D.

Associate Author of "A Manual of Psychological Medicine," &c.

ILLUSTRATIONS OF THE INFLUENCE OF THE MIND UPON THE BODY. Octavo. Price $4.00

The author shows very clearly in this book the curative influence of the mind, as well as its effect in causing disease, and the use of the imagination and emotions as therapeutic agents. His object is also to turn to the use of legitimate medicine the means so frequently employed successfully in many systems of quackery.

TIBBITS (HERBERT), M. D.

Medical Superintendent of the National Hospital for the Paralyzed and Epileptic, &c.

A HANDBOOK OF MEDICAL ELECTRICITY. With Sixty-four large Illustrations. Small octavo. Price $2.00

The author of this volume is the translator of Duchenne's great work on "Localized Electrization." Avoiding contested points in electro-physiology and therapeutics, he has prepared this handbook as containing all that is essential for the busy practitioner to know, not only when, but in EXPLICIT AND FULL DETAIL, how to use Electricity in the treatment of disease, and to make the practitioner as much at home in the use of his electrical as his other medical instruments.

VIRCHOW (RUDOLPHE),

Professor, University of Berlin.

CELLULAR PATHOLOGY. Translated from the Second Edition, with Notes and Emendations, by FRANK CHANCE, B.A., M.A., 144 Illustrations. $5.00

VAN DER KOLK (J. L. C. SCHROEDER),

THE PATHOLOGY AND THERAPEUTICS OF MENTAL DISEASES. Translated by Mr. RUDALL, F.R.C.S. Octavo. $3.00

WARING (EDWARD JOHN), F.R.C.S., F.L.S., &c., &c.

PRACTICAL THERAPEUTICS. Considered chiefly with reference to Articles of the Materia Medica. Third American from the last London Edition. Price, in cloth, $5.00; leather . . $6.00

There are many features in Dr. Waring's Therapeutics which render it especially valuable to the Practitioner and Student of Medicine, much important and reliable information being found in it not contained in similar works; also in its completeness, the convenience of its arrangement, and the greater prominence given to the medicinal application of the various articles of the Materia Medica in the treatment of morbid conditions of the Human Body, &c. It is divided into two parts, the alphabetical arrangement being adopted throughout. It contains also an excellent INDEX OF DISEASES, with a list of the medicines applicable as remedies, and a full INDEX of the medicines and preparations noticed in the work.

WYTHES (JOSEPH H), A.M., M.D., &c.

THE PHYSICIAN'S POCKET, DOSE, AND SYMPTOM BOOK. Containing the Doses and Uses of all the PrincipalArticles of the Materia Medica, and Original Preparations; A Table of Weights and Measures, Rules to Proportion the Doses of Medicines, Common Abbreviations used in Writing Prescriptions, Table of Poisons and Antidotes, Classification of the Materia Medica, Dietetic Preparations, Table of Symptomatology, Outlines of General Pathology and Therapeutics, &c. The Eleventh Revised Edition. Price, in cloth, $1.25; in leather, tucks, with pockets, ... $1.50

This manual has been received with much favor, and a large number of copies sold. It was compiled for the assistance of students, and as a vade mecum for the general practitioner, to save the trouble of reference to larger and more elaborate works. This edition has undergone a careful revision. The therapeutical arrangement of the Materia Medica has been added, together with other improvements of value to the work.

WILKS AND MOXON.

LECTURES ON PATHOLOGICAL ANATOMY. By SAMUEL WILKS, M.D., F.R.S., Physician to, and Lecturer on Medicine at, Guy's Hospital. Second Edition, Enlarged and Revised. By WALTER MOXON, M.D., F.R.S., Physician to, and late Lecturer on Pathology at, Guy's Hospital. $6.50

WILSON (ERASMUS), F.R.S.

HEALTHY SKIN. A Popular Treatise on the Skin and Hair, their Preservation and Management. Seventh Edition. . . $1.25

WILSON (GEORGE), M. A., M. D.

Medical Officer to the Convict Prison at Portsmouth.

A HANDBOOK OF HYGIENE AND SANITARY SCIENCE.

With Engravings. Second Edition, carefully Revised.

CONTENTS.

Chap. 1. Introductory — Public Health and Preventable Disease.
" 2. Food — Construction of Dietaries; Examination; Effects of Unwholesome Food.
" 3. Air: its Impurities; Unwholesome Trades.
" 4. Ventilation and Warming.
" 5. Examination of Air.
" 6. Water, Waterworks, Water Analysis.
" 7. Effects of Impure Water on Public Health.
" 8. Dwellings, Structural Arrangements, Dwellings of the Poor.
" 9. Hospitals; Plans of Pavilion, Cottage, and Contagious Diseases Hospitals.
Chap. 10. Removal of Sewage and Refuse Matter.
" 11. Purification and Utilization of Sewage.
" 12. Effects of Improved Sewerage and Drainage on Public Health.
" 13. Preventive Measures; Disinfection; Management of Epidemics.
" 14. Duties of Medical Officers of Health.
APPENDIX I. Excerpts from the various Public Health and Sanitary Acts.
II. List of Analytical Apparatus and Reagents, with prices.

Price $2.50

WARD (STEPHEN H.), M.D., F. R. C. P.

Physician to the Seaman's Hospital, &c., &c.

ON SOME AFFECTIONS OF THE LIVER and Intestinal Canal;

with Remarks on Ague and its Sequelæ, Scurvy, Purpura, &c.
Price $3.00

"Dr. Ward's book is of a purely practical character, embodying the author's experience, from his long connection as physician to the Seaman's Hospital. His accurate description of the diseases treated will amply repay the reader." — *Dublin Medical Journal.*

WILSON (ERASMUS), F. R. C. S., &c.

CONTAINING THREE HUNDRED AND SEVENTY-ONE ILLUSTRATIONS.

THE ANATOMIST'S VADE MECUM.

A Complete System of Human Anatomy. The Ninth Revised and Enlarged London Edition. Edited and fully brought to the Science of the day by Prof. GEORGE BUCHANAN, Lecturer on Anatomy in Anderson's University, Glasgow, with many New Illustrations, prepared expressly for this Edition.
Price $5.50

WEDL (CARL), M. D.

Professor of Histology, &c., in the University of Vienna.

DENTAL PATHOLOGY.

The Pathology of the Teeth. With Special Reference to their Anatomy and Physiology. First American Edition, translated by W. E. BOARDMAN, M.D., with Notes by THOS. B. HITCHCOCK, M.D., Professor of Dental Pathology and Therapeutics in the Dental School of Harvard University, Cambridge. With 105 Illustrations. . . . Price, in Cloth, $4.50; Leather, $5.50

This work exhibits laborious research and medical culture of no ordinary character. It covers the entire field of Anatomy, Physiology, and Pathology of the Teeth. The author, Prof. Wedl, has thoroughly mastered the subject, using with great benefit to the book the very valuable material left by the late Dr. Heider, Professor of Dental Pathology in the University of Vienna, the result of the life-long work of this eminent man.

WOODMAN AND TIDY.

A HANDY-BOOK OF FORENSIC MEDICINE AND TOXICOLOGY. By W. BATHURST WOODMAN, M. D. St. And., Assistant Physician and Lecturer on Physiology at the London Hospital; and C. MEYMOTT TIDY, M.A., M.B., Lecturer on Chemistry, and Professor of Medical Jurisprudence and Public Health, at the London Hospital. With numerous Illustrations. Preparing.

WELLS (J. SŒLBERG),

Ophthalmic Surgeon to King's College Hospital, &c.

TREATISE ON THE DISEASES OF THE EYE. Illustrated by Ophthalmoscopic Plates and numerous Engravings on Wood. The Third London Edition. Cloth, $5.00; leather . . . $6.00

This is the author's own edition, printed in London under his supervision, and issued in this country by special arrangement with him.

SAME AUTHOR.

ON LONG, SHORT, AND WEAK SIGHT, and their Treatment by the Scientific Use of Spectacles. Third Edition Revised, with Additions and numerous Illustrations. Price $3.00

WRIGHT (HENRY G.), M.D.,

Member of the Royal College of Physicians, &c.

ON HEADACHES. Their Causes and their Cure. From the Fourth London Edition. 12mo. Cloth. $1.25

The author's plan is simple and practical. He treats of headaches in childhood and youth, in adult life and old age, giving in each their varieties and symptoms, and their causes and treatment. It is a most satisfactory monograph, as the mere fact that this is a reprint of the *fourth* edition testifies.

WALTON (HAYNES),

Surgeon in Charge of the Ophthalmic Department of, and Lecturer on Ophthalmic Medicine and Surgery in, St. Mary's Hospital.

A PRACTICAL TREATISE ON DISEASES OF THE EYE, Third Edition. Rewritten and enlarged. With five plain, and three colored full-page plates, numerous Illustrations on Wood, Test Types, &c., &c. Octavo volume of nearly 1200 pages. Price . $9.00

WATERS (A. T. H.), M.D., F.R.C.P., &c.

DISEASES OF THE CHEST. Contributions to their Clinical History, Pathology, and Treatment. Second Edition, Revised and Enlarged. With numerous Illustrative Cases and Chapters on Hæmoptysis, Hay Fever, Thoracic Aneurism, and the Use of Chloral in certain Diseases of the Chest, and Plates. Octavo. Price $5.00

WALKER (ALEXANDER),

Author of "Woman," "Beauty," &c.

INTERMARRIAGE; or, the Mode in which, and the Causes why, Beauty, Health, Intellect result from certain Unions, and Deformity, Disease, and Insanity from others. With Illustrations. 12mo. $1.50

THE LATEST TEXT-BOOK

ON THE

PRACTICE OF MEDICINE.

Uniformly Commended by the Profession and the Press.

A HAND-BOOK OF THE THEORY AND PRACTICE OF MEDICINE. By FREDERICK T. ROBERTS, M.D., M.R.C.P., Assistant Professor and Teacher of Clinical Medicine in University College Hospital, Assistant Physician in Brompton Consumptive Hospital, &c., &c.

In One Volume, Octavo, of over 1000 pages. Price, in cloth . $5.00
" leather . $6.00

The Publishers are in receipt of numerous letters from Professors in the various Medical Schools, uniformly commending this book; whilst the following extracts from the Medical Press, both English and American, fully attest its superiority and great value not only to the student, but also to the busy practitioner.

This is a good book, yea, a very good book. It is not so full in its Pathology as "Aitken," so charming in its composition as "Watson," nor so decisive in its treatment as "Tanner;" but it is more compendious than any of them, and therefore more useful. We know of no other work in the English language, or in any other, for that matter, which competes with this one. —*Edinburgh Medical Journal.*

We have much pleasure in expressing our sense of the author's conscientious anxiety to make his work a faithful representation of modern medical beliefs and practice. In this he has succeeded in a degree that will earn the gratitude of very many students and practitioners: it is a remarkable evidence of industry, experience, and research. — *Practitioner.*

That Dr. Roberts's book is admirably fitted to supply the want of a good hand-book of medicine, so much felt by every medical student, does not admit of a question. — *Students' Journal and Hospital Gazette.*

Dr. Roberts has accomplished his task in a satisfactory manner, and has produced a work mainly intended for students that will be cordially welcomed by them; most of the observations on treatment are carefully written and worthy of attentive study; the arrangement is good, and the style clear and simple. — *London Lancet.*

It contains a vast deal of capital instruction for the student, much valuable matter in it to commend, and merit enough to insure for it a rapid sale.—*London Medical Times and Gazette.*

There are great excellencies in this book, which will make it a favorite both with the accurate student and busy practitioner. The author has had ample experience.—*Richmond and Louisville Journal.*

We confess ourselves most favorably impressed with this work. The author has performed his task most creditably, and we cordially recommend the book to our readers. — *Canada Medical and Surgical Journal.*

A careful reading of the book has led us to believe that the author has written a work more nearly up to the times than any that we have seen; to the student, it will be a gift of priceless value. — *Detroit Review of Medicine.*

Our opinion of it is one of almost unqualified praise. The style is clear, and the amount of useful and, indeed, indispensable information which it contains is marvellous. We heartily recommend it to students, teachers, and practitioners. — *Boston Med. and Surgical Journal.*

It is of a much higher order than the usual compilations and abstracts placed in the hands of students. It embraces many suggestions and hints from a carefully compiled hospital experience; the style is clear and concise, and the plan of the work very judicious.—*Medical and Surgical Reporter.*

It is unsurpassed by any work that has fallen into our hands as a compendium for students preparing for examination. It is thoroughly practical and fully up to the times.—*The Clinic.*

We find it an admirable book. Indeed, we know of no hand-book on the subject just now to be preferred to it. We particularly commend it to students about to enter upon the practice of their profession. — *St. Louis Medical and Surgical Journal.*

If there is a book in the whole of medical literature in which so much is said in so few words, it has never come within our reach. So clear, terse, and pointed is the style; so accurate the diction, and so varied the matter of this book, that it is almost a dictionary of practical medicine. — *Chicago Medical Journal.*

The author's style is clear, concise, and methodical.—*Chicago Medical Examiner.*

Dr. Roberts has given us a work of real value, and especially for the use of students is the book a good one. — *Lancet and Observer.*

TROUSSEAU'S CLINICAL MEDICINE.

COMPLETE.

In Two Large Royal Octavo Volumes.

EMBRACING ALL THE LECTURES CONTAINED IN THE FIVE VOLUME EDITION AS ISSUED BY THE SYDENHAM SOCIETY.

Price, handsomely bound in cloth	. . . .	$10.00
" " " leather	. . . . . .	12.00

Lectures on Clinical Medicine.

Delivered at the Hôtel Dieu, Paris, by A. TROUSSEAU, Professor of Clinical Medicine to the Faculty of Medicine, Paris, &c., &c. Translated from the Third Revised and Enlarged Edition by P. VICTOR BAZIRE, M. D., London and Paris; and JOHN ROSE CORMACK, M. D., Edinburgh, F. R. S., &c. With a full Index, Table of Contents, &c.

Trousseau's Lectures have attained a reputation both in England and in this country far greater than any work of a similar character heretofore written, and, notwithstanding but few medical men could afford to purchase the expensive edition issued by the Sydenham Society, it has had an extensive sale. In order, however, to bring the work within the reach of all the profession, the publishers now issue this edition, containing all the lectures as contained in the five-volume edition, at one-half the price. Below are a few only of the many favorable opinions expressed of the work:

"It treats of diseases of daily occurrence and of the most vital interest to the practitioner. And we should think any medical library absurdly incomplete now which did not have alongside of Watson, Graves, and Tanner, the 'Clinical Medicine' of Trousseau.

"The work is full of the results of the richest natural observation, and is the production of one who was enlightened enough to combine with new methods of investigation the vigorous and independent ideas of the old physicians whom he so eloquently magnifies. It is an extremely rich and valuable addition to the library of physicians and practitioners generally." —*London Lancet.*

"This book furnishes an example of the best kind of clinical teaching. It deserves to be popularized. We scarcely know of any work better fitted for presentation to a young man when entering upon the practical work of his life. The delineation of the recorded cases is graphic, and their narration devoid of that prolixity which, desirable as it is for purposes of extended analysis, is highly undesirable when the object is to point to a practical lesson."—*London Medical Times and Gazette.*

"The publication of Trousseau's Lectures furnishes medical men with one of the best practical treatises on disease as seen at the bedside. The conversational style adopted by the author lends animation to the work, and the translator deserves credit for having so well preserved the easy and ready style of the original." —*British and Foreign Medico-Chirurgical Review.*

"The great reputation of Prof. Trousseau as a practitioner and teacher of Medicine in all its branches, renders the present appearance of his Clinical Lectures particularly welcome." —*Medical Press and Circular.*

"A clever translation of Prof. Trousseau's admirable and exhaustive work, the best book of reference upon the Practice of Medicine." —*Indian Medical Gazette.*

www.ingramcontent.com/pod-product-compliance
Lightning Source LLC
La Vergne TN
LVHW020926110826
845150LV00004B/780

* 9 7 8 1 4 2 5 5 5 4 0 8 8 *